Quantum Leadership
A Textbook of New Leadership

Tim Porter-O'Grady, EdD, PhD, FAAN
Senior Partner
Tim Porter-O'Grady Associates, Inc.
Atlanta, Georgia
Associate Professor
Emory University
Atlanta, Georgia

Kathy Malloch, PhD, MBA, RN
President
Kathy Malloch Consulting Services
Glendale, Arizona
Faculty Associate, College of Nursing
Arizona State University
Tempe, Arizona
President
Arizona State Board of Nursing
Phoenix, Arizona

JONES AND BARTLETT PUBLISHERS
Sudbury, Massachusetts
BOSTON   TORONTO   LONDON   SINGAPORE

World Headquarters
Jones and Bartlett Publishers
40 Tall Pine Drive
Sudbury, MA 01776
978-443-5000
info@jbpub.com
www.jbpub.com

Jones and Bartlett Publishers Canada
2406 Nikanna Road
Mississauga, ON L5C 2W6
CANADA

Jones and Bartlett Publishers International
Barb House, Barb Mews
London W6 7PA
UK

This publication is designed to provide accurate and authoritative information in regard to the Subject Matter covered. It is sold with the understanding that the publisher is not engaged in rendering legal, accounting, or other professional service. If legal advice or other expert assistance is required, the service of a competent professional person should be sought. (From a Declaration of Principles jointly adopted by a Committee of the American Bar Association and a Committee of Publishers and Associations.)

Production Credits
Chief Executive Officer: Clayton Jones
Chief Operating Officer: Don W. Jones, Jr.
Executive V.P. & Publisher: Robert W. Holland, Jr.
V.P., Design and Production: Anne Spencer
V.P., Sales and Marketing: William Kane
V.P., Manufacturing and Inventory Control: Therese Bräuer
Acquisitions Editor: Kevin Sullivan
Manufacturing Buyer: Amy Bacus

Library of Congress Cataloging-in-Publication Data

Porter-O'Grady, Timothy.
    Quantum leadership : a textbook of new leadership / Tim Porter-O'Grady, Kathy Malloch.
        p. cm.
    Includes bibliographical references and index.
    ISBN 0-7637-3185-4
        1. Leadership. 2. Psychology, Industrial. I. Malloch, Kathy. II. Title.
    HD57.7 P666 2002
    658.49092—dc21

                                                    2002074424

Printed in the United States of America
07 06 05 04 03   10 9 8 7 6 5 4 3 2

The authors dedicate this book to Cathleen Krueger Wilson, RN, PhD, (1946-2000) nurse, therapist, consultant, colleague, and friend who first conceived the possibility of this kind of book on leadership. Her creativity and imagination in applying leadership to all venues of health service were an inspiration and a joy to all who knew her. Cathleen was a role model as nurse, mother, spouse, and friend and brought the full weight and energy of her person to her work and relationships. In death, as in life, she still serves to stimulate and encourage the best in all whose lives she touched.

Table of Contents

Preface ix

Acknowledgments xiii

Chapter 1—A New Vessel for Leadership: New Rules for a New Age 1
   Chapter Objectives 1
   Leading in a Fluid World 2
   Newton and Organizational Design 4
   Leaving the Industrial Age 5
   Change *Is* 6
   The Transition between Ages 7
   Leading Change 9
   Quantum Age Rules 13
   Conclusion 37
   Quiz Questions 38

**Chapter 2—Thriving in Complexity: Ten Principles for Leaders in
   the Coming Age** 41
   Chapter Objectives 41
   Chaos and Complexity and the Dance of Change 43
   Principle 1: Wholes Are Made up of Parts 46
   Principle 2: All Health Care Is Local 49
   Principle 3: Adding Value to a Part Adds Value to the Whole 52
   Principle 4: Simple Systems Make up Complex Systems 54
   Principle 5: Diversity Is a Necessity of Life 56
   Principle 6: Error Is Essential to Creation 58
   Principle 7: Systems Thrive When All of Their Functions Intersect
     and Interact 60
   Principle 8: Equilibrium and Disequilibrium Are in Constant
     Tension 64
   Principle 9: Change Is Generated from the Center Outward 67

Principle 10: Revolution Results from the Aggregation of
Local Changes 70
Conclusion 75
Quiz Questions 77

**Chapter 3—The Leader as Peacemaker: Managing the Conflicts of a Multifocal
Workplace** **79**
Chapter Objectives 79
Growth and Transformation 80
Avoiding Unnecessary Conflict 82
Identity-Based Conflict 89
Interest-Based Conflict 106
People and Behavior 111
Conclusion 113
Quiz Questions 114

Chapter 4—Living Leadership: Vulnerability, Risk Taking, and Stretching **117**
Chapter Objectives 117
Leadership Fitness in the New Millennium 118
Vulnerability 119
Power 120
The Cycle of Vulnerability 122
New Relationships 131
Complexity Communication 137
Collective Mindfulness 141
Strategies for Cultivating Leadership Vulnerability 142
Is There a Choice? 147
Conclusion 147
Quiz Questions 149

Chapter 5—Healing Brokenness: Error as Opportunity **151**
Chapter Objectives 151
Error in General 152
Errors in Health Care Service 156
Opportunities for Health Care Service 161
Health Care Leadership: Errors and Opportunities 164
Conclusion 182
Quiz Questions 184

Chapter 6—Emotional Competence: A Vital Leadership Skill **187**
Chapter Objectives 187
Underpinnings of Emotional Competence 188
Integrated Leadership 190
The Nature of Emotional Competence 191
The Emotional Risks of Leadership .202

The Benefits of Emotional Competence in Health Care 203
Developing Emotional Competence 209
Team Emotional Competence 213
Measuring Emotional Competence 216
Conclusion 218
Quiz Questions 219

Chapter 7—Toxic Organizations and People: The Leader as Transformer **223**
Chapter Objectives 223
Healing Is Our Business? 225
Toxic Behaviors 228
Ten Principles for Minimizing Toxic Behavior in Organizations 242
Conclusion 253
Quiz Questions 255

**Chapter 8—Transformational Coaching: Leading the Membership
    Community** **259**
Chapter Objectives 259
From Responsibility to Accountability 260
Transforming Work and the Transforming Worker 264
Evolution and Revolution 266
The Learning Organization 267
Organizing for Transformation 272
Dealing with the Lack of Time 273
The Leader as Revolutionary 277
Innovation Coaching 281
Making Integration Work 285
Hitting Problems Head On 290
Eliminating Firefighting Altogether 293
Conclusion 295
Quiz Questions 297

**Chapter 9—The Leader's Courage To Be Willing: Building a Context
    for Hope** **299**
Chapter Objectives 299
A Context for Hope 300
Will 301
Strategies To Facilitate Willingness 311
Relighting the Lamp 323
Conclusion 324
Quiz Questions 326

Chapter 10—The New Spirit of Leadership: Becoming a Living Leader **329**
Chapter Objectives 329
Chaos and the Call to Leadership 330

Self-Management and Creativity 334
Creativity and Innovation 337
Exercising the Spirit 345
Spiritual Intelligence: Ten Rules of the Road 349
Becoming Self 355
Listening for the Sounds of Change 357
Finding Spirit in the Chaos 358
The Compensations of Ignorance 359
Mystery 361
Synthesis and Synergy 362
Quiz Questions 365

Appendix—Quiz Answers 367

Index 369

Preface

Writing a book on leadership is a difficult and challenging task. Not that writing any book isn't difficult. The peculiarity of books on leadership, however, is that they can never be truly finished. Leadership is essentially a work in progress—a never-ending journey with facets and elements that add up to a broad and complex mosaic. Embedded in the leadership role are a host of behavioral, relational, interactional, and structural considerations that give form to the activity of leading. Research in each of these areas could line the shelves of libraries for generations. We submit that no one person could comprehend all that has been said and written about leadership, nor all the actions that have been done in its name.

Furthermore, as the world changes, new notions of how to advance the work of organizations and people emerge, new patterns of behavior develop, and these demand some level of explication and understanding. In fact, just like other segments of society, health care is going through the drama and trauma of reconceptualizing its work and priorities to take into account the new global reality and the most recent advances in technology. These advances are already bearing fruit and radically altering both the quantity and quality of life. And the changes yet to come will have an even greater impact than those that have already occurred.

For instance, the ever-increasing mobility of health services is creating a need to reconfigure these services and change the relationship between providers and those they serve. Accountability for choice and proper action are coming to rest more in the hands of the consumers, and health care leaders have the important job of enabling providers to alter their practices accordingly and to prepare consumers to assume the accountability that is being transferred to them.

A leadership book like this one serves as a snapshot, if you will, of the leadership role at a particular moment in time. In our attempt to identify and describe the right behaviors and strategies for the role, we have focused on the issues that are most representative of the current era. One of the earmarks of our era, of course, is the fast rate of change. Another is the obvious need for a new framework for the provision of health care services.

Health care leaders must push their organizations into this fray. They must be able not only to see into the darkness of the future but to live comfortably inside the potential—that risky, unsettled space between the present and the future. And because leaders cannot pull people into a future only they have conceived of, they must bring everyone to the table to shape the future through collective dialogue and concerted action.

In this book, we try to conceptualize the journey of health care and use the emerging images as a template to prioritize leadership skills and behaviors—those skills and behaviors that leaders need to employ to ensure their organizations are guided accurately and effectively. Our strategy is to first provide a glimpse into the future and then present some of the implications of the young sciences of complexity and chaos, thereby delineating the context of the leadership role at the outset of this new century.

There is simply no way that the changes in health care can unfold without a great deal of conflict. Most people assume that conflict in the workplace is bad and should be avoided. Nothing could be further from the truth. Conflict is a normal element of all interaction. Leaders must understand this and acquire the necessary skills to manage conflict in a way that yields the benefits that it is capable of delivering.

By handling conflict appropriately, leaders also will be better positioned to create a healing environment for providers as well as consumers of health care and undertake to heal a wide variety of emotional and spiritual injuries suffered by people as they struggle with the work of transforming the health care system. Building a healthy environment by being fully present and demonstrating compassion and accountability is a fundamental responsibility of the new leader.

Recently, a host of authors and researchers have reminded us that leaders must possess not just intellectual ability but emotional competence. After all, establishing and maintaining relationships is an essential part of leadership, and all relationships have an emotional component. To ensure that their relationships exhibit emotional maturity, leaders need to understand the nature of emotional competence and thus be able touch the emotional center in themselves and others. The value of emotional maturity for leadership is just beginning to be understood.

Behavior does not exist in a vacuum, and thus the context within which people interact and work together requires as much consideration as what they do. The enormous changes that are occurring, some of them very traumatic, are causing people to see themselves as awash in a sea of movement that does not make much sense. Staff members often fail to understand the direction in which their leaders are taking them and begin to lose hope and any sense that their work is meaningful. Leaders, in their actions, need to provide the foundations for hope and meaning and value. They must first find these things for themselves, then translate them into a language that others can comprehend and buy into.

Why are some leaders more successful than others at leading an organization through transformational change? Why are some able to create an environment of hope and calm despite difficult or even desperate circumstances? The answer can be found in the notion of personal willingness. Willing leaders are the co-creators of change. They recognize that no one person or no situation can take away their personal peace, joy, or sense of competence. They transmit these feelings to others in a way that encourages and enables them to embrace the new script and share in the writing of it.

Coaching people into the future they must live in requires special skills. Unlike in the past, leaders cannot simply force people into a mold or into compliance with demands that they played no part in setting. Allowing people to be investors, partners, and stakeholders in their own processes is a necessary talent for the new leader. Leading workers out of a toxic and perennially sick or stuck work environment is a part of this process. It requires the leader to understand the characteristics of neurotic and pathological organizations and those behaviors that prevent people and their organizations from embracing the changes they must adapt to in order to thrive in the new world of health care.

Finally, leaders must focus on the energy and spirit within to be innovative and grow and thereby act as models for others in their own search for meaning and value in what they do. But the ability to exhibit creativity, self-understanding, and personal growth is not obtained accidentally or without effort—it requires regular spiritual exercise, including periods of reflection, to develop. In the future, leaders, to sustain their effectiveness in the leadership role, will need to engage in spiritual work and increase their level of creativity.

Like others of its kind, this book is a work in progress. It is necessarily incomplete. There are already a host of good books on leadership, with more arriving on the bookshelves every day. They too are incomplete. What those individuals who want to learn about leadership must do is to see the myriad available resources on the topic as making up a single body of knowledge. Thus, if they want to improve their leadership skills, they should use this book as one resource along with others, understanding at the same time that the theory of leadership and its application will advance as more information becomes available.

The authors hope that the contents of this book will stimulate reflection and discussion. We think that it extrapolates in a defensible manner from current research and practices to newer ways of conceiving and exercising the leadership role. At this time, leaders are being challenged to take the next step in the journey toward better methods of leadership. Those whose lives they will affect have a right to expect the best that the leaders have to offer, especially as more is demanded of workers than ever before. We hope this book will play some small role in ensuring that those who provide health care services get from their leaders what they have every right to expect.

—Tim Porter-O'Grady and Kathy Malloch

Acknowledgments

A book of this kind cannot be completed without the support of a good number of people. First, I thank my co-author, Kathy Malloch, who committed full time and energy to this book and whose collaboration encouraged me. Thanks also go to Cathleen Krueger Wilson, whose vision and insight were the source of many of the ideas found in this book. I also acknowledge the many colleagues in nursing and health care who were both the subject source and the motivation for this type of book. Their encouragement kept the authors focused on writing a text that was both relevant and useful. Finally, I thank Mark Ponder, RN, for his support, partnership, and for being a sign to me that caring, loving, and nursing have nothing to do with gender.

—Tim Porter-O'Grady

Writing this book has been an experience that exemplifies the essence of complexity science. So many friends and colleagues have contributed to my development, and to them I am eternally grateful. A very important and special thank you is sent to Cathleen Wilson, who watched over the composition of this book from somewhere up there in the heavens. Thank you, Cathleen, for recognizing my potential and my frailties and for the strong mentoring that pushed me to places that I had not anticipated I would ever travel.

Thank you, Dr. Tim, for recognizing my potential also and for tolerating my shortcomings in meeting deadlines. Your invariably honest support is always affirming. I will treasure your guidance for many years. Most of all, thank you for your friendship and vital insight into the future of the health care system. You have challenged me to think and act in new and better ways.

Finally, my greatest thanks and recognition go to my husband, Bryan "Mallotchi," my very best friend and confidant, always encouraging me and tolerating my inconsistencies. Without his unconditional support, my work as a leadership advocate and healer would not be nearly as meaningful.

—Kathy Malloch

CHAPTER 1

A New Vessel for Leadership:
New Rules for a New Age

The hardest thing is not to get people to accept new ideas; it is to get them to forget old ones.

—John Maynard Keynes

Chapter Objectives

At the completion of this chapter, the reader will be able to

- Compare the characteristics of the Industrial Age with those of the emerging age.
- Enumerate the elements of quantum thinking and explain how it has influenced the journey into the Age of Technology.
- Assess the impact of quantum science and recent advances in technology on health care and clinical practice.
- Describe the implications of Age of Technology thinking on the exercise of leadership.
- Identify the different skill sets for leaders in the 21st century.

Nothing is the same—nor will it ever be again. Ours is a new age, filled with a host of inspiring and challenging opportunities that, just a decade ago, were the stuff of science fiction. Who would have thought that this generation would see the advent of fiber optics, satellite-based universities, genomics, lasers, and a host of technological innovations that boggle the mind and enthrall the imagination?

Along with these many innovations come the challenging adjustments we must make in order to live in this new world. Instant communication, boundaryless relationships, the globalization of economics and politics, Internet interaction, knowledge that exceeds our capacity to assimilate it—all are having a dramatic impact on every person's ability to thrive in the 21st century. For most of us, the changes have come so fast that we are unable to fully comprehend how they will affect us and are hard pressed to cope with their implications.

The pace alone—a pace simply unheard of in the last century—is enough to overwhelm even the most energized. As soon as we have the time to consider the particulars of the most recent changes, new changes are upon us and insinuating themselves into our culture. We do not even have the luxury of identifying their advantages and disadvantages and of considering their potential influence on our lives.

> **Key Point**
>
> *Communication technology has created a world without boundaries. We now must create our own boundaries in a way that produces a balance between the conflicting demands of our lives.*

Our society, for instance, is just beginning to understand the impact the Internet has had and will have on communication, business, and politics. Further, new elements of the Internet are already emerging to alter our lives and change the questions we are asking about what is passing before our very eyes. Yesterday's questions will not get answered because tomorrow has become today sooner than we ever could have imagined.

LEADING IN A FLUID WORLD

Leadership cannot be the same. Just as the underpinnings of our society are being radically transformed, so is the leadership necessary to guide people through life. The old models of leadership are no longer adequate to meet the demands of the times. When the world was slower paced and systems theory, complexity theory, and quantum theory were not as well formed or as influential, the nature and role of leadership were different. Even the operational realities of the workplace have changed to the point that work itself requires different skills and a different ethos (Exhibit 1–1).

The stable institutions of the 20th century are quickly unraveling as the framework for the new century gets constructed. Not only are the brick-and-mortar empires of the past breaking up, but work is being moved away from institutions altogether. The infrastructure of society is becoming less institutional and more information based, and the architecture of our places of work, service, and business is changing dramatically. Information structures are primarily relational and function horizontally, whereas most of our business structures have functioned vertically. Leading in a horizontal work culture is radically different from leading in a predominantly vertical work culture.

In the Industrial Age, organizations were primarily fixed, finite, and functional. Work in the Industrial Age was based on Newtonian principles, and from the beginning of the 20th century, when Fredrick Taylor laid down the foundations of scientific management, to the late 1960s, business organizations were structured mechanistically and hierarchically. Even the management theorists of the 1930s, 1940s, and 1950s did not radically alter organizational design. The worker was considered a subset of the work. Most training was gained on the job, and the apprenticeship model used for training was essentially

Exhibit 1–1 New versus Old Skill Sets

Knowledge Worker	Employee (Former Type)
• Conceptual synthesis	• Functional analysis
• Competence care	• Manual dexterity
• Multiple "intelligences"	• Fixed skill set
• Mobile skill set	• Process value
• Outcome practice	• Process practice
• Team performance	• Unilateral performance

hierarchical as well. The organization owned the work and set the rules. Communication and decision making traveled up and down the corporate ladder. The higher up the ladder, the greater a person's authority and autonomy. At the bottom were the workers who performed most of the functions—under the control of those who had moved "upward." Although attention was paid to both the work and the worker, it was barely reflected in the management structure and the application of leadership in organizations.

No longer. In the current world of work, it is not the organization that is owner of the work but instead the worker. The character of work changed substantially at the end of the 20th century—it became increasingly technical and complex—and now individuals usually have to be trained for jobs before they become eligible for them. Indeed, they are expected to arrive "on the run" and start contributing from the outset. Further, the organization's increased dependence on the worker has created a new power equation, shifting the locus of control from the organization to the worker.

In the Industrial Age, leadership meant being a good manager, guiding one's subordinates like a good parent, and directing their activities in the interests of the organization. The critical skills were those required for *planning, organizing, leading, implementing, controlling,* and *evaluating* (note the acronym constructed from the initials of these six words: POLICE). The ability to function well and undertake well-defined processes was the basis of every role. Good performance and a sense of responsibility were highly valued, strongly encouraged, and heavily rewarded.

> **Point To Ponder**
>
> *The worker is increasingly in control. The knowledge necessary to get work done is now mostly in the hands of those who do the work. Because the workplace is becoming more dependent on knowledge workers, a major shift in power and control has occurred, and the old structures are now in conflict with this new type of worker.*

So was compliance with the expectations of the workplace. Organizational leaders used vertical communication and command strategies exclusively to ensure that the workplace stayed focused and orderly and that the work was performed efficiently. They also refined hierarchical mechanisms and fostered congruence of workplace behavior in whatever way they could.

It was in this context that the first contemporary notions of leadership developed. A whole host of approaches to understanding leadership and acting as a leader emerged dur-

---

Group Discussion

We are living on the cusp of the transition between two ages, and life in the 21st century will differ substantially from life in the 20th century. The changes that will occur include changes in work and leadership. The group should brainstorm at least 10 changes that will occur in the new century and discuss their implications for leaders.

---

ing the century, and each one reflected prevailing notions of work and workplace organization (Exhibit 1–2). These various approaches helped create the current framework for leadership, both in the realms of action and of decision making.

NEWTON AND ORGANIZATIONAL DESIGN

Newtonian mechanics had a tremendous influence on 20th-century science *and* business. In particular, Newton's model of the physical universe influenced social theorists to view social relationships, roles, and work as highly mechanistic. In addition, entrepreneurs and organizational gurus constructed models of work in which work activities were highly compartmentalized, and they succeeded in spreading the use of these models throughout the world. As a result, work was generally designed with efficiency and effectiveness in mind, and special attention was paid to individual performance as a means of ensuring that the work was done as planned.

Also, 20th-century organizations focused on process under the assumption that, by constructing work processes properly, they would produce products and services of con-

---

Exhibit 1–2 Work Life Reality Shift

Old Reality	New Reality
• Scripted lives	• Own your script
• Unlimited resources	• Finite resources
• Fixed functions	• Tightness of fit
• Employee	• Stakeholder/member
• Fixed jobs	• Fluid roles
• Promotion	• Mobility

sistently good quality. Here again, the organizational literature reflected a reductionist model. The organizational gurus viewed organizations as being essentially the same as always, although differing in structure in minor ways and characterized by an increased degree of control over employees. As Peter Drucker pointed out, the cornerstone of most 20th-century organizations was control, as indicated by the "line and box" approach to configuring the workplace (Figure 1–1).

> **Key Point**
>
> *In the 20th century, the focus of work was on performing the right processes. In the 21st century, the focus is on obtaining the right outcomes.*

LEAVING THE INDUSTRIAL AGE

For the past 30 years or so, the standard models of work and the underpinnings of society have been undergoing a radical shift. The impact of our burgeoning technology has brought about a new construct for social structures and relationships across the whole human landscape. Quantum theory, developed and applied during the middle of the century, has helped create newer technologies that affect life from the molecular to the global level.

As an example, consider the computer chip, which has single-handedly altered human experience forever. Among other things, it brought about a whole new understanding of quantum principles and changed the very foundations of social life by connecting people in a new way. Further, we now live with the knowledge that everything is linked, and that events in one part of the universe have some kind of impact on what happens in other parts. Our understanding of the linkage between events is the basis for complexity science and

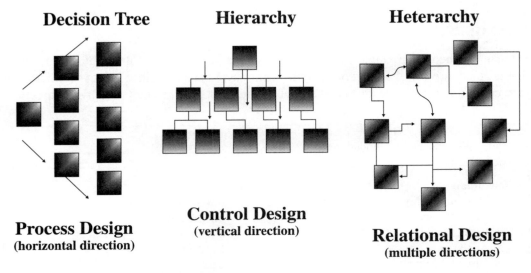

Decision Tree

Process Design
(horizontal direction)

Hierarchy

Control Design
(vertical direction)

Heterarchy

Relational Design
(multiple directions)

Figure 1–1 Changing Organizational Models

has led to changes in the conceptual foundations of the sciences and their social application (Exhibit 1–3).

In turn, these changes have raised the level of conflict surrounding basic issues ranging from the existence and nature of God to ethical and social norms. Claims that once seemed beyond question are now open to investigation and continuous challenge. New scientific discoveries have had substantial religious, philosophical, and ethical implications and have caused social discomfort among those holding traditional beliefs.

It is into this equation that organizational leaders are now thrust. The problem is that they too are experiencing the conflict endemic to the times. Most of them have spent the majority of their lives in the Industrial Age, just as everyone else has. They too are confronting newer realities with beliefs and practices acquired in the past. They too are struggling to make sense of the changes occurring worldwide. As an additional challenge, of course, they must not only engage with the changes but lead others in the effort to successfully adapt to them. Furthermore, the discoveries and innovations are occurring faster

> **Group Discussion**
>
> Health care providers at the beginning of the Age of Technology must be willing to leave some things behind (because they will cease to have value) and to take on some new things. List some of the practices, habits, rituals, or routines that need to be left behind and discuss symbolic acts or events that could be used to help let go of these formally.

than the rate of adaptation. As soon as one change is accommodated, another occurs, requiring a different response.

CHANGE *IS*

Quantum theory has taught us that change is not a thing or an event but rather a dynamic that is constitutive of the universe. People cannot avoid change, since it is everywhere, but they can influence its circumstances and consequences. In short, they can give it direction.

Exhibit 1–3 Conceptual Foundations

Newtonian	Quantum
• Mass production	• Envision the whole
• Compartmentalism	• Integration
• Reductionism	• Synthesis
• Analysis	• Relatedness
• Discrete action	• Team action

Schrödinger, a mid 20th-century physicist, used his famous "Schrödinger's Box" thought experiment to show that there are two prevailing realities operating at any given time, actual reality and potential reality. The former is the reality that currently occupies our immediate attention. Potential reality, on the other hand, although current and present, is not yet experienced. Being still potential, it is waiting for the right moment to become expressed and thus actual.

> **Point To Ponder**
>
> *A stop sign can be used to illustrate potential reality. When first seen, it notifies a driver to stop— but not immediately. The sign is a real object, a reality, and it does require a real response. The driver's preparation to stop is the first in the chain of actions, and it is this action that links the actual to the potential.*

Potential reality is the realm in which leadership takes form. The leader's role is to engage with the unfolding reality, perceive it, note its demands and implications, translate it for others, and then guide others into actions that will meet the demands of a reality not quite present.

In this transformational time between two ages, the leader's primary role is to live fully in the realm of potential reality. The leader is not so much an operational expert and problem solver as a good "signpost reader." To be effective, the leader will have to anticipate the path of change and then spell it out for those who are moving their own activities, knowingly or unknowingly, in the same direction as the change is taking.

THE TRANSITION BETWEEN AGES

Living at a time when the forces of change are converging, as always happens in the transition between ages, is especially difficult. The dynamics of a substantive change are moving in concert to create the underpinnings for a comprehensive transition from one way of living to another. This has occurred several times in human history. From the Middle Ages through the Age of the Enlightenment and the Industrial Age and up to the current era, which we might dub the Age of Technology (or the Information Age), historic indicators have presaged major shifts in human experience (Figure 1–2).

There is an important difference, though, between previous shifts and the one that is now occurring. When the previous shifts were viewed after the fact, their significance soon became clear, even if it was rarely apparent during the critical transition points. Nowadays, on the other hand, the period between predicting future changes and having to confront their unfolding is too brief to allow plans to be made to accommodate them. Indeed, today's leaders act as agents of change, but, like everyone else, they must also undergo the changes themselves virtually at the same time as they perceive them. Wholly new leadership skills are required to manage in this kind of a world.

Think for a moment about some of the ways in which the script of life is being rewritten for all of us:

- The Internet is currently the fastest growing primary business tool, and it is fundamentally altering how business gets done.

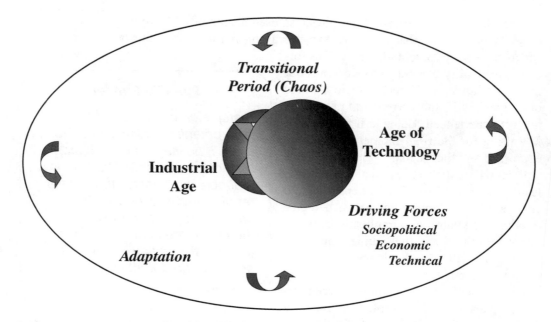

Figure 1–2 The Universal Cycle of Transformation. This illustration shows the dynamic and interacting forces of transformation.

- Fiber optics, in conjunction with satellite technology, have connected the world into a seamless communication network in which information can be transmitted instantly from any place on the globe to any other place.
- Information has thus become highly portable, and, given the developments in shipping, everyone has access to almost anything wanted or needed anywhere in the world.
- Each person has control over any relationship, personal or business, and can personalize any interaction within any context at any time and in any way he or she desires.
- Miniaturization has made it possible for people to be mobile and still remain connected to everything and everyone. Furthermore, it has made innovations in service, communication, information, and health care faster, easier, and less expensive to implement than ever before.

This is just a very small sample of the transformations that are occurring. And these transformations are only the beginning. Even so, they are having a major impact on our understanding, on the way we live and relate, and, of course, on the way we work.

Imagine the lives of our great-grandparents or even our grandparents and how different our lives are from theirs as a result of these technologies. Then consider the possibility that the children of current teenagers might never write or read as we have, interact and play as we have, relate to each other or travel as we have. And remember, it is this generation that will, not so long after we have retired, usher in the next stage of work.

Group Discussion

List dramatic discoveries and inventions that occurred during the past century and compare the way life changed as a consequence with the way life changed during the preceding millennium. Then discuss the changes likely to occur in the first decades of the 21st century, especially in health care.

In short, our generation is a transitional generation—the last generation of the Industrial Age and on the cusp of the Age of Technology. We are in essence the bridge between two ways of experiencing the world. What we do will lay the groundwork for a future that will look nothing like the world most of us know.

LEADING CHANGE

It is hard to believe that anyone today could be unaware that we are in the midst of a major social transformation—a transition to a new way of living and acting (Figure 1–3). The role of today's leaders is to encourage this transformation. Indeed, they must make a commitment to the journey and work hard to incorporate the changes in their lives in a very personal way. In other words, rather than simply suggesting that everyone and every-

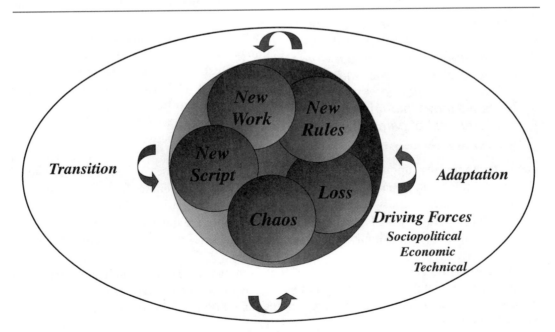

Figure 1–3 Universal Dynamics of Transformation. This illustration shows the continuous cycle of interacting processes that are the focus of the transforming work of leadership.

thing must change, they must lead by example. They must serve as witnesses to the changes and show others how to adapt to the changes in their own lives.

In the initial stage of this transformation, leaders must be able to show that the coming changes are critical and must, through their passion for movement, inspire responses from others. This is not the time for complacency but for truth telling and confrontation. In short, it is a time to persuade people that the changes could make a substantial difference in their lives and their work. Convincing people of this requires a level of honesty and directness once thought to be confrontational.

> **Point To Ponder**
>
> *The behavior of leaders must exemplify their commitment to sustain their own journey and to coordinate and facilitate the efforts of others to build a desired future.*

In the case of health care, the major transformation underway will lead to the end of the hospital-based, sickness-oriented model of service delivery. Our technologies will allow us to treat illnesses at an earlier stage and reduce the need for costly surgical interventions. As a consequence, not only physicians but nurses and other health professionals will need to make substantial changes in the way they practice medicine and provide services.

Leaders in health care must help people end their attachment to the kind of health care system they have become comfortable with. So many health professionals are mourning the loss of what is passing away or has passed away. In some cases, their sense of loss is understandable, but most of what is being mourned should not be retained or brought back. That was then, this is now. Some of the things that attracted many of us to health care have vanished for good. The question is not whether they will return, but instead how to adapt to the new circumstances.

> **Key Point**
>
> *Moving into a new age does not mean leaving everything behind. It does mean thinking about what needs to be left behind and reflecting on what does go with us as we move into an age with a different set of parameters.*

Health care leaders must try to engage others in the process of making their own changes. They must take whatever action is necessary to impress upon health professionals that this is a time of great mobility and of shifting foundations. In particular, they must call all stakeholders to the table to work out what must be altered and what must be introduced to fashion a new health care delivery system. A great tragedy will occur if health care leaders are unsuccessful in this task and allow the stakeholders to simply react to changes long since past. Complacency will guarantee failure.

Leaders may be victims of their own insights and past successes, which can cause leaders to use an outdated recipe for success as well as misleading measures of success. They must see the approaching challenges within the context of their becoming, not through the eyes of past triumphs.

Not only must leaders close the door on the passing age, but they must turn around and view the entire landscape in order to develop a workable vision of the future. Health care leaders often are too shortsighted, and their vision is too tenuous. The conditions that will determine the future of health care are vastly different from anything that has been experienced to date, and thus leaders need to construct a radical vision of how services will be provided in the new health care landscape. The impact of micronization, genomics, biotherapeutics, chemotherapeutics, and so on, is forever altering Western medicine (Exhibit 1–4), and the structures that support the provision of

> ### Key Point
>
> *The greatest impediment to future success is past success.*

Western medicine will also need to change. The bricks-and-mortar infrastructure and the current administrative and operational framework are no longer entirely relevant, and they will need to be adjusted in response to financial, political, and technological pressures. Imagine how painful that message is for the serious and talented men and women who have devoted their lives to building the current health care system. The requirement to tear it apart and begin anew is overwhelming to them, but they are called to this task by the changes that have occurred already and that suggest the direction in which health care is moving.

Health care leaders must be able to communicate to others their vision of the future and bring as much energy and commitment to the reformation of the health care system as possible. They need to capture the hearts and minds of all health professionals and other stakeholders in the health care system by being relentless communicators and forever challenging current ways of thinking and doing. They must push the walls of thought and work to ensure that the stakeholders are fully engaged in critiquing what they do, assessing the product of their work, and questioning whether what they are doing is congruent with the changing demands placed on them. Every stakeholder must continually examine the appropriateness of current work rituals and routines and determine what should be retained and what should be left behind as no longer relevant. The job of the leaders is to raise questions about the efficacy and effectiveness of current work routines and whether they are meeting new and emerging expectations.

The most important task of health care leaders is to communicate their vision, not so much by their words but by their behavior. If the leaders cannot respond appropriately to the demand for change, others will not be able to either.

Exhibit 1–4 Changing Medical Therapies

Old Therapies	New Therapies
• Surgery	• Lasers
• Salves and creams, drugs	• Microsurgery
• Accommodation	• Genomics
• Nothing can be done	• Pharmaceuticals
• Treatments	• Chemotherapy
• Enemas	• Radiotherapy
• Blood letting	• Synthetic products
• General supplements	• Specified supplements

Their next most important task is to anticipate the blocks in the way of substantive change. Implementing any planned modification requires the integration of numerous activities and people and thus faces many embedded obstacles. The most notable are elements of the organizational structure, which itself acts as insulation from the demand for change. One of the first jobs of a leader acting as a change agent is to diffuse the power of these elements and thus remove a large barrier to concerted and dramatic action on the part of the stakeholders.

Leaders must be aware that there are people who have devoted their lives to avoiding the prospect of change and that one person dedicated to blocking change can bring the entire change process to a grinding halt. Change avoiders or resisters must be identified, challenged, worked with, empowered, and placed in the midst of the change process so they do not impede the ability of the organization to thrive.

Because the transition from one age to another is a long-term process, leaders must continually set short-term goals in order to give stakeholders a sense of movement and accomplishment. The attainment of these goals allows the stakeholders to mark their journey forward and visualize and celebrate the process of change. It also gives them a moment of respite and reflection and helps them gather the energy necessary for the next stage.

> **Key Point**
>
> *The leader is an agent of change, responsible for providing others with a vision of change and ensuring that their response to the demand for change is appropriate.*

Leaders must look at change, not as an event, but as a journey—a never-ending journey. Every point of arrival, in other words, is also a point of departure. Therefore, leaders must carefully balance periods of effort and action with periods of rest and celebration so that the stakeholders will be regularly refreshed and reenergized to meet future challenges.

Finally, change is experienced on a personal level and a cultural level. And culture always rules. This truism must be solidly rooted in the mind of every leader engaged in transforming an organization. The task is to prove to the workers that the modifications will improve their work or the workplace. Today's workers are faithful, not to the workplace, but to their work. They know that they can take their skills elsewhere and be welcomed with open arms. The leaders must thus be aware of the demands regarding work that exist within the prevailing culture. Incorporating symbolic and cultural norms in the lan-

> **Group Discussion**
>
> Along with the nature of work, the characteristics of workers are changing. Discuss how the times are impacting the culture of the workplace and the characteristics of workers, compare the characteristics of new and old workers, and explore the issues that arise when both types of workers must perform together.

guage and process of change helps cast it into a form that the workers can understand and value. Every wise leader knows the political realities pertaining to a change process and adapts the process in light of them so that key stakeholders have their needs adequately met and can devote their efforts to implementing and sustaining the process.

QUANTUM AGE RULES

The new age, into which we are quickly moving, will be characterized by many new patterns and processes, as described below.

Linear Thinking Will Be Replaced by Relational and Whole Systems Thinking

Perhaps the most radical shift to occur will be the move away from mechanistic (Newtonian) and reductionist models of thought and research. In the 20th century, most research was based on vertical (or linear) processes. Quantum science, in contrast, has an affinity for complexity and chaos. The use of complex relational algorithms has lessened the former devotion to vertical processing, and relational and whole systems models now constitute a new foundation for scientific and business research. Because researchers are now capable of rapidly processing and relating complex arrays of data, they can use different processes for making decisions and creating new products and technologies, such as computer chips and pharmaceuticals.

Structure Is about Wholes, Not Parts

Our newly acquired capacity for discovering and understanding linkages and intersections has made it clear to us that at some level everything is interdependent. Further, our knowledge of the interconnectedness of everything has caused us to look differently, not just at the physical components of the universe, but also at organizations and human interactions (Exhibit 1–5). This is not to say, of course, that we always fully comprehend the nature of the interdependence between any particular elements.

The notion of fractals is critical for understanding the order that exists in chaos and for appreciating the impact of complexity on organizations and human behavior. The smallest level of a single organization and the most complex array of a large aggregated system containing the organization are connected inexorably through the power of fractals.

If you have ever looked at a hologram, which is a three-dimensional photograph of an image, you may have noticed that no matter what size section you focus in on, the entire image will still be present in the smaller piece. Holography thus can be used to explain the nature of fractals, for in a fractal the complete pattern is present in any component regardless of the level of detail or complexity. A tree is a good example from the so-called natural world, for its overall structure, including the trunk and branches, is similar to the branching pattern of each leaf.

Fractals have tremendous implications for organizations. From the smallest structural elements to the very complex patterns of behavior existing throughout an organization, the same patterns appear and are played out in precise detail. This fact implies that at every

Exhibit 1–5 The Language of Complexity and Chaos

New words from the science of complex systems describe a different world than we have grown familiar with. They express a whole set of dynamics that operate just outside our field of vision, yet they have a defining impact on our experience of life and the human journey in which we each play an important but not always known role. Some of the more unusual words include these:

- *Autopoiesis.* The process by which living systems continually seek to renew and reinvent themselves yet maintain their core integrity.
- *Autocatalysis.* A process in which information enters into a system in small fluctuations that continually grow in strength, interacting with the system and feeding back upon itself.
- *Dissipative structures.* Structures in which disorder is the source of order and vice versa. In this "dance" between order and disorder, old form ends and new form begins.
- *Strange attractor.* The activity of a collective chaotic system composed of interactive feedback between and among its various "parts" and evidencing "attraction" to its pattern of behavior.

level of the organization there exists a self-organizing capacity and that this capacity maintains a balance and harmony even in the midst of the most chaotic processes. To the extent that the balance and harmony are sustained, the organization's life is advanced. To the extent that they are upset or cannot be articulated, visualized, and acted upon at every level of leadership, the organization's actions will tend to impede its integrity and effectiveness. It is important, therefore, that the leaders of the organization be aware of the continuous and dynamic action of fractals in all organizational behavior and structure so that they can advance the consonance and value of the employees' activities and enhance the organization's ability to fulfill its mission.

Perhaps it is even more important for the leaders to recognize that, within the context of the fractals' dynamic action, their own actions have cascading and rippling implications in every other part of the organization. In fact, they should understand that no decision, action, or undertaking can occur any place in the organization without ultimately having an impact on every other action, decision, and undertaking. In addition, once they are cognizant of the web of interaction and interdependence that exists in the organization, the leaders will approach deliberation and decision making only with extreme care, caution, and thoroughness.

It is pertinent that issues of relationship and interaction, empowerment and ownership, have become increasingly implicated in our understanding of work. We now view individuals rather than organizations as owning work processes, and this change in our understanding has altered the relationship between workplace and worker. Further, by focusing on different descriptors in portraying how human dynamic systems work and how processes get sustained, we have created a new framework for considering design and function within the workplace and within the entire human community—and for considering what is and is not effective in the workplace and in relationships between people as well as for looking at issues of accountability, productivity, and value.

For example, no longer is it enough for leaders to assess the functional proficiency of individual workers as a way of determining whether a work process is fully effective and sustainable. Instead, they must also examine whether each worker's competence fits with the competence of the other workers. "Goodness of fit," not the individual proficiency of any single participant, leads to effectiveness and sustainability.

The Value of Work Is a Function of the Outcome, Not the Process

Our understanding of the value of work has undergone a change. In the past, the focus was on process, and the existence of a good work process was taken to be a sufficient condition of good service. We now recognize that process is not the only determinant of good service. Indeed, a work process gets its value from the purpose toward which it is directed (the desired outcome), and if the purpose does not inform and discipline the process, then the process can lose its value.

Work is not inherently valuable, despite the Judeo-Christian tradition. Consider how many people who have said that their work provided meaning in their lives found their lives pointless when the function and content of the work shifted. What they forgot is that work is not meaningful in itself but becomes meaningful when it fulfills an important purpose. People sometimes feel "burned out" when the meaning that should drive the work is sought in the work activity itself. When the work changes, they cannot cope because they experience not simply the end of a way of working but also an end of meaning. Their "how" has become their "why."

Process is not always connected to outcome and hence to value. Nurses and physicians, particularly, have a hard time understanding this. Sometimes their commitment to treating patients is not disciplined by the recognition that the value of any treatment activity lies in the final outcome. Indeed, they often provide health services in cases where there is little evidence that the services dependably result in a good outcome. Medical practice variance accounts for billions of dollars a year in health care expenditures. In the future, the connection between process and product—between particular treatments and their outcomes—must play a more significant role in the management of health care resources and the valuing of health services.

> **Key Point**
>
> *Competence is not about having skills but about using skills to achieve desired outcomes.*

> **Point To Ponder**
>
> *Work is not inherently valuable. Instead, it is valuable to the extent it fulfills a purpose. Therefore, the main focus should be not on the work itself, but on whether it achieves its ends.*

Technology Has Changed What People Do, How They Live, and Who They Are

When the technological advances of our own time are viewed objectively, they are difficult not to marvel at. Many inventions that first appeared in science fiction have been realized in the past few decades, and there are obviously many innovations yet to come, including some that will alter the very structure of life. Frightening as it may be, for the first time in human history we can control our own evolution and that of every other species on the earth.

Health care leaders need to realize that technology is transforming the very ground of health care for the first time since the development of germ theory. Genomics and related sciences are shifting the therapeutic framework for health care, probably for the rest of the century. How many of us are able to provide leadership in a postgenomic health care system? How many of us really know what that means?

Certainly, health care will become less dependent on the use of highly mechanical interventions, especially surgical interventions. Given the advances in bio-, chemo-, and pharmacotherapeutics, many conditions that required surgery can be handled more easily and less invasively through modern drugs. Even Alzheimer's disease will become a treatable illness before the end of the decade. The question is, what will be the implications of the switch to new therapeutic modalities, especially for the treatment of older persons and for the traditional institutional models of treatment (Exhibit 1–6)?

Leaders will have to grapple with these emerging realities and incorporate them into their own lives. Most people are finding it difficult, if not impossible, to see what the new technologies will entail for life in the 21st century, despite wanting to embrace them. They need help in grasping how the technologies will affect them and what adjustments they must now make to thrive in the coming age.

New Rules Will Apply in the New Age

Imagine not just learning to live within the context of a whole new set of rules but leading others to embrace them in their own lives and work. This is the fundamental leadership task—dealing with the same changes as everyone while helping others thrive in a new reality. What makes this even more challenging is that people are always inclined to reject the implications of the changes that are occurring.

Several late 20th-century innovations are still having a powerful impact on people's lives and on their relationship to health professionals and other service providers. These innovations include the Internet, wireless communication, fiber optics and lasers, and new drugs. The Internet, for example, not only has had an impact on global communications but has altered the way business is conducted. People can now shop without leaving home and even without any human contact whatsoever. They also can access a wide variety of information,

---

Exhibit 1–6 Seven New Age Imperatives

1. Open access to health information
2. Medicine/nursing based on genomics
3. Mass-customized diagnosis and treatment
4. User-specific insurance programs
5. Integration of allopathic and alternative therapies
6. Payment incentives tied to outcomes (quality)
7. Focused service settings for specific populations

including information that they once needed to visit a library or a professional expert to get. When people meet with their doctors, they might already have accessed health information from other sources and have questions and concerns that they want to discuss. The Internet, in other words, is helping to shift the locus of control from the providers of health services to the users, and it is also affecting the patient-provider relationship in other ways:

- Patients now determine the parameters of the patient-provider relationship, setting the stage for a different kind of interaction than has historically occurred.
- Patients need to develop partnerships with providers to sort through the available choices and pick the best. They need providers to act as educators willing to assist them in making health care decisions.
- Patients need help from providers both in verifying the accuracy of the data they have independently garnered from a host of sources and in interpreting the data.
- Patients are interested in options, not an order to undergo a particular treatment. They want to be able to consider a range of options within the context of their own personal values and priorities and choose the one option that best fits these.

Although the locus of control has shifted to the patients, they are essentially uneducated about health care. Still, ready or not, they now must take command of their own care and acquire whatever skills they will need to manage it. The current role of the providers is to

> **Group Discussion**
>
> In the transition between ages, consumers' expectations regarding their role in health care decisions and processes are changing. Discuss the changes and describe the role of health professionals in helping consumers develop the insights and skills they need to manage their own health effectively. Also discuss the dangers to consumers from making their own decisions as well as the actions that health care leaders can take now and in the future to mitigate the dangers and ensure that consumers become accountable decision makers.

ensure that the patients not only have the proper tools and skills but actually succeed at managing their own care. Consequently, providers are having to alter their priorities. Rather than always intervening medically and giving care themselves, they now frequently help their patients make proper health-related decisions and learn how to perform necessary self-care tasks. To an extent, they are becoming health service agents, assisting their patients in getting whatever equipment or services they and their patients have determined are needed or desirable.

Health Care Will Be Provided Earlier Than in the Past

Over this next century, bio-, chemo-, and pharmacotherapeutics will come to dominate the health services landscape. Because technology will be able to assess a person's physiology in ever greater detail, diseases will be identified sooner than they are now, and diagnostics will make it possible to predict with high levels of accuracy a person's degree of risk for particular diseases and conditions and provide preventive treatment before symptoms manifest.

The question for the health professional is, how will the improvement in diagnostics alter the practice of medicine? In the past, medical and nursing interventions generally required the recipients to be hospitalized. The therapies of the future will require much less hospitalization and will hardly impede the patients' normal routines. The main goals of health professionals will be to provide the right therapy at the right time and educate people about their life processes, their health, their choices (including medical and lifestyle choices), and the risks associated with each choice.

> **Key Point**
>
> *People no longer have to undergo a hospital stay to obtain most medical services. More than 50 percent of medical treatments do not require hospitalization, and by 2010 that figure will rise to over 70 percent.*

The largest two groups of health professionals, nurses and physicians, have much to accomplish in the next two decades if they are to successfully make the transition to the new era. Their clinical roles will change substantially during this period, and getting these groups to converge around a new way of delivering services will be a challenging and tumultuous experience for health care leaders. They will require extreme diligence as well as a skill set that will stretch their resources to the limit. To design the future, they will have to understand the current landscape and how it differs from the familiar territory of past experience.

The Context in Which Leadership Is Applied Is Undergoing Changes

From deconstructing infrastructure to confronting "new age" workers, leaders have a new set of tasks before them—tasks they are not fully prepared to address. For most leaders, their understanding of the nature of leadership was formed in the early and middle 20th century and reflects outmoded models. During the last third of the century, newer models of leadership and its application have emerged. These models are based on new ideas about organizational structure and managing people and processes (Exhibit 1–7).

In the past, organizations were built on the Newtonian principles of mechanistic functioning, compartmentalization, and vertical control (Exhibit 1–8). The dominant theme of Newtonian thinking is that the universe is simply one vast machine. In fact, Newton saw the universe as a sort of giant clock that could be explained in mechanistic terms, and he and his followers took the goal of physics to be the discovery of the laws that supposedly govern the parts of the universe (material particles and the bodies of which they are constituents). Almost all of the scientific progress of the late 19th century and first half of the 20th century was grounded in Newtonian concepts.

The kind of mechanistic explanation favored by Newtonians has not been able to account for human behavior and other patterns of activity in the universe, however. In the

Exhibit 1–7 The Major Tasks of the 21st-Century Health Care Leader

- Deconstructing the barriers and structures of the 20th century
- Alerting staff about the implications of changing what they do
- Establishing safety around taking risks and experimenting
- Embracing new technologies as a way of doing work
- Reading the signposts along the road to the future
- Translating the emerging reality into language the staff can use
- Demonstrating personal engagement with the change effort
- Helping others adapt to the demands of a changing health system
- Creating a safe milieu for the struggles and pain of change
- Enumerating small successes as a basis for supporting staff
- Celebrating the journey and all progress made

early decades of the 20th century, questions were raised about the adequacy of Newtonian physics to explain the incongruous and "messy" underpinnings of the universe. Biology, perhaps, has offered the best evidence that not everything works mechanistically and that the universe is rife with chaos and incongruities.

Quantum theory and other more recent scientific theories have had a large impact on theories of leadership. Many of the elements of traditional leadership grew out of a Newtonian framework, especially those focusing on hierarchical control. Indeed, organizational leaders during the 20th century tended to rely on vertical hierarchies and compartmentalization of activities in order to manage people and productivity, and the structures of their organizations reflected this tendency. The rise of quantum theory and the new appreciation of complexity and chaos as the foundational characteristics of the universe have changed our views of science and life (Exhibit 1–9). Many writers mistakenly believe that all that has occurred has been a shift in focus from physics to biology, but this way of looking at the matter itself reflects a kind of compartmentalism. Rather, what people are beginning to understand is that all elements of the universe are a part of a broad system of intersections and relationships.

All of our current theories of leadership are challenged by the major shifts in scientific thinking noted above. What were once thought to be the foundations of leadership are now being subjected to further exploration and clarification. Hierarchy and order, for instance,

Exhibit 1–8 Newtonian Characteristics

- Vertical orientation
- Hierarchical structures
- Focus on control
- Reductionistic scientific processes
- Top-down decision making
- Mechanistic models of design
- Process-driven action

Exhibit 1–9 Quantum Characteristics

• Multifocal characteristics	• Center-out decision making
• Nonlinear structures	• Complexity-based models of design
• Focus on relatedness	• Value-driven action
• Multi-systems scientific processes	

are no longer seen as requisites for leadership, and the rules governing relationships and interactions within organizations have been forever altered. Further, it is now recognized by some that the patterns of relationships in an organization are just as important as the relationships themselves or what lies within the related elements. Leaders must understand and apply these newer notions if their organizations are to thrive internally and externally.

Group Discussion

Describe the core concepts of Newtonian thinking and how these concepts were manifested during the 20th century. Consider, for example, how social institutions and structures reflected the commitment to Newtonian thinking and how Newtonian thinking influenced the leadership role.

Leaders Must Replace Traditional Leadership Models with Models That Reflect the New Framework

The current literature on leadership contains a large array of concepts that suggest a whole new framework for action. Foremost among these is the concept of complexity and the view that everything is related. This view entails that the interactions between the parts of a system are critical to the system's productivity and ultimately its sustainability. The main leadership task, then, is not so much to manage function or work but instead to coordinate the elements (e.g., the workers) and facilitate their relationship at every organizational level.

Leaders must maintain a panoramic view of the world to discern the direction their efforts should take. Their ability to see intersections, relationships, and themes is what ensures that the organization will undertake the activities it needs to in order to thrive.

In the Industrial Age, leaders were concerned most of all with function and operation. The work was compartmentalized, and the focus was on the activities of the individual employee. The employee's work life was regulated by a set of job obligations, and by meeting these obligations the employee was able to advance upward, receive better pay, or obtain other rewards. A performance evaluation system might be in place to assess the employee's proficiency, and any rewards given to the employee would be based on the quality of the work, not on whether the work had made a difference to other employees or the organization as a whole. Work processes have historically been treated as having more value than their outcomes.

In the new age, the ordering will be reversed. The most important question will not be "What have you done?" but "What difference did it make?" The former question reflects the Judeo-Christian tradition that work is inherently valuable, whereas we now view work as valuable to the extent it achieves the purposes toward which it is directed. Consequently, leaders need to consider the relationship between the work, the worker, and the purpose of the work as a dynamic that continuously drives value. Further, they need to understand that the relationship is cybernetic, which means that each element supports and feeds the others in a seamless connection.

Although the relationship between process and outcome is clear, it is not always direct. There are many circumstances and variables, including inherent and contextual influences, as well as unplanned factors embedded in the process, that affect the relationship between each of the elements of the work and the outcome of the work. These variables interact with the work process and influence both the process and the outcome. It is here that complexity plays its part.

The new age commitment to focusing on process from the perspective of outcome creates havoc among health professionals. Leaders must be fully aware of the professionals' intractable attachment to process and the functional activities that make it up. People generally come to prize particular work activities once they become expert at and are rewarded for doing them. They find it a challenge to adjust or even eliminate what they do in the face of a lack of evidence that it produces anything meaningful or sustainable. Indeed, simply getting folks to the table to discuss the product of their activities can be difficult. Yet, this is what leaders must do if they are to change the content of the work and make it more meaningful.

> **Key Point**
>
> *In the emerging age, a large part of the leadership role will involve facilitating the transition to a new way of living and working. Leaders will increasingly devote their energies to helping others adapt to the new rules for thriving in the world of work.*

Group Discussion

Explore the notion of goodness of fit between outcomes and the processes. In particular, discuss how a leader's expectations regarding staff would likely change if the leader looked at processes not independently but from the perspective of their outcomes. As part of this discussion, describe what steps the leader could take to get staff to focus on product (outcome) rather than function (process) and what changes would occur in the provision of health care services as a result.

Everything Is Part of One Comprehensive System

Formerly, it was believed that three types of functional relationships existed. Any two things in the universe were independent of each other, they were interdependent, or one was dependent on the other but not the reverse. In the quantum age, however, we realize that all things are interdependent (Exhibit 1–10). That is, all things are tied together in a wide variety of refined and sometimes inexplicable ways, some obvious and some all but invisible at any level of observation.

Leaders now must carry out their tasks with an awareness of the relatedness of processes, actions, behaviors, and functions. Nothing acts independently, nor adds to the viability of an organization independently. Every element interacts with every other element in some way, and all the elements together constitute a complex mosaic of movement and intersection. When looked at as a whole, the picture the elements present—and the information they impart—is entirely different than when they are viewed separately. Indeed, looking at the parts independently of each other may lead one to draw conclusions that might actually impede the progress of a whole process or prevent its completion, with lasting and perhaps limiting results.

To help the readers adopt the proper perspective, this book discusses the principles of complexity and chaos theory and explains how chaos can affect work, relationships, organizations, and interactions. It also discusses many of the new skills and talents that leaders must acquire as well as new metaphors and terminology better suited to describe work-related interactions and processes. By attaining a deeper understanding of the implications of systemness and complexity, leaders will relate to and interact with others in new ways and be challenged to develop a new foundation for their role as leaders.

A New Understanding of Planning Is Needed

In the Industrial Age, it was believed that everything should be outlined and planned down to the smallest detail. The expectation was that by planning future activities with

---

Exhibit 1–10 Interdependence

In nature everything is interdependent. There is an ebb and flow between all the elements of life. Leaders must see their role from this perspective. Most of the work of leadership will be managing the interactions and connections between people and processes. Leaders must keep aware of these truths:
- Action in one place has an effect in other places.
- Fluctuation of mutuality means authority moves between people.
- Interacting properties in systems make outcomes mobile and fluid.
- Relationship building is the primary work of leadership.
- Trusting feeling is as important as valuing thinking.
- Acknowledging in others what is unique in their contribution is vital.
- Supporting, stretching, challenging, pushing, and helping are part of being present to the process, to the players, and to the outcome.

great specificity, an organization could respond to the current situation accurately and effectively. Henry Mintzberg (1994) has stated that most of the largest companies in the world were really only able to accomplish 20 percent of what they had originally planned to do. Think of the resources devoted to planning that garnered virtually no return on investment.

When a plan is constructed, the future looks a certain way at that moment in time, and the context at that moment creates the foundation for what is perceived. However, since change is constant and the universe is forever in a state of chaos and creativity, the context is shifting rather than stable. The reality at the planning stage quickly gives way to a new reality that could not have been anticipated at the planning stage. And of course this cycle is continuous and never-ending, making it impossible ever to plan with broad certainty.

> ### Key Point
>
> *Chaos is an essential constituent of all change. It works to unbundle attachment to whatever is impeding movement. Chaos challenges us to simultaneously let go and to take on. It reminds us that life is a journey of constant creation.*

Leaders now must incorporate the vagaries of complexity and chaos into the process of anticipating and planning for the future. Detailing the specifics of some future state is no longer a viable means of planning. Discernment and signpost reading are better skills to have than are those related to defining and direction setting. Leaders must realize that no real-time insight is sustainable, nor is it entirely accurate. It is simply a reflection of the particular point a person or organization is at in their continuous and relentless unfolding and becoming.

A good leader is one who can read the signposts suggesting that a change is imminent and can discern the direction of the change and the elements indicating its fabric. The good leader synthesizes rather than analyzes and views the change thematically and/or relationally, drawing out of it what kind of action or strategy should be applied—the response, that is, that best positions the organization to thrive in the coming circumstances.

For a leader to act as a strategist nowadays means not detailing the organization's future actions, but translating the signposts of change into language that has meaning for those who must do the work of the organization. Translating the signposts into understandable and inspiring language is more critical than almost any other strategic task. It is vital that a change have implications for those who are doing the work. Another way of saying this is that it must have meaning to them within the framework of their work activities so that they can commit to it, which they must do if they and the organization are to adapt to the change successfully. The leader's job is to describe the change in a way that allows the workers to understand its value and how it will affect their own efforts.

In this new era, leaders need insights about contextual themes rather than step-by-step guidance on how to implement a minutely defined vision. They must understand that their organization is on a journey and that they need to continuously peruse the landscape for guidance rather than create a list of steps through which the organization will move on its way to a preset future. Becoming aware of the themes and undercurrents and reading the contextual signposts regularly is a wiser and more effective strategy for the new age leader than laying out a itemized plan that may or may not correspond with future conditions.

Swarmware and Clockware Need To Work Together

Kevin Kelly (1998) coined two terms, *clockware* and *swarmware,* to describe contradictory forces that must work together to create meaningful action and a thriving workplace. Clockware is the rational and structured process framework; it is ordered, vertical, rational, purposeful, and organized. Swarmware, on the other hand, consists of the disparate intuitive, sensed, inherent processes at work just under the surface of all action. Swarmware is as essential to the effectiveness of a system as clockware. Overdependence on either one will prevent the system from adapting to the demands of change and keep it from thriving.

> ### Point To Ponder
>
> *Good leaders know how to integrate the rational and the intuitive, for both are equally important. They conflict with each other but also complement each other. Consequently, leaders must think clearly and rationally while at the same time remain sensitive to the underlying flow of change.*

Historically, leadership has emphasized rational and operational science skills and functions at the expense of intuition and feeling. In most workplaces, the former, seen as more "masculine," are prized, whereas intuition and feeling, often viewed as "feminine," are taken to be less applicable in the hard-driving corporate world.

Even in health care, caregiving and relational behaviors were viewed as okay for nurses and doctors but as having no place in the business end of service delivery. The principles of quantum, chaos, and complexity theory, however, entail that failure to incorporate these behaviors into the operations of an organization—in addition to rational, hard-driving, objectified behaviors—will reduce the organization's viability. Too much of the rational and hard driving can alienate people and distance them from the work process, reducing their energy, their creativity, their commitment to the organization, and their ability to perform their jobs effectively.

Simply being capable and competent in form and function is not enough; leaders must also exhibit the ability to balance a complex range of skills and system resources in order to develop the employees' capabilities and grow the organization. They must know how to create a balance between means and meaning and enter into the relationship between all the elements at the personal level and at the organizational level. Incorporating their vast array of behaviors and skills into the mosaic of interactions creates resonance between the functional and the relational, both of which are essential for developing and maintaining the vitality of person and system.

Leaders Must Find the Right Balance

Weighing the various structures and influences in a work system and finding just the right mix of elements is a challenging job. Yet that is exactly what leaders must learn to do. And they must learn to do it with a minimum of artificial supports and structures.

The infrastructures of most of the health care system are so burdensome and complex that they actually interfere with the ability of organizations to do what they are designed to do. Because of overstructuring, most organizations would not know how to live without the structural elements that encase every function and activity in the system.

In the new age, we must come to realize that there should be just enough structure to support the integrity of the organization and not an ounce more. The more structure an organization has, the more structure it serves and the more resources are drawn away from the system. Structure is actually an enemy of work and effectiveness. Under the rubric of "good order," structure drains the energy and creativity out of a system and obstructs relationships and interactions necessary for the system's functioning. It ends up crippling the system's ability to do its work and to fulfill its purposes. The goal of an organization's leadership should be to reduce structure as much as possible.

Structure is like information, in that both can easily be overvalued. Information clearly should play a role in decision making. Yet there will never be enough information to make a decision guaranteed to be the right one in the circumstances. Furthermore, an organization can strangle itself with data in the effort to know everything pertinent to a critical decision before making the decision. Leaders need to accept that they will never know enough to guarantee the correctness of their decisions and that information is simply a tool that offers a glimpse of relevant factors at a given point in time. Because conditions are constantly changing, too much dependence on information can lead to poor decisions just as easily as a total lack of information can.

For information to be valuable, its quantity is not as important as its relevance, and its quality is not as important as its timeliness. Leaders must know how much information is enough, what its focus is, what it

> **Point To Ponder**
>
> *Information and data are tools for decision making. Since information can be collected ad infinitum, the critical issue, for a leader facing a decision at a given moment, is whether there is enough information to make an informed decision. Of course, the circumstances determining the amount and type of required data can change. In other words, information needs are dynamic and not stable.*

indicates, and what its bearing is on the decisions that need to be made. They also must know when the limits of information have been reached and when its application requires discernment, deliberation, and judgment.

At every level of activity, there is a complex pattern of irregularity. Quantum scientists call this pattern a *fractal*. Fractals are embedded in every element and process of life. While complex, they exert an influence on order and chaos in the universe and are evident in the action of planets and stars, plants and animals, even the beat pattern of a human heart. Our understanding of fractals and their application to organizations flies in the face of every organizational model. These models, including the organizational charts and job descriptions associated with them, are part of a concerted effort to exclude from organizational life the disorder and chaos that lies just below the surface. Yet no matter how rigorous the structure, the chaos bursts through and creates confusion and discord, making nonsense of efforts to control it.

> **Group Discussion**
>
> In a fractal, the whole is replicated in each part. Each branch of a tree, for example, shows the same pattern as the whole tree, as does each leaf. Again, the indentations and projections in a few feet of shoreline may mimic those in a 100-mile stretch of coastline. Apply the notion of a fractal to organizations, groups, and teams. For instance, how does the notion of a fractal apply to the design of an organization? To the relationship between leaders? To roles? How does it apply to the organizational chart for a health care system?

It is impossible to codify all the activities in an organization. How many health care facilities now have so many policies and procedures in place that they sit on the shelves neglected until the next accreditation visit? It is simply not possible to codify all the elements, interactions, and relationships necessary for the care of human beings. The vagaries of the human condition militate against creating a format or structure that sets adequate behavioral or procedural parameters for treating medical conditions. The foundations of action lie in the principles of care and service, but while the principles are constant, the context within which they are applied is not.

> **Key Point**
>
> *The leader is a primary facilitator of the journey to a new way of working. The leader's role is to keep people on the journey and help them understand what that means to them.*

Here again it is the relatedness between factors that should drive a leader's response. Since the elements, behaviors, and variables affecting action are uncertain, the leader's task is to achieve as much balance as the circumstances will allow. And since this balance is fluid, the leader must act to adjust it in response to changes in the circumstances, including internal and external influences. The leader is always interpreting, explaining, adjusting, and applying the issues and dynamics affecting the character of the work and the integrity of the workplace.

Besides being an explicator of chaos wherever necessary, the leader must be present to the staff in a way that assures them of connection, understanding, and experience. The leader must show that he or she is as vulnerable to the vagaries of circumstance as anyone else and can live with chaos comfortably and knowledgeably. Still, it is difficult at best to deal with chaos. People fundamentally love order and want their leaders to deliver stability and "normality." Despite this fact, leaders, rather than insulating people from their innate disorder, must instead help them to embrace it, understand it, and develop the personal skills necessary to cope with it.

Chaos and Paradox Are Always at Work

Even at the fundamental levels of life, chaos is hard at work. Creatures as small as one cell are constantly undergoing accidental modifications that give them a better chance of thriving. It is a basic requisite of all life to be able to adapt to changing conditions. The demise of the dinosaur is a good example of what happens when living beings fail to adapt.

The age we are fast entering is vastly different from the age we are leaving. Science and technology are altering every aspect of our lives. Our challenge is to embrace the new circumstances and then sort out their implications and applications as we go. For the person who says, "I don't want to learn about computers and how to use the Internet," the best response may be to say, "Die, it will be easier on you." Although facetious, that piece of advice reflects an element of truth. Technological advances and the challenge of adapting to them are not going to go away.

In the coming age, leaders will be called upon to tell the truth, teach coping and adaptation skills, and learn new skills and apply them in new ways and in new settings. The infrastructure that generated past leadership roles is disappearing, and the new circumstances will demand new roles and challenge everyone to respond to a whole new set of questions.

Furthermore, the new age will open up the door to uncertainty and a general lack of "rightness." The prevailing principles will be open to interpretation and will be applicable in a host of ways. No one response to a change or answer to a question will be clearly best. There might be many correct responses depending on the cultural and intellectual context. Leaders will have to respect the diversity embedded in every condition or issue (Exhibit 1–11).

The techniques for finding common ground, for sorting through the various landscapes representing the diversity inherent in each issue, are now required by every leader. Also required are consensus-building and group process skills, for leaders have the job of getting people to come together around issues and help them determine appropriate responses within the context of their own roles. This is a challenge that cannot be met by establishing standardized job procedures or rules.

Exhibit 1–11 Paradox

There are many paired elements of life that appear contradictory but at a deeper level are in fact complementary. These include the following:
- Chaos and order (there is order in all chaos and vice versa)
- Creativity and tension (tension leads to creativity and creativity causes tension)
- Conflict and peace (conflict is necessary to peacemaking, containing in it the elements upon which peace must be built)
- Difference and similarity (difference seen at a great distance appears as an integrated whole)
- Complexity and simplicity (complexity is simply the visible connection between aligned simplicities)

Leaders must develop an affection for risk and for the edges of agreement and understanding. They must be able to "push the river" so that the mental models people bring to the resolution of concerns or the determination of strategies and actions are shifted or even fundamentally altered. There is nothing worse in deliberation than using a mental model or frame of reference that does not fit the circumstances. As we move inexorably into the new age, we must try to understand its characteristics within the context of its becoming rather than the past. Peter Drucker said it best when he suggested that we must all close the door on the Industrial Age and simply turn around.

> ### Key Point
>
> *All decisions and actions are rife with risk. Risk cannot be eliminated and should not necessarily be decreased, for courses of action that possess great value tend to be associated with higher risk. What is important to determine is not whether the risk can be eliminated, but whether the level of risk is appropriate for the actions undertaken and, if so, what strategies can accommodate the risk.*

It is in turning around that we begin to confront the inadequacies of our historic mental model. We begin to see the future unfold within its own context rather than one we bring to it. We look over the landscape of our becoming and are stimulated to go to those places that least fit our prevailing mindset and that challenge what we understand and the language we bring to the journey.

Leaders need to be called out of certainty into experimentation. They must take smaller steps and let the consequences of each step suggest the best direction in which to move next. It is in the steps of experimentation—of testing and evaluating—that their direction and its appropriateness can be discerned most easily. Finally, leaders stand to gain most information about what is viable and sustainable by bringing a variety of testing procedures together and using them jointly.

Pay Attention to the Informal Network

In every organization there is a formal structure and process and an informal network. This network is primarily relational and carries most of the information about how people in the organization think or feel and what their sentiments are regarding almost anything in the system. It is as vital and valid a part of the system as any other, and it requires attention because, among other things, it typically contains essential pieces of the dynamic that have been overlooked or missed as well as the "undiscussables," issues that are too sensitive to lay on the table and opinions that do not reflect the prevailing point of view. Embedded here too are some of the most dynamic notions of what should happen or what should be done.

All elements of the system, whether formal or informal, are a part of the dynamic of change in the organization. Each can be a vehicle for action and even transformation. Leaders need to pay notice to all the informal pathways and networks of communication and relationship, from hallway conversations to lunchtime discussions, from whispered comments to sarcastic asides—each plays a role in the complex web of interactions necessary for sustaining the organization. Taking an opportunity to hear, communicate, or interact is never inappropriate. All means are legitimate and deserve attention. Each, when joined with the others, contributes to discovering the state of the organization and determining the proper actions to take in order to strengthen it.

Simple Systems Are Linked To Create More Complex Systems

The universe consists of a web of simple and discrete networks that cannot survive or function without some intersection and interaction with each other. Complexity is the sum of simplicity. Each needs the other to thrive. Simple systems seek each other out in a mysterious dance of self-organizing and join with each other at appropriate intersections to configure a larger whole. Called *chunking,* this process is similar to fitting pieces together from a child's erector set to build a structure. Each element has its own purpose and meaning, but its purpose remains unfulfilled until it interacts with the other elements.

The implication for human organizations and behaviors is that all things begin with the simple. Sustainable change rarely originates at the top of a system; instead, it usually starts at the center and works its way outward. For instance, the purpose and meaning of a service organization are generated by the staff closest to where the services are provided, which is also the organization's source of development.

Leaders need to understand that sustainability comes from where the organization lives out its life—the point of service. Here the pieces of the organization come together to fulfill the organization's purpose. Here is where providers and clients come together to live out the processes toward which the organization's infrastructure and operations are directed.

Although leaders profess to recognize the importance of the point of service, the design of many organizations does not reflect the point of service's key role. The organizational

Group Discussion

Karen Weiss, RN, is the head of the nursing department in a medical clinic. The staff members like her because she can get things done and keep things moving. Although she has a highly developed sense of order, recent changes are making it harder for her to stay "in control." She feels as though things are getting ahead of her and she is losing her touch. Others also are not as satisfied with her performance as they were. Discuss the following questions: What is the real issue in this case? How is Karen's need for control in conflict with the principles of complexity? Who has accountability for decisions? Should Karen change her manner of leading? If so, how should she change it, and what does she need to do in order to change it? How does Karen make sure that staff are more involved in decisions that affect their own lives?

hierarchy typically strangles the dynamics of the system and creates an artificial and unsustainable framework for decision making and action taking. Individuals not at the point of service take responsibility for strategy, policy, and direction setting and, by so doing, remove the authority to act from its rightful place. It is a universal principle that the further away from the point of service a decision about what goes on there is made, the higher the risk, the greater the cost, and the lower the sustainability. Sadly, many organizations increase their risk and their costs and fail to attain their objectives as a result of failing to incorporate this principle into their way of doing business.

Staff, in constructing the correct complex-relatedness and infrastructure, must be free to "chunk" from their center and create linkages with the strategic, financial, and support structures that facilitate their work. Here again, tearing away much of the intervening infrastructure and the organizational layers and compartments serves to free the organization to enter into the more fluid and variable relationships it needs in order to provide health care. The simple essential components can then be joined by those who own them to other essential components to construct a web of intersections and resonating connections that hums with life and meaning.

The operation of a computer perhaps best exemplifies these forces at work. Software code has defined functions but must interact with other pieces of data before it has utility for the computer user. A certain segment of code may be said to have application value, but it must interact with other segments before this value can be realized. In other words, each segment has value in virtue of its contribution to the whole.

Learning occurs in the same way. Simple concepts lead inexorably to other simple concepts, and when they are all ultimately tied together, the learner understands the interdependence of different simple processes and thereby achieves knowledge. Furthermore, the learner recognizes that knowledge, rather than valuable in itself, is valuable to the extent that it can be applied in action.

What complexity teaches us about knowledge is that it is not so much a capacity as a tool. It has relevance at a particular moment or in a specific situation. A shift in the context, an increase in understanding, or new information affects the elements of knowledge and challenges the person to "move on" and adjust what is known, valued, and applied. In fact, there is an endless dynamic comprising the aggregation of knowledge, the letting go of what is no longer valid, and the reaching out for what is next in the endless journey of learning. The critical point here is that what is relevant or irrelevant, adequate or inadequate, at any given time is not the whole of a person's knowledge but rather pieces or elements of knowledge (chunks). The person moves in and out of these chunks and in so doing alters the relationship between them and the whole complex of knowledge.

> **Point To Ponder**
>
> *Knowledge traditionally has been viewed as something that one possessed. Today, however, it is viewed as a utility—something not possessed but accessed. People who want to use knowledge should know how to access it, how to use it, and when to let it go.*

Good leaders understand this and are able to use it in the interests of others and of the organization. They never get so attached to any specific item, process, or activity that they treat it as permanent and/or unchanging. Each item, process, or activity is part of a mosaic and comes and goes depending on the demand for it at various times. Good leaders know to let go when that is appropriate and to take on and adjust when that becomes necessary. Furthermore, they know that the organization's complex and chaotic circumstances require them to keep an eye on the larger picture and read the changes that are occurring or about to occur and make the necessary adjustments at the appropriate time.

Good leaders know that a complex system works when the simple systems work. If something is wrong at the point of service, the system as a whole will be affected. Since the interdependence between simple components is so "tight" in an effective and viable complex system, any break in the simple (or local) systems will lead to breaks at all levels of the complex system. It is by ensuring the effectiveness of the simple systems that good leaders facilitate the integrity and efficiency of the whole system (Figure 1–4).

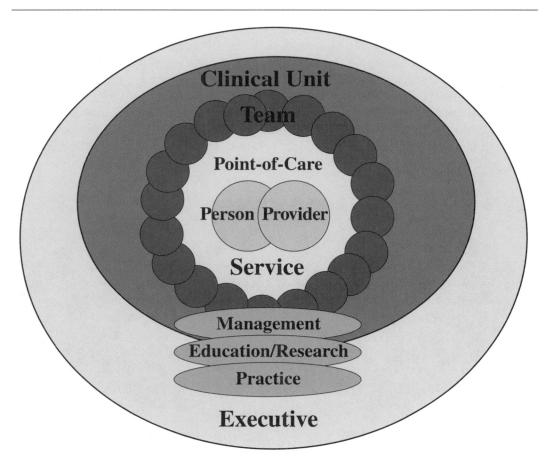

Figure 1–4 Point-of-Service Systems Design

Systems Do Not Compete with Each Other but Simply Seek To Thrive

Chaos theory and quantum theory hold that competition is anomalous. Still, the current literature on organizations and their management contains numerous discussions of the viability and importance of competition.

All living systems seek to thrive. At a fundamental level, they are not concerned with each others' survival unless it is somehow related to their need to thrive. Adaptation is not about competition between the fittest but about survival of the fittest, and the survival of a system is more dependent on its inherent adaptability to its environment than on anything else. To thrive, the system must have beneficial interactions with its environment and must also have the capacity to adjust to the prevailing conditions quickly and effectively. A system is fundamentally in competition with *itself,* not with anyone or anything else (Figure 1–5).

The concept of being in competition with oneself is generally foreign to capitalistic ways of thinking. Still, even capitalism treats competition as fundamentally a personal exercise—a contest between oneself and others for profitability and success. What it does not always recognize is that whether success is achieved has less to do with one's competitors than with one's adaptability, creativity, energy, and commitment to succeed. In other words, the pursuit of success should be viewed, not as a contest with others, but as a personal effort to give one's best and thrive in the environment one has chosen to live in.

In the coming age, persons and organizations increasingly will be challenged to adjust to the new context and the new rules. Those that thrive will be those that can read the signposts and apply the new rules to their own lives or their own operations. Organizational leaders will need to learn the fundamentals of thriving in the new age. They must make a diligent effort to keep up with the transformations in technology, global communications, information infrastructures, and social conditions. Here again, reading the signposts

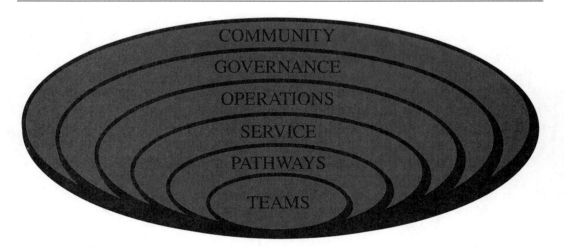

Figure 1–5 Structural Integrity and Interdependence: Functional Components of a Health Structure. Each component of the structure acts on and in concert with other components, all of them working together to advance heath care.

becomes a very important skill. Paying attention to indicators, monitoring innovations, experimenting with new and unfamiliar approaches, and living comfortably with the ambiguity and "noise" of change are all essential skills for the great leaders of the future.

The Compression of Time Will Affect How Work Is Done

There simply cannot be a leader anywhere on the earth who has not noticed the not-so-subtle change in our sense of time and space. Most people now in the work force have noticed how time has speeded up and how radically its quickening has affected the content and flow of work. Leaders can turn anywhere and hear others in the organization suggest that there simply is no time to do all that is required. Leaders themselves are aware of how very little time they seem to have to meet what appears to be an increasingly large set of demands.

Technology, including the prevailing methods for purchasing and shipping material goods, is primarily responsible for the compression of time and work. For example, LASIK surgery, a type of corrective eye surgery, takes only seven or eight minutes; Internet grocery stores deliver groceries within two hours of the placement of the order; and communication by e-mail is virtually instantaneous. Quick transmission of information and quick delivery of goods and services are increasingly normal in our global society.

The need for hierarchy—for many layers of decision making and management—has all but disappeared from the business world. In the late 1980s and early 1990s, business leaders reconfigured their organizations to eliminate management structures that had long been part of organizational culture. The goal for organizations was to become nimble and fluid, and whatever impeded their achievement of this goal was either cast off or reconceived.

Health care organizations are today going through a crisis similar to the one that existed in the business community 10 years ago. There is too much "bricks and mortar" infrastructure in place to support a delivery system that has all but disappeared, and this infrastructure is now an impediment to the system's survival. Changes in technology, service structure, clinical models, consumer demand, and health care economics are conspiring to create a need for health care organizations that possess the same fluidity and nimbleness formerly required of businesses. The chaos currently being experienced in the system arises from the conflict between the requirement for a radical shift in design and service and the continuing commitment of leadership to the outmoded infrastructure. The myriad stakeholders in the health care industry—nurses, doctors, hospitals, pharmacists, and so on—are struggling to hold onto

> ### Key Point
>
> *There is never enough time. Technology has compressed time so that what once was enough is now insufficient. Leaders must help others see their work from the perspective of compressed time. For example, now that clinical interventions require less time than previously, practitioners and patients must shift their expectations to fit the narrowed time frame.*

their piece of the health care pie without realizing the pie is now being sliced in an entirely different way.

The compression of time is inexorably working to reconfigure the context for health care and restructure its framework without the consent of the participants. Health care leaders must now focus on interpreting external demands and translating them into internal actions. They are being called into the chaos of creativity in order to produce a good fit between the new framework demanded and the infrastructure that must be constructed to support it.

> ### Point To Ponder
>
> *Over the next decade, as health care services and interventions become more mobile, organizational leaders will be engaged in the deconstruction of the institutional infrastructure of health care—the bricks and mortar.*

Much of the current work of health care leaders involves deconstructing health services. The current infrastructure must be largely deconstructed so that it can be replaced by newer models of service and support. Leaders must perform a range of activities in reconfiguring health care to fit the coming age, when space and time will be further compressed, services will be more fluid and more highly mobilized, and the locus of control will shift from the provider to the user. The changes that will occur include these:

- The hospital bed will cease to be the main point of service. During the next two decades, the number of hospital beds will decline by about 50 percent.
- The service structure will be decentralized. The health care system will deliver small, broadly dispersed units of service.
- Services will increasingly move out of the hospital. More than 70 percent of the medical services currently provided in hospitals will be provided in clinics and doctor's offices by the end of this decade.
- The core practices of the professions will be substantially altered. The institution-based, late-stage services that once predominated are being replaced by high-intensity interventions that do not require hospitalization, and these interventions will transform the roles of the various health professionals.
- Users of health services are becoming more accountable for their own health. Providers now have the major job of helping to transfer the locus of control for medical decision making and life management to individuals who have never had it and do not yet know what to do with it. Their work over the next two decades will include educating the users of health services and assisting them in acquiring the necessary skills.

For the deconstruction of health services to be effective, leaders must know that this transformation is taking place and agree to lead the effort. The conditions are already in place, but the work of making the change meaningful and feasible has yet to be done. If a leader is opposed to the transformation or is unable to acquire the necessary skills, then both the leader and the transformation will suffer.

One responsibility of leaders is to help others mourn the loss of what is passing. For example, many of the reasons that led people to enter the health professions no longer apply. Despite this, health professionals often continue to believe that the reasons are still valid or refuse to acknowledge that their idealization of the past might be keeping them from embracing the future, to their own detriment.

One way to aid health professionals in mourning their losses is help them enumerate these losses and determine what they must let go in order to obtain the skills and master the roles needed to function in the new health care system. Each person must give a voice to his or her own losses and symbolically let them go so as to be able to turn in the direction of change and innovation and meet the coming challenges. By doing this, the person becomes free to explore the changes and ultimately design a personal strategy to accommodate them.

> ### Group Discussion
>
> Twenty years ago, the average length of stay in a hospital was about 5.7 days. In the coming decade, the average procedure will require a stay of only 4.5 hours or less. These two facts indicate the extreme shift in the nature of clinical services. Discuss how the new service model will change the way health care providers work. What tasks will have ceased to possess value? How can leaders convince staff to abandon old practices that are no longer relevant? And what are the implications for patients?

Death is part of the cycle of life and is a requisite of all change. Not everything in the universe that thrives will continue to do so. When circumstances change radically, some formerly vigorous systems will fail. In some cases, the demands are beyond the system's capacity to adapt; in other cases, the changes call for a new work format that cannot be achieved simply by altering some of the characteristics of the workplace.

Leaders are obligated to help those things that should diminish or die to do so quickly. They are expected to make it clear to the staff that the process of bringing something to an end is as necessary as any other organizational process. A part of the tough work of helping necessary change along is changing staff attitudes about the permanence of work. Employees do get stuck in their rituals and routines. Their attachment to these routines may be the only point of security they have in this fast-paced world. What they might not know is that holding onto practices that are no longer relevant endangers their ability to succeed in the future. Leaders must "truth-tell" to keep staff in mind of the fact that work effort and function are transitory and that attachment to the work itself may be the greatest impediment to their own success and that of the system.

Leaders must keep their eyes fixed on the work and on how changes might impact the ability of staff members to do the work. The function of work will continually change, and attachment to work routines simply slows the individual's adaptation. A refusal to adapt does not diminish the demand for change; it just makes the adjustment to the change increasingly more difficult for the individual.

All Change Ultimately Makes Good Sense

As Stephen Hawking has eloquently stated, "Change is." Chaos, complexity, and change are not things but forms of dynamic activity. According to Hawking, they are the only constants in the universe. They will never cease, for their end would be the end of everything. Perpetual dynamic movement is what underpins every action and process. This aspect of reality is less understood and less often made use of than physical laws, but it exists nonetheless.

> **Key Point**
>
> *Change is.*

Leadership is mainly concerned with adapting to change, and all the leadership functions and activities outlined in this and other contemporary leadership texts are informed by this understanding. In fact, theorists are inclined to be less definitive than formerly in their statements about the attributes of leadership and in their recipes for leadership success. Instead of being guided by an unchanging set of principles, leaders need to be fluid and adaptable, for their role changes in concert with the changing conditions.

Leaders are aware that it is in the pursuit of meaning that the direction of a change can best be discerned. They continually look past the real and the present toward the unformed and potential to better evaluate the present and the direction of transformation. The subtle themes and ebbs and flows that lie just beneath the surface of events and experiences have more to say to leaders than do the events themselves.

Leaders know that much of what is seen and experienced is a metaphor for the operation of the infrastructure of change. The chaos so often represented in the change process is a cover for an explicit and elegant order that can only be perceived by focusing on the whole rather than the parts. Indeed, looking only at the individual parts makes it almost impossible to see the integrity, order, and beauty embedded in an elegant web of flow and linkage.

Leaders are motivated by the connections that give meaning and value to the current and the real (Exhibit 1–12). The rules that guide the journey of change are both simple and complex, and the full set is not fully comprehensible all at once. An important task for any leader is to discern the predominant operating variable impacting the journey at any given moment. Using insight, the leader is able to apply the value it represents and use it as a window for viewing the next factors, principles, or interacting forces pushing toward the next step in the transformation.

Leaders are forever caught in the potential. It is their ability to thrive in the potential that distinguishes good leaders from the rest. Good leaders are always on the edge of chaos, looking over the horizon, looking just beyond the precipice, and they are able to read, interpret, and express what they discern there. Their real gift is their ability to walk back to where those they lead are living and translate what they have seen into a language that has force and meaning for those who can hear it. They then have the job of getting behind the staff and pushing them into their own conceptualization and definition of the emerging reality, allowing the staff to own what they see and act on it in a responsive and viable way.

Exhibit 1–12 Motivated versus Unmotivated Leaders

Unmotivated	Motivated
• Focus on the present	• Focus on the potential
• No time for the work	• New kind of work
• Things are getting worse	• Things are different
• Cannot do the work any more	• New mental model for work
• No one knows . . .	• How can I get to know . . . ?
• It is too much for one person	• Share the work
• This too shall pass	• It is a journey I lead
• Doing more with less	• Doing different work differently

CONCLUSION

Leadership skills are learned skills, and their mastery requires neither magic nor a high level of intellectual capacity. Leaders emerge in a wide variety of circumstances and reflect a broad range of talents and personalities. There is no one pattern of behavior or personality type that is most suitable for the leadership role. In short, leaders come in every size and shape.

What leaders must possess is the ability to understand the vagaries and complexities of human interactions and relationships. In their role as leaders, they must take into account chaos and complexity as these do their work and create their inimitable patterns of adaptation and growth. Good leaders live in the edgeland between now and the next and are able to engage folks in the journey of the whole across the landscape of a preferred and optimistic future.

Leaders in the coming age will need new skills as well as new insights about leadership and the preferred methods of "journeying." These skills and insight can be learned, adapted to current conditions, and applied in a variety of ways to meet the demands of the journey. In their application, an individual may come to discover the leader in him- or herself, feel the excitement of leadership work, and catalyze others in the journey of discovery and advancement.

REFERENCES

Kelly, K. 1998. *New rules for the new economy.* New York: Viking Press.

Mintzberg, H. 1994. *The rise and fall of strategic planning.* New York: The Free Press.

SUGGESTED READINGS

Briggs, J., and D. Peat. 1999. *Seven life lessons of chaos.* New York: Harper Perennial.

Cameron, J., and M. Bryan. 1992. *The artist's way.* New York: Putnam.

Fulmer, W. 2000. *Shaping the adaptive organization: Landscapes, learning and leading in volatile times*. Chicago: AMACOM.

Hock, D. 1995. The chaotic organization: Out of chaos into order. *World Business Academy Perspectives* 9, no. 1: 5–18.

Holland, J. 1998. *From chaos to order*. Reading, MA: Helix Books.

Holland, J. 1995. *Hidden order*. New York: Addison-Wesley.

Kelly, S., and M.A. Allison. 1999. *The complexity advantage*. New York: McGraw-Hill.

Wheatley, M. 1996. *A simpler way*. San Francisco: Berrett-Koehler.

Zimmerman, B., C. Lindberg, and P. Plsek. 1998. *Edgeware*. Irving, TX: VHA, Inc.

Quiz Questions

Select the best answer for each of the following questions.

1. For the past 30 years we have been leaving what age?
   a. the Middle Ages
   b. the Age of Technology
   c. the Information Age
   d. the Industrial Age

2. What is the primary vehicle moving us out of the past age?
   a. economics
   b. technology
   c. satellites
   d. politics

3. As we get closer to fully living in the new age, the pace of change:
   a. quickens
   b. slows
   c. becomes unstable
   d. stays about the same

4. Adaptation means:
   a. adjusting to the current reality
   b. accommodating the emerging reality
   c. bringing the past reality forward
   d. living fully for today

5. Autopoiesis is a process in which:
   a. living systems seek to continually reinvent themselves
   b. living systems leave behind forms they do not like
   c. living systems maintain their stability throughout each change
   d. living systems end themselves because they have no other role

6. Accountability is a matter of:
a. using good work processes
b. acting responsibly
c. performing efficiently
d. achieving desired work outcomes

7. Systems thinking identifies which of the following as an essential characteristic of all systems:
a. codependence
b. predictability
c. interdependence
d. incrementalism

8. Chaos is essential to all change. The primary purpose of chaos is:
a. to confuse people enough to make them change
b. to challenge people to see clearly the changes that are coming
c. to cut people's attachment to the past and engage them in the "noise" of change
d. to get people to identify the characteristics of a particular change and to respond specifically to these characteristics

9. The primary role of the leader during a time of great change is:
a. to help people embrace change and engage with the change efforts of others
b. to explain the kinds of changes people can expect
c. to keep people from experiencing too much pain during the change process
d. to push people into necessary changes and help them cope

10. Chaos theory and complexity science require leaders to alter their understanding of how change works. To develop a new understanding of change, leaders must first see their role in relationship to:
a. the changes that are occurring in the workplace
b. the whole system and its place in the change process
c. the staff's issues and their responses to the demands of change
d. the challenges that lie ahead in implementing new changes

CHAPTER 2

Thriving in Complexity:
Ten Principles for Leaders in the Coming Age

To everything there is a season,
And a time to every purpose under heaven.

—Ecclesiastes, 3:1

Chapter Objectives

At the completion of this chapter, the reader will be able to

- Analyze the key characteristics of complexity and their impact on the leadership role.
- Evaluate personal characteristics and their fit with the leadership skills needed in the coming age.
- Formulate personal goals for adapting to the leadership role in the presence of chaos and complexity.
- Summarize the principles of complexity and describe their practical implications for the leadership role.
- Apply the principles of complexity theory to the personal exercise of leadership.

Not only is this a time of great change, but change is now experienced in a different way. The introduction of quantum theory and the subsequent application of complexity and chaos theory to human organizations have altered the nature of leadership forever. In particular, leaders must become aware of the implications of complexity theory for the leadership role and for the processes associated with transforming work and the workplace, since the principles of complexity theory will largely determine how best to help others own their own change, undertake the right change processes, and understand the new rules of engagement in this postindustrial age.

All over the world people are being overwhelmed by their work, the pace of change, the limitations on their time, and the endless advance of technology. Health care especially seems to be experiencing severely increased demand and severely decreased resources. The pace of change is so rapid that many health care leaders have left the field and many health professionals are considering whether to follow. Several factors are operating to create this situation:

- *Change is endless.* In the "good old days," it seemed as though changes came in an ordered fashion and with enough time between them to allow people to adjust to the new demands. Indeed, because changes came so rarely and moved so slowly, people almost believed they created them rather than responded to them. Today, changes come so quickly that it is difficult to know when one change ends and another begins. Further, five or more changes may be unfolding at one time, and because people must deal with these changes simultaneously, they often do not know how they are doing or if any of the changes are sustainable. They may be confronted by so many changes and may be making so many changes that they wind up changing the changes. Stephen Hawking has stated that "change is," by which he means that change is a constant. Change is not a thing but a dynamic, a context for everything that happens in the universe. During a time of transition, forces converge to make it possible for many changes to actually occur simultaneously. What is most striking about the nature of change today is the large number of forces converging and the large number of changes unfolding at the same time.
- *Information is remarkably more available than in the past.* Previously, the amount and kind of information needed at work was rarely readily available. Today, the vast amount of data on hand makes it very difficult to separate out what is relevant and valuable. The goal is not simply to find the right information but to find it at the right time in the right form. Indeed, too much information is just as much a hindrance as too little. Making good decisions is still a matter of choosing the data carefully. Further, this is the information age, which means that information is the key to sustaining integrated activities. The importance of information has in turn affected the content and manner of decision making. Clinicians, for example, rather than depending solely on principles and human judgment, now must draw from increasingly complex categories of information in their decision making.
- *Knowledge is now a utility.* In the 20th century, knowledge was treated as a possession. One had knowledge or gained knowledge. The process of learning was essentially a process of "stuffing" facts into one's head. As a result of this process, the knowledgeable person possessed knowledge and could draw from it when necessary. Today, however, the quantum perspective has led us to see knowledge as a utility. Because so much information is available, no one could ever have sufficient capacity to acquire all the knowledge he or she will need. Thus, the focus has shifted from possession to access. To use knowledge appropriately, people must be able to access the right knowledge at the right time in the right way for the right purpose, apply the knowledge wisely and well, and then let the knowledge go when it is no longer relevant. The current challenge for leaders is to recognize that knowledge is a utility and to develop the skills needed to access knowledge in the fundamentally new context for knowledge management.

• *Technology is changing the character and content of the service relationship.* There is virtually nothing that has changed the circumstances of life as radically as the application of new technologies. Most of us are confronting technologies that we read about in science fiction novels and assumed we would never live to see. Twenty years ago, the average length of stay for hospital services (the only health care services available) was around 5.7 days. Today, the average length of stay for high-tech services is around 4.5 hours. What a dramatic change for the providers and users. All the characteristics of service have been impacted by technology. Procedures once done only in a hospital under close supervision can now be done in a clinic or even at home. Laser therapy, CT scanners, portable anesthesia, just to name a few, are signs of the radical shift occurring in the delivery of services. The shift is still in its formative stages, with much more to come as a result of improvements in pharmaceuticals and the application of genomics.

The above list merely indicates the dramatic changes that are affecting health care. Further, the pace of change is not likely to slow any time soon. The quantum, complex, even chaotic nature of change as the convergence of forces periodically brings about an age of transition, and that is exactly what we are living through now (see Figure 1–2).

CHAOS AND COMPLEXITY AND THE DANCE OF CHANGE

The interacting and intersecting character of complexity draws all of us into a web of relationships and understanding that will ultimately change our way of living. From strange attractors to webs of influence and relatedness, the elements of complexity theory are altering the rules of work and interaction by giving us a deeper understanding of the relatedness of things and the role of change and discernment in human progress.

The strange characteristics of complexity are embedded in human activities as well as physical processes. A thing at one level of reality is affected by everything else at all other levels. Sometimes the causal process can be readily seen and understood. In most cases, however, it not transparent and requires special knowledge to be understood. In addition, because of the connection between all elements of any process, the observation of the process has an impact on what takes place, as attested to by the wave-particle duality of electrons, which exhibit wave characteristics or particle characteristics depending upon the experimental arrangement.

> **Key Point**
>
> *Understanding complexity is a requisite for understanding relationships. Complexity science teaches us that everything is related at some level.*

The impact of leadership often depends on the amount of time the leader spends living in the potential. Using Schrödinger's cat, the famous thought experiment intended to illuminate the difference between actuality and potentiality, we can understand the importance of leaders applying the principle of the potential to their own role.

Actual reality is the state in which most of us live; it is where we perform our actions out of awareness of the present. We live actively in the present and attempt to meet the demands that lie right in front of us and that define our experience in current time and space. Potential reality, though just as real and current as actual reality, has different characteristics (Exhibit 2–1). Living in the potential means being aware of a reality that is not present but is inevitable because of the prevailing circumstances. A good example is the standard stop sign placed at intersections. When a driver sees the sign, he or she understands what it means and is willing to respond to it appropriately. However, the driver does not stop immediately, because that would be an inappropriate (or *untimely*) response. The sign is a symbol of potential reality in play; action is inevitable but does not occur instantly.

Leaders are good signpost readers. They understand what the signposts are saying about the journey but act on them only as the circumstances dictate. Their ability to anticipate what actions will be needed, through accurate reading of the signposts, is one of the keys to being a good leader. It is also what is meant by living in the potential (Figure 2–1).

How many organizations have been led by people who live so thoroughly in the actual that they are unable to anticipate events far enough ahead of time to allow for an effective response? How many organizations merely react to one crisis after another because the power of the potential was never incorporated into the leadership role in a way that would allow it to be applied properly and at the right time?

Living in the potential requires leaders to recognize that they are managing a journey and thus need a specific set of skills. Leaders who have been raised on the 20th-century model of leadership tend to focus on the goal or endpoint and implement activities that will get people to that goal. In a chaotic period, when deconstruction is occurring at the same rate as construction or even faster, the dust of change makes it difficult for leaders to even see the goal. Instead, they must read the signposts of change, explain to others what they mean, and engage these others in activities that will move the organization in the direction indicated by the signposts. Two skills are critical here: the ability to read where the change is occurring and

> **Point To Ponder**
>
> *How many leaders realize that their primary work is to help others deal with the changes that affect their lives and their work? Living in the potential for change is focusing on the "journey" of work rather than the "events" of work. It is this journey that should be a leader's primary focus.*

Exhibit 2–1 Actual versus Potential Reality

Living in the Actual	Living in the Potential
• Focus on the present	• Inclusion of coming events
• Living the experience now	• Seeing the work as journey
• Focus on good process	• Focus on good outcomes
• Key is work quality	• Key is right results
• Emphasis on current activity	• Read "signposts" of change
• People focus on own work	• People focus on team

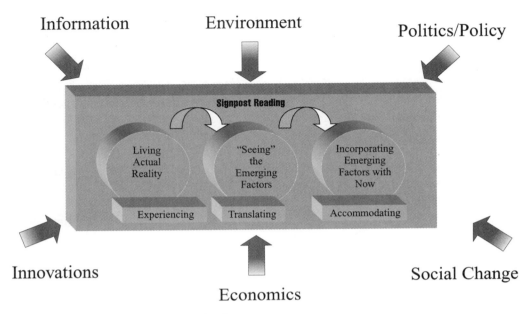

Figure 2–1 Seeing the Journey into the Future

determine the right responses and the ability to anticipate the next signpost early enough to evaluate current progress and determine this signpost's relationship to the next one. In short, leaders need to fluidly respond to current demands and changing circumstances, remain open to the messages carried by longer term indicators, and act in accordance with these messages.

Group Discussion

Sue Craft loves the details of managing her department and tends to focus on the staff issues of the day. There does not seem to be a problem beyond her abilities, and follow-up is her specialty. Sue has noticed, however, that more problems than usual are emerging. Although she is not certain where all of them are coming from, a lot more changes are originating "up there" than usual and creating more daily problems. She is beginning to feel overwhelmed. Discuss the options that are available to Sue for dealing with the increase in problems. In doing so, consider the following questions. Is her focus on the problems that arise daily appropriate for someone managing a department? How might her leadership role be altered to help her handle the large number of changes being handed down by the higher levels of management? How might Sue change her orientation to be better in touch with future issues?

Many leaders get sucked into the concerns of daily work (actual reality) to such an extent that they lose sight of the potential. When leaders focus their energies on daily activities, they are not able to discipline these activities in the light of imminent influences or circumstances. In many if not most organizations, the ability of leaders to engage their own future at the right time is frequently compromised by the fact that they never saw it coming. All eyes are on the activities of the moment, which consume everyone's attention and prevent anyone from seeing the emerging shifts and circumstances that will ultimately affect the organization's ability to thrive.

Many authors, from Nicholas Negroponte (1995) to Kevin Kelly (1998), have delved into the dynamic of complexity to make it understandable and applicable to human enterprises. They have arrived at certain principles as well as a number of insights about the coming age and how to navigate through it. The remainder of this chapter consists of a presentation of rules that will be helpful to leaders as they consider the leadership role and separate out the activities that best match the demands in the new world of work.

PRINCIPLE 1: WHOLES ARE MADE UP OF PARTS

Wholes are made up of smaller units that are always interacting with each other to sustain the whole.

In the 20th century, all that managers had to do was focus on the units of work for which they were responsible. They were evaluated within the context of their own units of service, and if they did well in those units, managed the work force well, and advanced productivity and profitability, they were rewarded and sometimes even promoted.

In a systems mindset, any service unit is looked at as a part of a broader context that gives the unit direction and purpose. A unit does not simply provide services independently of its relationship to other parts of the organization. Each unit, at some level, is required to ensure that what it does fits well with the activities of the other units. According to systems theory, the fit between the components of a system is as critical as the work of any one component.

> **Key Point**
>
> *Leaders need to be focused on issues of "fit." They live in the "white space," the connections, most of the time and are constantly attempting to see where the intersections are and how they facilitate the work of the system.*

The most common problem in systems is that a unit and the people that make it up often get co-opted by their work and their intentions. Because they live their work and relationships within the context of the unit, they forget that whatever they do has a broader frame of reference that must be taken into account in assessing the viability of their work.

An organizational leader must always keep the focus on the organization's broader purpose. The leader's role is to ensure that there is a goodness of fit between the activities of those at the point of service and the overall work of the organization. This takes considerable doing, especially when the leader is also paying attention to the kind and quality of work done at the point of service. The leader's presence at the point of service can cause the leader to get caught up in the day-to-day activities of the service and forget the ultimate goals toward which these activities are directed.

Leaders have the responsibility to see and live "systemness." The difference between institutions and systems is significant (Exhibit 2–2). In institutions, most of the work is compartmentalized and organized vertically, which, together with the focus on process, creates a clear separation between the various loci of the work. Because the focus is on results at the point of productivity, special roles are created in order to address the issue of fit. Yet those responsible, from managers to specialty engineers, are not located where most of the work is done, and those who do the work are instead engaged in the tasks to be done and the processes to be undertaken.

Group Discussion

Systems are different from institutions. Systems thrive on relationships and intersections, and models of systems reflect relationships rather than control. Discuss the effect that a systems orientation would have on the design of a health care facility. Draw an organizational chart to reflect relationships instead of functions, including relationships to its community, other services, other health systems, and so on. Finally, discuss the differences between leading a facility that is a system and leading a facility that is an institution.

In most organizations, the organizational chart speaks volumes about the structuring of work and the value placed on it. Lines and boxes enumerate the various functional capacities expected within the context of each role. The reporting infrastructure is critical to the structuring of work, and clear lines and patterns of interaction are important—but only with regard to communication about work activities.

Exhibit 2–2 Systems versus Institutions

Institutions	Systems
• Unilateral interests/goals	• Multifocal interests/goals
• Nonaligned	• Strong alignment of stakeholders
• Driven by self-interest	• Mutual interests
• Focus on structure/function	• Focus on relatedness
• Highly competitive	• Outcomes driven
• Survival focused	• Centered on thriving
• Vertically integrated	• Horizontal/vertical linkage

Workers at the point of service generally are not concerned with value, linkage, and integration. Instead, they are busy performing the routines of daily work and perfecting these routines so that the work gets done effectively and within the allotted time frame. As a result, they often view the work as more important than its purpose and become caught up in the politics and process of work, impairing their ability to embrace change and adjust their activities in response to new demands.

In systems, on the other hand, the real work of management and leadership is to refocus work and place it back into its appropriate context. To do this, however, leaders must avoid being equally co-opted by the work and thereby prevented from identifying its relationship to other factors that influence it.

Many of the problems in organizations arise from the inability of leaders to think and act horizontally. In other words, leaders must be able to see the whole and characterize each of the units of work within the context of its contribution to the whole. They must also be able to see how the units work together to advance the purpose and value of the whole.

In essence, leaders, regardless of their location, see all work from the perspective of the system. Indeed, they analyze each work activity in terms of the function it plays in achieving the purpose of the whole, and their role is based on the system's imperatives and how the work activities operate in concert to achieve them. At the same time, the structure of the system enables the leaders to see and act out of systemness and keep in touch with the demands of the whole, although their ability to do these things is compromised to the extent that the infrastructure is not in place.

Systems are more biological than mechanical. They are the sum of all the dynamics that drive them. Therefore, they are best viewed as a set of relationships rather than components. In systems, the intersections between the elements are as critical as what goes on within any single element. The goodness of fit between the actions and processes of a system is what ultimately creates the fluidity that is the system's essence. Goodness of fit is much more important than any element by itself. Effective leaders always examine the activities of the members in order to determine their goodness of fit. One of their challenges is to bridge the dichotomy between the workers' focus on good task and their own focus on good fit.

Leaders and staff need to recognize that no one person can make a sustaining contribution though his or her own efforts alone. While an individual's efforts can achieve incremental improvements, the sustainability of these improvements depends on the degree of interface between the individual's efforts and the consolidated efforts of the whole. The ability of leaders to make this fact clear to the staff is critical to the effectiveness of their activities.

> **Point To Ponder**
>
> *Everything in our society reflects a vertical orientation, including organizational hierarchies. Leaders now must complement vertical thinking, which is about control, with horizontal thinking, which is about relatedness. Both are necessary, yet leaders, because of the prevalence of vertical thinking, must at this time concentrate on building horizontal connections.*

As noted, work is not inherently valuable. Instead, its value lies in its purpose, and the efforts of leaders should reflect this reality. Yet decades of process and functional orientation at every organizational level have made a belief in the value of work a fundamental part of every worker's belief set. Just observe the reaction of health care workers to the myriad work-related changes that in their view prevent them from effectively doing the activities with which they have become most familiar. In addition, many workers are mourning the fact that they are no longer performing the tasks they had come to know so well. What they have forgotten is that many of these tasks have been made obsolete by changes inside and outside the organization, and leaders now have the major challenge of reintroducing staff, as well as other leaders and managers, to the concept of system and then convincing them of the importance of fitting the organization's work to its changing purposes.

During the 20th century, the various health care disciplines, out of a need to find meaning in their professional work, tried to define themselves and to devise and promulgate practice parameters. Indeed, one of that century's achievements is the contribution of the health care disciplines, from nursing and medicine to pharmacy and nutrition, to the improvement and elaboration of health services, leading to a broader and more complex array of services than at any time in human history.

Today's challenge for the health professions is to make their boundaries more fluid and to renegotiate their roles in order to create a comprehensive continuum by better integrating the health services they provide. The professions now must find what connects them together rather than focusing on what separates them. In other words, here again the components (the professions) must converge to address the whole (the public's health). Further, the technological tools now make it possible to do this—and also make it necessary, at least if the health professions are to ensure the health of people over their ever-increasing life spans.

Group Discussion

Discuss the health care professions as they are currently configured and predict their likely future. Are they going to be able to function effectively in the 21st century as they now exist? If not, how will they have to be revised in order to remain relevant in the new age of health care?

PRINCIPLE 2: ALL HEALTH CARE IS LOCAL

The integration and effectiveness of health services depend on local relationships, not centralized authorities.

Everyone has heard at least once that all health care is local. As Martin Buber would have said, all health services are provided within the context of the "I-Thou" relationship: someone provides a service, someone receives it. Through this fundamental human equation, care and healing emerge, and everything from structure to equipment, competence to relationship, is reflected in it. When two or more parties interact, the result is always an intimate exchange of expectations, conversation, and action. From a systems perspective, most of the other components of the system converge at some level to support this exchange, and those that do not ultimately will impede it.

The function of structure in a service system is twofold: (1) to ensure the integrity of the system and the ability of its components to work in concert to achieve its ends efficiently and effectively and (2) to facilitate the work of the system. In health care, the purpose of a health system is to address the needs of the community. The system, of course, cannot serve its community without also serving individual members of the community at the point of service; although at the governance level, the system serves the community as a whole. Both levels—the point-of-service level and the governance level—are essential, and each supports the other.

The main implication of the principle above is that each element of the system must serve to empower those at the point of service and allow them to provide care to the community through their individual acts (see Figure 1–4). In an effective system, 90 percent of the critical decisions are made at the point of service, and the life of the system is always primarily lived out there as well.

An effective system has no more structure than is absolutely needed for its work. When unnecessary structure exists, it tends to suck resources and work away from the point of service. The more structure a system has, the more likely the system will support its structure rather than its services, the more money the structure will cost the system, the fewer the resources the system will have available, and the less able the system will be to thrive and fulfill its purpose.

In a system, everything operates from the center out. Systems are organic in shape and design, and the most obvious configuration for a system is a circle. That this is so indicates that systems are more about relationships and intersections than about anything else. Systems possess flow and fluidity and are more dynamic than static. They encompass interactions and relationships in a continuous and vibrant interplay that results in the fulfillment of their purposes. All the activities of a system work together to help the system adapt to changes, meet its goals, and ensure its survival.

Every system take its life from the places where it intersects with the greater community. In particular, a health services system is directed toward advancing the health of the community in which it is located, and there is obviously a tight relationship between the system and the receivers of its services. The system must therefore make sure that its services reflect the community's culture. The leader's role is to see to it that the purposes of the system and the needs of the community are congruent and that everything the system does is directed toward meeting those needs in a culturally appropriate manner.

Key Point

All health care is local. A system operates from its point of service outward. If a health care provider is not directly giving care to a patient, he or she is serving someone who is.

All other components of a system are intimately connected to its center—the place where it carries out its mission. It is at this place, the point of service, that the provider and the receiver of services meet, the community is served one member at a time, the life of the system is expressed, and the value of the system is realized. All the system's other components should be configured to support the activity at its center.

The point of service is also where the majority of conflicts occur and where a poor structure has the largest impact. If the processes at the point of service are not structured with goodness of fit in mind, the system will begin to break down. Eventually, its purpose will become lost and its ability to thrive will be compromised.

The vast majority of the work done by the leader of a system involves building sustainable relationships and keeping the system intact and on course. Because a system is a membership community, it can easily lose sight of its purpose and forget what its real work is. The leader seeks congruence between its purpose and the work of its members, and in doing this the leader faces the challenge of overcoming the ever-present conflict between personal and collective agendas. The leader must keep aware that the system is a membership community and remind others of this fact as well. A good leader realizes that the system's survival depends on the dance between good structure and good process, the members' focus on the product of their work, and the positive impact the system has on those it serves.

A good leader also ensures that the structure of the system does not impede the system's fluidity and flexibility—its ability to quickly adapt to changing conditions. To do this, the leader must revise the structure as the system grows in order to position the system to better serve the community. The leader must also always be sensitive to the tightness of fit between the system's structure and its purposes, for the structure has the potential to obstruct the work processes rather than support them. When the structure does act as an obstacle and draw to itself unnecessary resources, it must be reconfigured.

The point-of-service workers must be able to act so as to meet the demands of the culture of those they serve. For example, they should have few constraints placed on their ability to make decisions and construct appropriate service arrangements and processes. Of course, their actions should be informed by principles and practices worked out in advance by the stakeholders at the point of service.

The configuration at the point of service must at some level reflect the character and content of the work. Here the issue of differentiation becomes critical. Each population-based service configuration is unique since it represents the characteristics of the specific population served. The 20th-century addiction to sameness must be overcome. The rules that govern the functioning of each service must be derived from the service's relationship to those served, not its relationship to the

> **Point To Ponder**
>
> *Culture rules. The point of service is driven by the culture of the patient population, and the system is driven by the culture of its community, which gives it purpose, and the culture of its members or workers, who give it focus. These constituencies converge to drive the system to thrive.*

prevailing structure of the system. Although structure is critical at other places in the system, it is not appropriate at the point of service, for here the culture of the population is more important than the needs of any other element of the system.

The above makes clear the importance of the point of service and the need for structural independence and functional liberty at the point of service. Each point-of-service worker has an obligation to ensure that the decisions and activities that unfold there are congruent and that each is informed and disciplined by the system's purposes and direction as it addresses the needs of the community. Furthermore, the decisions made at the point of service should predominate because they give form to the work of serving the community one person at a time. Out of this dynamic—consisting of the interplay of the system's purposes with the worker's decisions and activities—comes the seamless and symbiotic relationships between the system and the workers that create the place where the system lives out its purposes and makes a difference in the lives of those it serves.

> **Group Discussion**
>
> The point of service drives about 90 percent of the decision making in a healthy and effective system, and therefore most of the decisions should be made by the workers located there. The Ritz-Carlton Hotel is well known for allowing its point-of-service workers to make service decisions to enhance the guests' experience. Discuss the effects on a health system of moving 90 percent of the decisions to the point of care. What impact would this have on the authority structure of the system? What changes would have to occur to make the transfer of decision-making power sustainable? How would staff have to change to manage the additional decision-making power?

PRINCIPLE 3: ADDING VALUE TO A PART ADDS VALUE TO THE WHOLE

Anything that adds value to any part of a system adds value to the whole system. The sustainability of the system requires the aggregation of numerous additions of value.

In the Industrial Age, assessments of value were often based on volume. The most common measure of the value of work, for instance, was the quantity of work done. Even the language of health care reflected a volume orientation: nurses, physicians, and other health professionals, as they said, wanted to do the "most" they could do for their patients. The processes associated with work were viewed as almost more important than the work's purpose, and there was almost a sense that the activity of providing health care was inherently valuable. The orientation toward process was almost sacrosanct, and much attention, even in the quality movement, was devoted to establishing good processes for delivering services.

Although process is vital, it does not itself create or add value. Work processes are always disciplined by and gain their meaning and value through the purposes toward which they are directed. Any activity, to be meaningful, must at some level advance some purpose; otherwise, the worker is taking value away. Even if the worker does nothing, the action of doing nothing is actually drawing value away because the purpose could have been advanced by some activity—an activity that is not being performed. Work, then, either adds value or reduces it. It adds value when it advances the purposes of the work, and it takes value away when it does not advance these purposes.

In a true system, all activities, roles, and functions, no matter how large or small, have value. Each, when working in concert with the others, does something to advance the system's purpose and has an impact on the system's vigor and viability. It is for this reason that careful selection of every role in the system is essential to the system's ability to thrive. This ability depends in part on the goodness of fit between roles and functions, not simply on the roles and functions themselves.

The triadic relationship between purpose, person, and performance is the cornerstone of any measure of vitality in any kind of system. The effective leader understands this relationship almost intuitively. It is so embedded in the dynamics of the system that almost nothing can be accomplished if it is not used as a framework. The whole is a reflection of the fit between its parts—of the

> ### Key Point
>
> *Everyone in a system is obligated to add value to the system. Everyone is doing something, even if it is negative. If someone is not adding value, he or she is taking away value.*

congruity and resonance of the many functions that make up its infrastructure. As these elements join in a seamless dance of intersection and interaction, each individual element becomes invisible, but all of them together, at least in a true system, work so harmoniously and are so tightly interwoven that they are perceivable only as a whole. In a noneffective system, the parts and pieces are easy to see because of their incongruence and lack of flow or fit and because they appear out of context. Rather than contribute to the whole, they draw resources, energy, and attention away from the whole, impairing its integrity. They can cause a system to break down and fail to achieve its purpose.

Leaders must operate out of an understanding that each element of a system is a microcosm of the system. To lead any one element, a leader must direct his or her vision from the whole to the part rather than the reverse. The focus should be on the whole system and on how the element contributes to the integrity and action of the whole. From this perspective, the leader diagnoses the element and evaluates its goodness of fit with the other elements. The leader also attempts to keep value, which depends on the congruence of work, quality, and resources, at the center of everyone's sense of relationship to his or her work and to the workplace (Figure 2–2).

The leader is always aware of the connection between the elements of the system and the fluidity and "tightness" of the intersection between elements, where the life of the system is most evident. Questions related to interface, connection, integration, communication, and interaction are the driving concerns of the leader. If there are problems in a system, even if they originate in inadequate or failed processes, they are ultimately expressed in brokenness between the elements and in their failure to exhibit the flow, seamlessness,

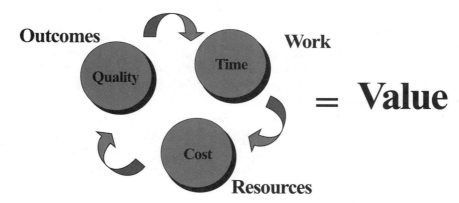

Figure 2–2 Creating Sustainable Value: Balancing the Value Equation

and linkage essential throughout the system. For the system to advance, individual contributions must be woven together in a way that achieves substantive consonance.

PRINCIPLE 4: SIMPLE SYSTEMS MAKE UP COMPLEX SYSTEMS

Simple systems combine with other simple systems to form more complex systems. Complexity grows incrementally through the interconnecting of smaller, simpler systems (called chunking).

To understand complexity, one needs to look for the simplicity that lies at its center. Everything is related to everything else in some way or other. This concept lies at the center of any understanding of how systems operate and thrive. The task of a system's leader is to delineate the linkages and intersections between all elements of the system. The leader identifies the common elements present everywhere in the system and those unique contributing elements that are located at critical places in the system and contribute to the effectiveness of the whole.

Every element of a larger system is a system itself. It has its own simplicity, complexity, and chaos. If the component system is viewed only as something simple, its fit and contributing purpose remain invisible. They are disclosed when the system is seen in the appropriate context (i.e., as part of the larger system).

Each component system abides by the same rules as the larger system. The compo-

> ### Point To Ponder
>
> *A leader who is head of a particular service or department always sees his or her role from the perspective of the whole system. In fact, the best way to look at matters is that the leader is leading the whole system from the perspective of the particular service or department. It is each leader's commitment to the system that gives the leader, no matter where located, focus and a framework for the expression of his or her role.*

nent system must have fluidity, fit, and integrity, and its parts must intersect and operate in a way that advances its contribution and value. It is the component systems' substantial and continuous interaction—what Kevin Kelly calls clumping—that maintains the integrity of the larger system.

With regard to component systems, there are two basic requirements. First, each must have well-integrated components itself and function well internally. Second, it must intersect and interact with other related systems in order to make up the larger system and ensure its effectiveness (Figure 2–3). In the past, leaders have not always paid attention to these requirements. Many organizations have suffered from the narrow focus of leaders who concentrate on their area of responsibility to the detriment of other component systems and the enterprise as a whole. Even reward systems sometimes encourage people to excel at the expense of others, destroying relationships, obstructing interaction, and skewing the distribution of the available resources. Whole organizations are held hostage to these

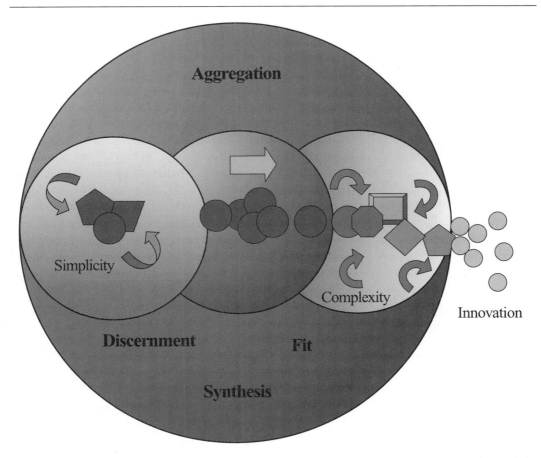

Figure 2–3 From Simplicity to Complexity: Aggregation across the System. The actions of the processes (discernment, synthesis, fit, and aggregation) intersect and interact to build and sustain the system and support innovation.

Group Discussion

Sam Casey, as head of his department, has consistently looked out for the interests of his department and its staff. Occasionally he has had to fight other departments to get what he wanted for his own. According to him, that is all part of being a good leader. Discuss whether he is right. Among other things, consider Sam's approach from the perspective of systems thinking. What problems are his approach likely to create? What advice could Sam be given to help him improve his leadership? How should a departmental leader balance the system's needs and the functional needs of the department?

highly unilateral decision makers and never fully achieve their potential. The glue of trust is never established, precluding the level of productivity that can result from a truly resonating system.

Every leader of a component of a larger system must ensure that it operates effectively. The effectiveness of a component system, however, cannot be achieved simply through having an internal locus of control. For example, in an organization that provides health services, although the point of service drives the content and culture of the entire organization, the point of service must also reflect the obligations and operations of the entire organization. Each smaller system should mirror the larger system, although it will be refined through its specific manner of representing it. Anyone who comes directly to the smaller system should see a picture of the whole system, including that system's mission, service, quality, and outcomes, all of which should be manifest in the smaller system's work.

Too often, health care organizations have components that do not fit together well. Think how typical it is for people seeking health care services to get asked the same questions over and over again as they move through the system. From admissions to treatment, a patient may face five or more points of query simply because the components do not interact sufficiently to eliminate the need for them. The cost of allowing simple systems not to operate smoothly together has never fully been measured.

PRINCIPLE 5: DIVERSITY IS A NECESSITY OF LIFE

Diversity is essential for life. Only where diversity is present can the ability to thrive be assured. Diversity makes chaos visible, as it pushes systems to forever adapt to changes in their environment.

It is common wisdom, at least if you believe the literature on leadership, that conflict should be avoided and that processes must be in place to reduce conflict in a system to a minimum. Unfortunately, nothing could be further from the truth.

Diversity is the visual manifestation of the chaos that exists within all systems. That chaos is the energy that arises from the conflict between the elements of a system as they intersect to create the conditions necessary to the system's adaptation. Diversity is a characteristic of the endless dance of design and configuration as the elements confront each other and sort out a way of fitting together.

In creating an effective and meaningful workplace, leaders must attend to a number of issues. First, they must understand that diversity is necessary for a system to thrive. Kelly (1995) uses *heterogeneity* to refer to the essential element in the movement and adaptation of any system, but whatever the word, a wide range of views and roles is essential for determining the direction the system should move in and for establishing the common ground necessary for leading the participants and elements in that direction. Homogeneity is the enemy of success because it represents the unilateral, the stable, the inert. Missing from homogeneity is the conflict between elements and their sorting and reconfiguring around ever-changing circumstances as the system keeps rhythm with the environment within which it must thrive.

The presence of conflict indicates that a system is healthy and energetic. It enables the leader of the system to see the differences that exist and challenges the leader to sort through them in order to determine what they are saying to the organization. Embedded in these differences are the many indicators and varieties of influence that, when viewed together, tell the leader where the organization is, what the issues are, and what the organization's responses might be.

> **Point To Ponder**
>
> *Homogeneity is the enemy of truth. If everyone says the same thing and thinks the same way, no issue will be explored in sufficient depth and breadth to discover the truth. Heterogeneity is essential to the search for truth. It allows for the kind of deep and broad examination from which truth can emerge.*

The leader must recognize that his or her main work is interpreting present activities in light of their potential to create the future. The future does not simply happen. Each future moment is part of a flow of activities whose completion lays the foundation for the next set of activities and the next moment. Each moment encompasses indicators of the next moment and of the changes that will occur. To influence the future, therefore, the leader must be able to see the vortex of conflicting and converging elements that are together working to bring about the future.

The leader must be able to harness chaos through its visible conflicts and divergences, for these reveal the direction of any changes that are occurring. It is for this reason that the leadership role in today's world is more that of gatherer than director. In the old Newtonian model, the leader of an organization was expected to determine the organization's endpoint and then direct the organization toward it through personal influence. Nowadays the leader's strategy should be to engage with the diverse components of the organization in order to determine the right direction to move it. In doing this, the leader should capitalize on the strengths and skills, insights and wisdom, that are located in these diverse components. It is only by embracing the diversities and conflicts within the organization that the leader will be able to discover the actions most likely to keep the organization thriving.

Here both the value and meaning of conflict become especially important. Conflict is a vehicle for discerning the proper direction for the organization to take. In particular, it is the strongest indicator of where to begin the work of determining the most appropriate actions at any given time. The leader both honors the essential differences that exist and uses them to reach clarification. These differences include cultural differences as well as the diversity of insights, opinions, and skills possessed by members of the organization. No one person has all the knowledge and abilities necessary to adequately "see" the patterns of diversity and chaos. It is only through processes that actualize the disparate potentials present in the full range of participants that the signs of change and its themes can be

---

Group Discussion

Charles Frederick has been the chief operating officer of a health clinic for two years. He is nice enough but hates to have his views or leadership questioned. Therefore, although he hires bright people like himself, he wants people who think like him so he will not have to fight to achieve his goals. In time, his staff have come to understand this and have stopped offering different insights and points of view. Discuss what happens when leaders hear only what agrees with their own thinking. What is missing from the decision making in such a situation? What are some of the problems that arise? Among other issues, what are the effects on accountability?

---

found. A good leader is able to tap into this diversity by using effective methodologies. Through dialogue, for example, the leader pulls out the premises, themes, and signposts that indicate the best direction for the organization to move and the actions most likely to lead it in that direction. The goal, in short, is to build collective wisdom upon common ground.

PRINCIPLE 6: ERROR IS ESSENTIAL TO CREATION

Both random error and conscious error are essential to the process of creation. In fact, error underpins all change.

Historically, leaders have been taught that error, especially in health care, is harmful and must be avoided at all costs. What we have come to understand is that error is an essential constituent of change. Further, it can be used as a measuring device to indicate where people are currently located on the pathway to some desired endpoint. Therefore, leaders need to value error as a useful leadership tool.

Error is present everywhere in the universe. It is embedded within systems and contributes to their adaptation and thriving. Error indicates where a system has to adjust to new circumstances. It forces people to stop a process of change long enough to assess the situation and make the necessary modifications before resuming the process. It informs the agents of change where they are and what is happening. It alerts them to a change in conditions or a breach in the process or a demand for a response. Error indicates where the system is in relationship to a process or initiative. It alerts people to the convergence of the variables that led to the mistake or flaw and that demonstrate its presence or its impact on the flow of events.

Error is essentially a teacher. At varying levels of complexity, error indicates a break in the confluence and congruity of processes in a way that causes participants to note the break, assess the situation, and take action. Although some errors are certainly undesirable, such as those resulting in death or severe damage, even they serve as indica-

> ### Key Point
>
> *Error is essential to all progress. Far from being a deficit, error indicates where someone is on the journey. The only unacceptable error is the error that is repeated.*

tors of problems and as incitements to action. They teach, inform, advise, warn, and alert by showing that the current circumstances vary dangerously from the norm. They point dramatically to important lessons and ensure that the lessons are in fact learned.

Error plays a critical role in learning and in developmental activities. It is when error fails to teach that the negative energy embedded deep within it begins to operate and create problems. The only inappropriate error is the error once repeated. An error's repetition indicates that the relevant lesson remained unlearned (Exhibit 2–3).

Error, as a constituent of change, can be used by a leader to better evaluate a change process and determine the best activities for advancing the system and preventing the same mistakes or flaws from recurring. The leader's attitude toward error in general determines how he or she will address individual errors. If the leader values error as a tool, then he or she will tend to use each individual error as a guide to improving performance. If the leader treats error solely as a cause for punishment, then individual errors will never be able to serve as indicators of problems and as stimulators of corrective action, to the organization's detriment.

Of course, some errors must be controlled for. Life-threatening or risk-intensive errors must be managed in a way that reduces their incidence and impact, even though these also have the capacity to teach. They cannot, however, be eliminated entirely. The leader must remember that there is a randomness to error and that all the good planning and control in the world will not eliminate every mistake and defect. Errors can be reduced by a high degree of management and control, as shown by the redundancy approach to airline con-

---

Exhibit 2–3 Mistakes versus Errors

Mistakes	**Errors**
• Are nonrandom	• Are random
• Are repeated	• Are repeatable
• Do not result in learning	• Contain lessons
• Impair sustainability	• Foster sustainability

struction and operation, which compensates for inherent error by making multiple options available to respond to the errors that do occur. The whole airline industry is built on error management, which accounts for the fact that the level of risk from errors in flight is lower than the risk present in any other business activity.

> **Point To Ponder**
>
> *Risk can never be fully eliminated. Indeed, risk should be viewed as a resource that simply requires good management. It is inherent in all human activity and must be accommodated in any plan. Planning for error makes room for risk and provides the space to learn from it.*

Health care organizations also have a large capacity for reducing risk from errors, but more attention could be paid to risk and error systems in these organizations. Indeed, many errors and risks are not discussed and may even be ignored or overlooked because of the legal implications of exposing clinical errors. In recent years, however, the unacceptable level of risk resulting from medication and medical procedure errors has brought about a renewed interest in risk reduction and error management activities. Increasingly, health care leaders are using error as a tool in managing behavior and as a vehicle for change rather than as a cause for disciplinary action. Consequently, they and other leaders would do well to become familiar with the new science developing around the management of human error.

PRINCIPLE 7: SYSTEMS THRIVE WHEN ALL OF THEIR FUNCTIONS INTERSECT AND INTERACT

Systems thrive when the full range of their functions intersect and interact in a continual dance of relationship and transformation.

Newton once described the universe as a great machine. Einstein said it was more like one great thought. His point was that nothing in the universe is mechanical or organized in a machinelike structure.

Systems science has taught us that the universe operates as a set of interacting forces and interdependent relationships. There is nothing in the universe that is not in some way acting on or interacting with something else. Because interdependence is an essential characteristic of systems, the leadership role in a system is critically different from the leadership role in institutional models of organization.

Traditional theories of leadership—those that informed the work of leaders and organizations in the 20th century—reflect both linear and vertical thinking (Exhibit 2–4). This mechanistic and highly structured approach to leadership favored the use of compartmental and definitive work structures and processes to organize and codify work and its products. Workers were considered subsets of the work and were organized and treated accordingly. Much of what defined work was both developed and owned by the organization.

In the latter part of the 20th century and the beginning of the 21st century, the very foundations of work and the workplace began to change. Newer models evolved because of the advent of computers and information technology and their impact on every aspect of soci-

Exhibit 2–4 Linear versus Lateral Thinking

Linear Thinking (Industrial Age)	**Lateral Thinking (Age of Technology)**
• Vertically oriented	• Multidirectional
• Hierarchical	• Horizontal
• Mechanistic	• Whole oriented
• Reductionistic	• Integrative
• Compartmental	• Intuitive
• Controlling	• Relational

ety. Knowledge work became increasingly important to the workplace, and organizations now require substantial knowledge capacity. The emergence of the knowledge worker changed the relationship between the worker and the work and also between the worker and the workplace. In today's world, workers typically acquire the skills and knowledge needed for a certain type of work in an academic setting rather than in the workplace.

Workers also have become much more mobile because their skill sets have much broader utility than previously. Knowledge has become a resource in extreme demand, to the point where it is in essence a scarce resource, and consequently workers now are more important to the workplace than the workplace is to the workers. Because knowledge has great utility and transferability, workers have many more employment options.

While the worker was changing, so was the workplace. In local enterprises as well as global entities, the organization and design of work have been radically altered. Organizations at all levels have had to create tight, efficient, nimble, and quickly adjusting work units in order to thrive in the more fluid, horizontal world of wireless communication, fiber optics, and other highly sophisticated technologies.

In this new world of intersections, interactions, interdependencies, and horizontal

> **Point To Ponder**
>
> *Advances in technology have made work more portable. Knowledge workers, because of their high-level skills, have gained substantial control of the work they do and have also become more mobile. Unlike the previous generation of workers, they are not faithful to the workplace. Instead, they are faithful to the work, moving anywhere the opportunity to do it appears.*

linkage, the entire infrastructure of work has been altered, as has our understanding of the mechanics necessary to facilitate effective work. The movement from institutions to systems has created a foundation for a new characterization of work and the worker.

Systems encompass closed and open components. Closed components are predictable, efficient, and ordered. They are the parts of a system that are constant and remain unaffected, at least directly, by external influences. The open components are adaptable and change in response to the demands of the environment. All functions and relationships in a system interact with and are dependent on the intersecting actions and processes in the system. Components such as production, service, management, governance, support, and locus of control are all included, according to common understanding, in the set of system functions. Of course, the relationship between the elements of process and outcome as well as the relationships between structural and process components are complex and ever changing. In a complex system, no one element remains intact as other elements adapt to internal and external forces or lead the process of adapting to these forces.

It is this constant wave or flow of change and adaptation that operates as the undercurrent of every system. The action never stops. The leader of a system, always aware of this movement and the constant exchange of energy between all the components, looks for the drivers and receivers of action and change. The leader's attention must be on the ebb and flow of the cycles and the vortex of change as the system interacts with external sociopolitical, economic, and technological forces. The object is to discern the effects of these forces and to judge what actions will maintain the system's integrity, adaptability, and viability.

The leader of the system, of course, cannot perform these tasks unilaterally. All the leaders of system components must be made aware of the processes and skills necessary to manage systemness and of the interacting elements that make systems thrive. Any system will be negatively impacted if a single leader acts in the best interests of his or her component and without consideration for the impact of his or her behavior on the integrity of the whole. Such a leader actually holds the system "hostage" to the component.

Component-centered behavior is common in traditional organizations. Various units, services, or departments of an organization might operate over long periods of time at the expense of other parts of the organization, especially if great sums of money can be produced as a result. However, component-centered behavior is not sustainable. The day finally will arrive when the organization will have to pay substantially for the unconnected behavior, and the organization's ability to thrive ultimately will be threatened.

Every leader of a system component must recognize that his or her proper role is not simply to make the component thrive but to help make the whole system thrive. The leader's main attention will of course be on the component, but ensuring the fluidity, interface, connectedness, and flow of the full range of system components is that leader's real work.

Many theoretical approaches have emerged over the years to try to define the structure and processes associated with an organization's work. From bureaucratic theory through the human relations school, the contingency and resource dependent approaches, and the strategic, population, and institutional models, theorists have written extensively on how and why organizations function as they do. According to the complexity approach, any element described by any of the above theories may act at any given time in an organization, and the interaction of forces will tell the leader how the organization is behaving and what the implications of its behavior are for its work and its transformative journey. Every system must possess structure and cultural foundations and must be able to respond flexibly to the environment and relationships, create value, improve itself, and interface directly with the external processes that influence its future. In other words, each theoretical approach contributes at some level to our understanding of how systems operate and how to make them effective.

Biological metaphors frequently have been used to characterize the activities of systems, and each metaphor can provide leaders assistance in focusing on the functions and rela-

Group Discussion

The Industrial Age saw the emergence of a whole host of schools of leadership thought. Discuss the various approaches to leadership advocated by these schools (e.g., bureaucratic, human relations, behavioral, contingency, and situational). Then reflect on the type of workplace that is emerging and discuss the implications for leadership style. As a help, consider which approaches to leadership might be appropriate or sustainable in the new age of work.

tionships that must work in concert. The analogy of a hologram also has been presented as helpful. In each part of a hologram, regardless of how many times it has been divided, the whole is always present. In this analogy, a whole system is reflected in each of its parts, and the cybernetic relationship between the whole and each part is critical to both. The role of the leader, on this account, is to keep focused on the "hologram"—the constant interchange between the parts and the whole and the impact of the parts on each other and on the operation and integrity of the whole.

The leader must pay special attention to the points of interaction between the various components, for there lie most of the action, energy, and noise of the system, as well as most of the relationship, goodness-of-fit, and workflow problems. Because of the intensity of the dynamics there, sometimes problems and issues are not resolved or are "turfed" outside the locus of accountability that exists at these connective points. Examples include physicians taking their problems to the "administration," managers letting relationship problems "hang," staff members refusing to deal with other staff members because the interactions would be too painful, and so on. Indeed, most activities, perhaps as much as 90 percent, reside at the point of service and the intersections between the service positions. Because

> **Key Point**
>
> *The primary job of a leader is to manage relationships and interactions, mostly at the intersections of the system. Seeing the organization holographically (i.e., in three dimensions) can help the leader detect the interactions and processes that occur there.*

these locations are where the work of a clinical system gets done, most of the issues affecting the work arise here. The problems are exacerbated if they are not resolved where they arose.

As principle 7 states, the thriving of a system depends on the intersecting and interacting of its functions and actions. The best metaphor here is that of a continual dance of interaction. The leader's role is to act as choreographer and ensure that the parties and the parts resonate with each other in a seamless flow to sustain the energy of the system.

PRINCIPLE 8: EQUILIBRIUM AND DISEQUILIBRIUM ARE IN CONSTANT TENSION

There is a constant and permanent tension between equilibrium (stabilizers) and disequilibrium (challenges). This tension is essential to life and reflects the fact that disequilibrium is the universe's natural state.

Although it is normal for the universe to live on the edge of its own chaos, a certain amount of stability is necessary for change and for taking action. The role of the leader in this delicate equation is to find the points of stability and use them as places where evaluation and action can occur. The notion of variation is central to the balance between stability and instability. Agents of change (e.g., individuals, families, businesses, communities, countries, and computer programs) interact continuously on the variables and elements affecting events and direction of movement. Through use of their skills, knowledge, mental and physical properties, and location, leaders, among other agents of change, are able to take the best path to achieving improvements.

Leaders understand the dynamic interaction between stability and change and walk the narrow way between them with consciousness and purpose. They understand as well that absolute and continuous stability is synonymous with death. Recognizing this, they know the value of chaos and the necessity of harnessing it to improve the circumstances and processes of work and productivity.

People do not make change. Instead, like disequilibrium, change is universal. This fact is at odds with the usual desire of people for stability and quiet in their personal lives. Leaders understand both the prevalent human wish for stability and the universe's tendency toward the creative and the chaotic. They know that they must develop strategies for addressing the conflict between equilibrium and disequilibrium—strategies that take into account both the environment and their own goals. Further, they know that not all strategies work as planned, and they periodically evaluate every strategy in use to make sure it is having the effect desired and revise it as necessary.

> **Key Point**
>
> *In systems language, stability is another word for death. Absolute stability is the absence of life. The leader always walks a tightrope between stability and chaos, tending to favor the latter.*

Time and shifting circumstances, often in part created by earlier strategies, have an impact on the chance of success of current strategies and on the formation of future strategies. A strategy that has stood the test of time can suddenly become unavailing. Changes in people and conditions can converge or act independently to influence what will work and what will not. Leaders must understand that wide variation in the effectiveness of a strategy over time is normal, and they must keep this fact in mind as they attempt to lead change and help people adjust to the inevitable adaptations that are a constant part of life.

The fluctuating effectiveness of strategies is one reason that measures of success are so critical to making judgments about what works. By using structured approaches to evalu-

Group Discussion

Margie Smith likes to have all of her ducks in a row. She believes that good order indicates good leadership. Her office is clean and orderly, and her life is highly structured. Margie hates when people clutter up their lives and are unable to think logically or act rationally. She works hard to make sure that her staff know what she expects and do everything as she thinks it should be done. Recently, though, the pace of change has picked up, and new programs and technologies are being implemented faster than Margie can handle. She has become less orderly, less comfortable, and, at times, short with staff. She occasionally speaks negatively about some of the changes, she has asked her supervisor whether the rate of change could be decreased, and she has even begun to think about looking for another job, one that would give her more control. Discuss what Margie needs to do to cope better. What changes should she make in her role as leader? What is the chaos she is experiencing trying to tell her? Is changing jobs going to be an effective solution to her current discomfort?

ating success, leaders can better determine what is working, what is not, what is shifting, what is emerging, and what adaptations need to be implemented. Measures do not have to be perfectly accurate, they simply have to say something about where changes are occurring and what adjustments are indicated. In a complex system, an apparently "wrong" outcome is as significant as a "right" measure might be. In other words, in the chaos of change, it is as important to know the "wrongs" as it is to know the "rights."

Changes in people or populations may create a need for changes in process and approach. A change may alter people's circumstances, even their behavior, resulting in a need to alter the strategy or approach for the next stage of change. For example, people are affected by using the Internet, and thus those who use the Internet will likely require a process and mechanism of change that accommodates their new "position" as Internet users. If the approach to change does not accommodate the fact they have become Internet users, the adaptations implemented will have limited success. In general, the changes undergone by people must inform the strategy used by leaders to guide further evolution.

Leaders look to people as both indicators of change and vehicles of change. While any leader is interested in changing people, he or she must be aware that these very people are a source of their own change by being a source of learning and adaption for each other, by acting as recipients of change or improvement, and by being part of an environment that is itself always in transition. A good leader is aware that the people with whom she or he works are virtual experts on their position and condition relative to a desired or needed adaptation. Looking at this population, the leader determines where it is in relation to any given change and uses it as a template for evaluating measures and indicators of change. The general behavior of a population will always influence its specific behavior, just as any specific behavior might inform the leader about the best methods for altering the population's general behavior. For example, if a population uses a specific tool, such as a wireless palm device, for managing personal information and communication, it will more easily adapt to using such a device for communication, documentation, and interaction in the clinical setting. People's individual behaviors serve as both signposts and templates for broader and further adaptation in other settings and circumstances. Thus, as noted, leaders must be good signpost readers and translators and must use their interpretive skills to facilitate further change and adaptation.

Leaders must also understand that complexity and chaos represent energy. Although they do not generate the energy, they harness it in support of a particular form and direction. This energy is always swirling in human circumstances—it never stops. Leaders discipline the energy, driving it in a direction that results in desirable or congruent changes. The interaction between energy and effort is what gives the changes their form, and it is the substance that can be defined and measured.

A leader must be able to discern the interaction patterns in the energy and flow of a change, for these patterns are most indicative of the context and content of the change. The interaction between forces, agents, and environment is the substance of the change and informs the leader about appropriate responses. The leader is looking for the convergence of these forces and elements. The "story" that they contain, when well read, tells the leader what responses are likely to lead to specific outcomes or products. From this set of responses, the leader selects those that are likely to move the system in the direction that is needed or desired.

Not all selections will be correct. The leader will choose an ineffective response as often as an effective one. Here again it is not the selection that is critical to the change process but what the effect of the selection tells the leader and what the leader's response is. When a strategy is correct and does result in a preferred behavior or condition, adaptation is said to have occurred, and this adaptation forms the foundation for the next change. For example, particle beam CT scanners were highly successful as diagnostic tools, yet they also formed a foundation for improvements and refinements. Electron-beam whole-body CT scanners currently provide more detail and accuracy and have broader diagnostic and clinical utility, but these scanners could not have been developed until the earlier scanners had been devised and used. Adaptations often build on previous adaptations. In fact, all adaptations are temporary and merely serve as the foundation for future adaptations.

> **Key Point**
>
> *The leader lives in the space between action and potential, anticipating the next step and translating the process for others.*

Leaders are constantly aware of the intense interaction of complexity. This interaction is often represented in a chaotic vortex of energy that on the surface looks undecipherable. Yet when critically "read" and put into context, it often reveals the "stuff" that will ultimately influence the next stage of change. Leaders are always pushing up against this potential energy, and the good leaders are those who can translate it (context, systems, processes, and structure) into a concerted action. When this action is joined with other related actions, the entire set creates the foundation for meaningful change. This can be viewed as a process of harnessing complexity. Through understanding and using complex interactions and intersections, through recognizing that all this is clothed in chaos, good leaders act to create the future.

PRINCIPLE 9: CHANGE IS GENERATED FROM THE CENTER OUTWARD

Change moves from the center of a system to all other parts, influencing everything else in the system.

Every system has a unique life that defines its meaning and value and gives it an individual character. Within the system are all the activities that create a balance between the work of the system, the internal demands, and the external demands. Because every system is part of a larger system, there is an ever-evolving dance of interchange between the activities inside the system and between the system and the larger system it is part of (Figure 2–4).

The "center" (i.e., the point of service) is where the system lives out most of its life, and the workers at the point of service are especially critical to its ability to adapt and thrive. There are, however, many components of a system that contribute to its integrity and allow

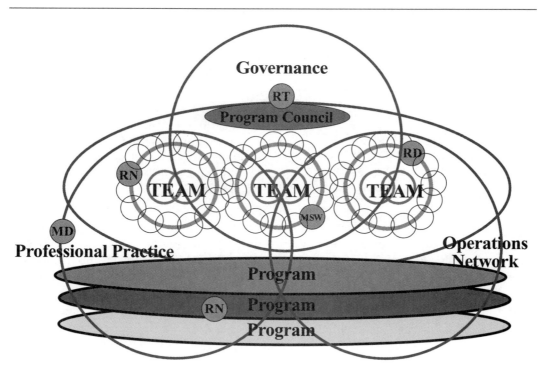

Figure 2–4 Out of Simplicity: A View of a Complex Health System. Beginning with the patient and provider (team), the whole system brings its components together to support the work of advancing health care.

it to function and adapt, and many types of personnel, from managers to staff, play a role in advancing the work of the system.

In a service system, the value of the system is determined by the character and content of the services on offer. The services have value when they are provided in a manner that satisfies those who use them. In addition, the services contribute to the system's ability to thrive by spreading the notion that the system provides high-quality services. Even more than the activities of marketing and business planning, the delivery of the services themselves creates the system's reputation, and thus the people who deliver the services are critical to the ability of the system to thrive. They are in fact much more critical to the system than any other single role or factor, although this statement should not be taken as denigrating the value of any of the intersecting roles that make up the system.

No service system can be sustained if the point of service does not deliver. Although this truth is easy to state, in many, if not most, service organizations, the power, independence, flexibility, and locus of control necessary to respond immediately and appropriately have been designed out of the system. These organizations have a vertical array of controls and hierarchical structures and processes that obstructs the making of decisions where the pertinent issues most often arise (i.e., at the point of service). The ascending ladder of control moves the authority for decision making away from the point of service, and the further away the locus of authority is, the less likely the decision will meet the need that motivated it. In a typical example, a physician on a unit who has a problem with a staff member might take the issue to the administrator to make sure that the highest level of authority is brought into play. The only difficulty is that if the problem is to be solved permanently, the solution must involve those who are located where the problem arose, and so action on the solution must be returned to the point of service.

Key Point

A system will thrive only if those at the point of service own the decisions that are made there.

Systems develop dynamic and cyclical patterns. In a typical pattern, there is a core or centerpoint where the pattern either originates or culminates. The mosaic of activities ultimately builds on or supports the centerpoint (Exhibit 2–5). In a service system like a health care organization, all structure that is sustainable builds on the service configuration, and the system's sustainability depends on the degree of congruence between the prevailing service structure and the supporting structures. If the system is well designed, most of the organizational configurations advance the freedom of activity and judgment at the centerpoint (i.e., point of service). If they do not, they increase the chance that the supporting systems will become the centerpoint and will therefore draw energy away from the proper locus of control and create a framework that will demand attention and resources that should be focused on the point of service.

The more the focus of a service system is drawn away from the point of service, the more expensive the structure of service becomes. Consistent with Taguchi's rule, the further away from the point of service a decision about what happens there is made, the higher the cost, the greater the risk, and the lower the sustainability of the outcome. In a system

Exhibit 2–5 Mosaic of Decision Making in a System

Point-of-Service Decisions	**Unit or Service Decisions**
• Individual	• Coordinated
• Service driven	• Support based
• Judgment based	• Standards driven
• Highly variable	• Resource related
Team-Based Decisions	**System Decisions**
• Team defined	• Integrated
• Group standard	• Collective
• Protocol driven	• Direction setting
• Agreement based	• Resource generating
	• Support systems based

in which those responsible for structuring the system are not dedicated to enabling the locus of control to remain at the point of service, the tendency is for more and more decisions to move away from the point of service and for more infrastructure to be built to compensate for the lack of control there. In addition, the more infrastructure that is built, the more extensive the lack of control becomes. The cycle of compensation continues until there is so much infrastructure that the cost of supporting it exceeds the cost of providing services.

The leader of a service system is always laboring to fully comprehend the essential interactions between the system elements and assess the degree to which those interactions facilitate the work going on at the center of the system. The leader also must assess the degree to which the system's configuration supports the openness and ownership of decisions and actions at the point of service and the amount of compensation

> **Key Point**
>
> *When any system has too much structure, it begins to support the structure rather than accomplishing its objectives. Unnecessary structure draws resources away from the system's services and interferes with its ability to do its work. The same holds true for unnecessary management.*

necessitated by inappropriately made decisions. The leader judges the level of skills at the point of service and looks at the support structures necessary to ensure that the level of competence there is at the right level and in the right configuration to meet the needs of those served. It is not just what the leader knows about the people, the services, or the system that matters, it is also what the point-of-service workers know.

The effectiveness of the system is directly related to support that exists for the ownership and application of decisions and actions at the point of service. In addition, if the structure at the point of service supports decision making and action at the point of service, less infrastructure must exist at other levels of the system to compensate for the lack of control there. Thus, the leader, knowing that financial and professional costs are paid when the locus of control shifts to other places in the system, must ensure that most decisions and actions remain at the point of service. A shift in the locus of control will cause the decisions to poorly fit the specific situational needs of the services and their providers. It also will obstruct the provision of competent, skilled, high-quality services and the workers' sense of ownership over the work.

The leader is fully involved in setting up and assessing the adequacy of the support structures of the overall system. These structures must be configured in a way that does not take from the point of service what belongs there. So also must the functions of strategic, operational, and service support be configured in a way that allows them to be understood and implemented there. The goodness of fit between the contextual activities of the strategic and support systems is vital, because all the processes that unfold in the structure of the overall system must ultimately contribute to the provision of services. The translation of these processes is critical to the database of the point-of-service workers and informs their decisions and actions. The leader acts as moderator of the relationship between those in the strategic and support systems and those at the point of service.

PRINCIPLE 10: REVOLUTION RESULTS FROM THE AGGREGATION OF LOCAL CHANGES

Revolution (hyper-evolution) occurs when the many local changes are aggregated to inexorably alter the prevailing reality (called the *paradigmatic moment*).

Most changes that occur are evolutionary; that is, they happen in a steady and regulated process over a period of time—most often over a very long period of time. As Darwin pointed out, the evolution of species is a dynamic process in which the living creatures best able to adapt to the changing environmental circumstances survive and thrive.

A revolution, on the other hand, is a dramatic, almost instantaneous, change in conditions, and it presents living creatures with the challenge of adjusting quickly enough. In a revolution, many events converge to create a situation in which life can no longer be lived in the same way.

Point To Ponder

The only difference between revolution and evolution is the time and pain it takes to make a sustainable change.

A revolution usually will occur in a system when the components jointly make enough of a demand for significant change. This demand is usually a result of the components being acted upon by the external or internal environment or by sociopolitical, economic, or technical transformations. In order to thrive in the face of the demand for change, the system must quickly alter its structure and behavior in such a way as to operate as effectively as it did in the previous circumstances.

Much of what is happening in health care is revolutionary in nature. The very foundations of health care are being transformed by the impact of new technologies, whether in the realm of computers and the Internet, robotics, pharmaceuticals, or genomics. Technological advancements are so pervasive and influential that, in concert, they are fundamentally altering health therapeutics as well as the delivery of health services. In particular, health services are less "bed based" than they were, the structures of hospitals and other health care organizations are being radically transformed, and providers must seek new ways of offering services.

Group Discussion

New sciences such as genomics and complexity science, advances in older sciences such as pharmacology, and technological developments are conspiring to change the health services format. What is currently in place will be largely deconstructed, and newer structures and models will now need to be conceived. Brainstorm the myriad changes dramatically affecting health care at this time. After listing these, discuss how they will alter the design of health services. What might some of the new designs be and how will they change the use and location of health care providers in the health system?

The role of health care leaders is to focus on the implications of the revolutionary changes occurring, including the implications for the behavior of those who work in the health care field. Health care leaders must help other health care professionals to adapt to the changes and must position health care organizations to continue to thrive. They must discern the new roles, processes, and behaviors that will be necessary for future success.

The current transformation in health care is attended by changes in other conditions that will challenge the ability of health care organizations to keep doing business in the same way. For instance, the environment will require these organizations to reconfigure supporting structures and finances, for the older configurations will become severely stressed in a way that threatens them. A further threat is presented by the fact that, while the supporting infrastructure of economics, policy, and work is being revamped, the still existing structures and behaviors will be even less effective than previously.

Here again, the leader of a health care organization must recognize the critical nature of the shift and undertake the dramatic and sometimes perilous process of quickly revising structure, processes, and behaviors to become more congruent with the emerging demand (Figure 2–5). Besides reading the signposts of the change accurately, the leader must begin to create a sense of urgency about the change in the minds of those who will live in this new world. The issue creating the drama and suspense is whether everyone's responses will be timely and appropriate. The leader must move people quickly through mourning the loss of established rituals and routines and raise the stakes for thriving and advancing the work in the context of a new set of parameters.

In a time of revolution, all the principles of adaptation and complexity management come into play. The leader's ability to apply these principles and bring the elements of complexity and chaos together will determine whether the organization thrives. As an

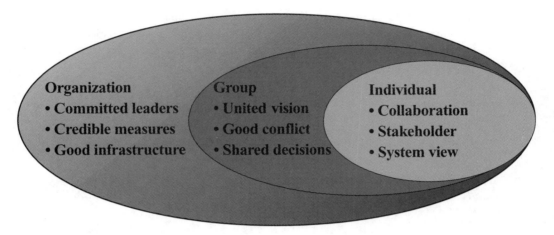

Figure 2–5 Organizational Levels and Associated New Age Characteristics

agent of change, the leader knows that there are a variety of "agents" in a system that can stimulate action or change. The leader is always looking for how these agents act to create the critical events that lead to an adjustment or a transformation.

The leader also knows that there are a variety of choices and strategies that can create a good fit between the demand for an adjustment and the response. The leader looks for the relationships in the demand for change. By paying attention to the themes and mosaic that best demonstrate the flow and impact of the patterns, the leader can facilitate the making of good decisions and the undertaking of effective actions.

Key Point

Leaders are agents of change. They bring the vision and context of change to the stakeholders so that the latter can develop the content of change.

There is both substance and artifact in all change. The leader's role is to sort through the options and determine which elements are evidentiary and which are simply "noise" representing the change itself. The leader does not discard the artifacts of change but instead determines their value and uses them either as tools of change or symbols of the journey itself. These artifacts may tell the participants where they are in the journey and may also provide help in getting through the journey's various stages.

Testing the way of the transformation is as important as any other activity. Although many things that occur during a revolution are important, equal amounts of "stuff" are unhelpful or even obstructive. Furthermore, it is important to determine where the system is in the process of change—what has been accomplished and what has yet to be done, what the deviations are and what the successes are as well. Consequently, a means of measurement is needed so that the agents and strategies selected can be validated against the distance traveled and so that the expectations can be compared with the reality (Figure 2–6).

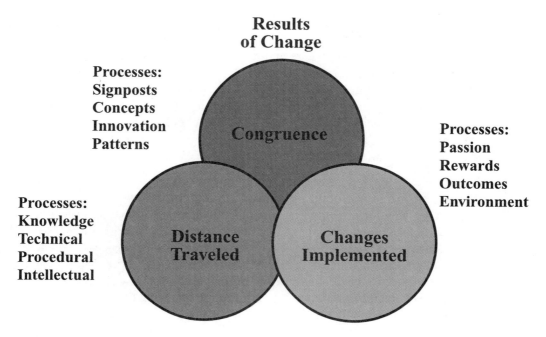

Figure 2–6 Evaluating Transformation. Each of the processes is applied to determine or confirm the results of change and the sustainable movement of the system.

Exploration and experimentation are essential elements of any major change. The context is often significantly different from what was previously experienced or lived, and as the context changes, so too do the rules. Both the journey and the way of living that results from the journey are so different from the past that previous experience is inadequate to meet the new demands. The script gets written as part of the journey itself. This means that most of the change agents are learning about the change at the same time as they are leading the adaptation to it.

Choosing strategies that fit the circumstances is not always easy to do. Because the ground is shifting as people are trying to learn to live on it, the leader must have an open attitude regarding what is to be discovered there. The leader must base his or her understanding of what is meaningful and sustainable on the journey thus far and how it has been experienced. The leader's experience forms the database for the next stage of the journey.

At the same time, the leader is experimenting with actions. Not knowing what the sustainable or valuable actions are until they are applied, the leader recognizes that there is an element of risk that must be embraced. All actions are prone to error. Indeed, the very risk of error advances the opportunity for learning and adaptation. Any particular error may contain the answer to a problem or at least be a signpost that could not be discerned in any other way, making the error a tool for the evaluation of direction and goodness of fit.

In short, the leader sees everything within the context of systemness. All elements of a dynamic system are related and interact with each other, and the interactions, when aggregated, are what create the conditions for the system's adaptation and ability to thrive. When internal need and external conditions converge, they create the demand for change and adaptation.

The leader sees systemness everywhere and recognizes that he or she can play a major role in the system's ability to adapt and improve (Figure 2–7). Whether the leader plays such a role largely depends on the leader's ability to anticipate, live in the potential of change, and embrace each change at the right time. In addition, the leader must realize that he or she is an important change agent and must always act out of that understanding.

To ensure that the system adapts appropriately to changes and continues to thrive, the leader needs to keep in mind the following:

- The leader must apply both the skills of exploration and those of exploitation and know when to apply each skill set.
- The leader must know which processes accommodate and use inherent variation and which processes maintain stability and good order throughout a period of change, and the leader must then use these processes appropriately. Some level of inherent stability and some normative forces help to reinforce adaptation, and yet innovative and creative solutions and strategies are often embedded in the chaos and variance. In other words, both stability and variability are essential for adapting to change.
- Knowledge of the inherent interactions of elements in the system can direct the leader to build on those intersections that bring coherence, integrity, and trust into the system. These features of systemness can enhance people's ability to change and adapt quickly and well.
- All strategies have consequences. The leader must determine the appropriate strategies for guiding the system in the right direction. The implementation of these strate-

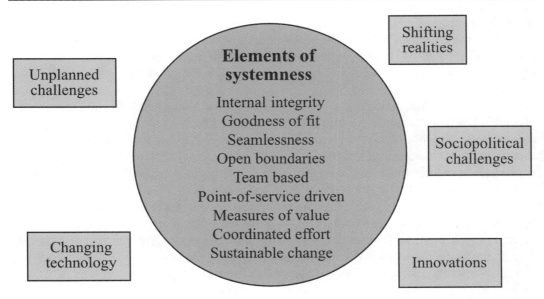

Figure 2–7 A System and Its Context. The system is "seen" through the continuing presence of its elements as they are acted upon by the external forces that make up the system's context.

gies must take into account that random influences may lead to valuable insights not available in any other way.

- Systems are membership communities. They operate through the consent of their members. The relationship between the members, including their communication with and support of each other, is as critical as any other factor for ensuring sustainable adaptation.
- Failure can be an important measure of direction and change. It should not, however, be an uncontrollable factor and should operate within the context out of which it emerges. Small changes should not contain large failures. If they do, that indicates that the associated strategies are ineffective or misconceived.
- The team is the basic unit of work, and the relationship between the core members drives all successful change. Here is where change gets lived out and applied. The interaction, relationship, and competence of the team members are essential to the viability of the team's work and the sustainability of the system. In human systems, all else exists to support the work of this unit.
- Small changes lead to big changes. Further, all changes affect the system as a whole, either individually (evolutionary change) or in the aggregate (revolutionary change). It is not possible to affect any part of a system without ultimately impacting the whole system.

CONCLUSION

The above presentation of principles is neither exhaustive nor fully developed. It should, however, alert readers to the fact the leadership role in the Information Age must operate on different concepts and ideas than those common in the Newtonian-inspired Industrial Age. Leaders must review the adequacy of their skill sets in light of the realization that the era of unilateral and vertical orientation of functions is quickly passing.

Dramatic and dynamic changes are continuing to impact the leadership role. To understand this role in the new age of work, leaders must learn about quantum principles and how they are to be applied. They must also become adept at understanding biologic metaphors, which are much stranger tools of thought than the old machine- and building-based metaphors. Permanent structures are no longer good models for work, especially in health care, and the type of architectural infrastructure characteristic of the coming age is information infrastructure. Leaders must now devote their full energy to pulling people out of work and service models that no longer operate efficiently and placing them in a context that demands thinking and acting in radically new ways.

It is interesting to note that, in recent times, people have not become more isolated. In fact, the opposite has occurred. Human beings have more potential for relationship and connectivity than at any time in history. The tools of connection and communication are creating linkages that were once only dreams. Living in this kind of a world, however, brings its own set of challenges and requires a different way of relating and behaving.

Leaders have an obligation to move people and structures into the new framework for work and leisure. To do this, they need a different mental model, new tools and skills, and a genuine desire to move both themselves and others into the new age. They need new knowledge, true enough, but they also need excitement so encompassing that others can see it and feel it, be energized, and develop the hope and enthusiasm necessary for creating a sustainable future.

When all is said and done about leadership—and these days much is said about it—what is important for each leader is to engage with and embrace the script of life and to get others to do the same so that the conditions of life are improved. Through discernment and exploration, design and formation, experimentation and application, leaders can help foster the richness of experience that enhances the quality of life for all. It is the effort to make life better and the chaos out of which improvements emerge that give form to the leadership role. It is the process of discerning and drawing from the complexity of all systems the simplicity that lies at their center and applying that simplicity to the lives of others that give critical substance to the work of every leader.

REFERENCES

Kelly, K. 1995. *Out of control: The new biology of machines, social systems and the economic world.* New York: Perseus Publishing.

Kelly, K. 1998. *New rules for the new economy.* New York: Viking Press.

Negroponte, N. 1995. *Being digital.* New York: Knopf.

SUGGESTED READINGS

Hesselbein, F., et al. 1997. *The organization of the future.* Drucker Foundation Future Series. San Francisco: Jossey-Bass.

Gryskiewicz, S. 1999. *Positive turbulence.* San Francisco: Jossey-Bass.

Hawking, S. 1988. *A brief history of time.* London: Bantam Books.

Holland, J. 1998. *From chaos to order.* Reading, MA: Helix Books.

Kelly, S., and M.A. Allison. 1999. *The complexity advantage.* New York: McGraw-Hill.

Zimmerman, B., C. Lindberg, and P. Plsek. 1998. *Edgeware.* Irving, TX: VHA, Inc.

Zohar, D. 1990. *The quantum self.* New York: Quill–William Morrow.

Zohar, D., and I. Marshall. 1994. *Quantum society.* New York: William Morrow.

Quiz Questions

Select the best answer for each of the following questions.

1. Change can be defined as a dynamic rather than an event. This means that change is:
   a. cyclical
   b. periodic
   c. timely
   d. continuous

2. Complexity science is based on a new understanding of the operation of the physical world. This understanding is referred to as:
   a. Newtonian physics
   b. quantum mechanics
   c. universal science
   d. the Einstein principle

3. The new age has been ushered in by a number of converging forces. The three main forces converging are sociopolitical, economic, and:
   a. technological
   b. international
   c. scientific
   d. commercial

4. Systems are dynamic entities driven more by relational elements than by functional processes. In this way they resemble:
   a. biological structures
   b. business structures
   c. social structures
   d. information structures

5. In a healthy system, 90 percent of decisions are driven by:
   a. the top of the system
   b. the bottom of the system
   c. the point of service
   d. the managers

6. According to complexity theory, anything that adds value to a part of the system adds value to the whole system. One of the implications of this principle is that:
   a. each part of the system drives the work of the whole system
   b. the whole system is the only legitimate source of sustainable value
   c. all real value derives from the work of the people in the system
   d. anything that adds value to a part of a system adds value to the whole system

7. In complexity theory, *chunking* is:
   a. the support provided to a complex system by the operation of simple systems
   b. the formation of a complex system by the incremental aggregation of interacting and interdependent simple systems
   c. the operation of a complex system consisting of independent parts
   d. the dynamic relationship between independent simple systems

8. Diversity is essential to change because it:

a. creates the variety required by change
b. accentuates the similarities that exist through change
c. makes chaos visible and underscores the need for adaptation
d. highlights the difficulty of reconciling differences

9. Error is also essential to change. Not all errors are acceptable, however. Those to be avoided are:

a. system-based errors
b. errors in judgment
c. repeated errors
d. human errors

10. Systems are driven by different rules than functional institutions. The cornerstone of systems design consists of:

a. relationships and intersections
b. functions and actions
c. policies and processes
d. rules and regulations

11. The leader of any system, in order to ensure the system's vitality, needs to pay special attention to which of the following:

a. stability
b. chaos
c. form
d. function

12. Revolution in a system occurs when:

a. the pace of evolution is insufficient for the necessary changes
b. things cannot continue to operate in the same way
c. violence is introduced into the system
d. many local changes occur at once

CHAPTER 3

The Leader as Peacemaker: Managing the Conflicts of a Multifocal Workplace

Cooperation is the thorough conviction that nobody can get there unless everybody gets there.

—Virginia Burden

Chapter Objectives

At the completion of this chapter, the reader will be able to

- Recognize the key principles of conflict resolution in dealing with a wide variety of conflict-based issues.
- Apply conflict management principles and processes in the everyday exercise of the leadership role.
- Distinguish between normal conflict management and the management of differences.
- Formulate personal insights regarding how to apply conflict management skill-sets as part of the leadership role.
- Distinguish between identity- and interest-based conflict and describe the best approach to dealing with each type.

Conflict is often looked at as a negative aspect of reality, yet it exists everywhere, from the foundations of life to the complexities of social interchange. The challenge presented by conflict is that it is often rife with pain and violence. However, that it frequently has those features is evidence of our inability to see conflict as normal and to develop mechanisms for managing it well. Because it is so much a part of the human experience, we would do better to learn the dynamics of conflict and incorporate its management into our human skill-set. This chapter treats conflict as normal and offers a range of techniques and methodologies for managing it in such a way as to ultimately achieve purposeful action and improved relationships. The emphasis is on developing skills for facilitating the use of conflict as a tool for promoting good interaction and advancing relationships. The chapter also outlines the difference between interest- and identity-based conflict and describes the processes used to address each.

Conflict is normal. It is present in every human relationship. It is a sign of the Creator's commitment to diversity and in fact represents diversity in action. It is the dynamic content of diversity, and human conflict is essentially diversity being worked out in the human community.

> **Key Point**
>
> *Conflict is normal. The challenge is to know what it is when it happens and what to do about it when it is recognized for what it is.*

Conflict should never be avoided. Instead, it should be embraced as a fundamental part of human interaction. Conflict is the most frequent dynamic in human relationships. And yet it is the most misunderstood and misused element in the whole arena of communication and interaction.

Embracing conflict is easier said than done, of course. A particular instance of conflict can involve a significant emotional overlay that adds stress to the interaction. This emotional component takes the conflict to a level of intensity that is uncomfortable and often destructive. At higher levels of intensity, the process of being in opposition becomes its own end, and the purpose and product of the conflict disappear in the dust raised by the process. The emotional component creates so much unpredictable and untenable content that most people simply back away from the conflict, unable to figure out how to deal with it or cope with its pain.

Fear and avoidance of conflict are main causes of the problems that can arise when a conflict occurs. Another cause is ignorance of the processes of conflict management. When a person becomes embroiled in a conflict, many feelings rush to the surface and begin to be expressed in one form or another, until eventually the person is dealing with feelings rather than the conflict that generated them. As a result, the original reason for the conflict can get lost in the interaction and may even be forgotten, replaced by another reason. In this scenario, ending the conflict amicably will not resolve the underlying problem, which has the potential to bring about another skirmish. The cycle can continue indefinitely, building layer upon layer over the underlying problem and making it ever harder to discern.

GROWTH AND TRANSFORMATION

All conflict provides a dynamic opportunity for growth and transformation, and leaders should treat conflict as simply another tool of good leadership. Peter Drucker has often said that 90 percent of leadership is addressing human behavior issues. A good proportion of this 90 percent involves addressing issues that have some form of conflict at their base.

The secret of good conflict management is simple, but the process is not. The secret is to get the parties in conflict to discern the root issues and mutually agree on actions to be taken. Actually building an effective process to accomplish this goal, however, is a complex task.

Conflict management takes into account that people differ in a whole range of ways and that factors as broad as culture, race, gender, social status, and income group and as specific as personal beliefs, family position, mental health, intelligence, and emotional maturity all can influence the onset and process of a particular conflict (Exhibit 3–1). It also takes into account that typically the parties to a conflict are unequal in some way, that one party may have a substantial advantage over the other (e.g., the lion's share of power). If a satisfactory outcome is to be obtained, the conflict management process must create equity at the table. It must utilize a mechanism that closely reflects the character and content of the conflict and moves it toward a mutually agreed resolution. This mechanism must be able to take into account the sources and contextual components of the conflict as well as the content elements. It must also address the power equation so that any unevenness can be accommodated and the process can unfold in a balanced and fair way.

> **Point To Ponder**
>
> *About 90 percent of the average leader's responsibilities involve dealing with human behavior and human interaction. Given that this is true, why do leaders spend so little time learning how to resolve the issues that arise out of human dynamics?*

Leaders, to do their job well, must acquire basic conflict management skills. Most lack these skills or have failed to master them, and, as a result, in many organizations a whole range of conflicts fester and grow. The possession of well-honed conflict management skills has become even more important owing to the increasingly interdisciplinary nature of the workplace, since the calling into question of historical relationships can easily give rise to conflicts.

Nurses have an additional set of concerns regarding conflicts and their resolution. In some ways, the history of nursing parallels the history of the women's movement, includ-

Exhibit 3–1 Sources of Conflict

Environmental Sources	Individual Sources
• Cultural	• Ego
• Nationality	• Personality
• Religion	• Identity
• Class	• Intimate relationships
• Economics	• Beliefs
• Politics	• Perceptions
• Society	• Perspectives
• Resources	• Education
• Race	• Position and role

ing the subordination and powerlessness experienced by both women and nurses (most of whom have been women). Recently, the education of nurses and other health profession-als has gone far toward creating intellectual and role equity, but long-standing medical practices and legal constraints on the scope of practice for various health professionals make these professionals, including nurses, uncertain of the agendas of physicians and administrators and skeptical of the processes that have been employed to resolve conflicts between the professions. In the view of nurses, the relationship they have had with physi-cians and administrators has historically been one-sided and biased against them, and their sense of being ignored or even silenced has not created a good foundation for building equitable relationships and resolving conflicts, to say the least.

Indeed, nurses are sometimes inclined to engage in passive aggressive, hostile, uncoop-erative, or avoidance behavior, even if the consequences are damaging to themselves. Part of the explanation is that they have not always been able to avail themselves of the matu-rity that comes with development, dialogue, conflict resolution processes, and some level of success. Another part may be the fact that the practice and service delivery models in use generally do not require nurses to interact at a high level. Most nursing work is de-signed to be performed by independent nurses or nursing teams assigned to defined groups of patients. This type of work involves little work sharing and keeps nurses from the vital interactions that would develop their relational skills. The conflicts between nurses and between nurses and other health professionals fall into the category of identity-based con-flicts, and their ultimate resolution requires, among other things, reconstructing the rela-tionship between nursing and the other professions.

Group Discussion

It has been said that health care is both risk adverse and conflict ad-verse. Discuss this claim. First, consider whether it is indeed true that health professionals avoid conflict to an unusually high degree. To reach a conclusion, it may be helpful to look at the following ques-tions. Does the structure of health care services create unusually clear lines of demarcation between people? Is the hierarchical nature of health care services a promoter or preventer of conflict? Are there fewer or more personality issues in health care settings than in other settings? How does the physician's role and position affect the inci-dence of conflict?

AVOIDING UNNECESSARY CONFLICT

Because conflict is an essential component of human interaction, trying to create con-ditions in which conflict is completely absent is pointless. Leaders instead should devote themselves to managing conflict, which includes preventing unnecessary conflict. Some of the conditions that help prevent unnecessary conflict are described below.

An Environment of Open Communication

It goes without saying that creating a climate of openness and trust is an excellent way to facilitate work and relationships. Although some leaders believe that tightly controlling work creates the fewest problems and that a "tight ship is the best run ship," that is not true for the normal activities of work. Leaders must realize that the relationship between the members of the work team is the most critical factor influencing the extent to which the conflict becomes a way of life. A sense that there is nothing that cannot be dealt with, that there are no "undiscussables," is essential to avoiding unnecessary conflicts.

The leader of an organization has enormous influence over the organization's culture. The leader's personal style of relating to and communicating with others sets the tone for the workplace, and it does not take long for others in the organization to discern what is acceptable and what is not. The leader's behavior toward staff and his or her responses to the stressors and challenges of the job create the model of acceptable conduct and act as the framework for what topics can be approached and what behaviors are appropriate.

> **Key Point**
>
> *An environment that abounds with "undiscussables" is an environment that breeds mistrust and unnecessary conflict.*

Groups become very skilled at seeing and noting the permissible and the political. Group members know what they must "go around" to get things done. What cannot be dealt with openly and directly is addressed secretively and behind closed doors. It is when open communication is absent that the infrastructure of conflict begins to take form and processes leading to irresolvable differences begin to emerge.

Congruence between Organizational and Professional Work Goals

A good way to prevent conflict is to ensure that the goals of individual workers and the goals of the organization support each other. It is commonly understood that complementary goals prevent conflict and competitive goals generate conflict. The history of the work in America is rife with instances where organizational goals and processes were at odds with the goals and expectations of those doing the work and where conflict sprang up as a result.

When there is goal congruence, people are more open, cooperative, engaged, and supportive and less angry and frustrated. When everyone is clear about expectations and processes and there is a supporting structure that contributes to the meeting of expectations, less conflict is generated.

Of course, congruence between goals is not always possible. Therefore, people must be given the opportunity to disclose what the differences are and how they are affected by these differences. If the reasons for the differences and the character of the differences can be made clear, people will find them easier to accommodate or accept. In addition, they will find them easier to accommodate or accept if they understand that all issues and situations are transitional and all relationships operate within the context of the human and relational journey (Figures 3–1 through 3–5).

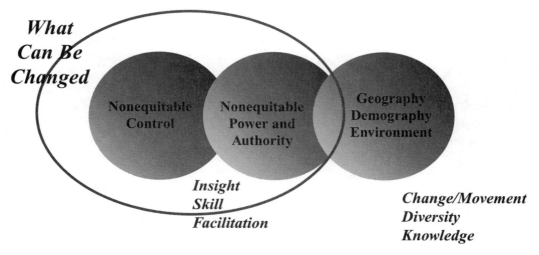

Figure 3–1 Structural Conflicts

Managing Conflict Productively

Leaders should devote more resources to the task of recognizing sources of conflict soon enough to handle disputes in the right way at the right time than they should devote to avoiding conflict. Following are some rules for handling conflict appropriately and productively.

Time and place can play a role in diffusing or inflaming a conflict. For example, if a conflict arises in public, the wise leader will act to remove the parties to a private place where the issues can be dealt with directly and freely. In many cases, a conflict will first reveal itself at a critical or stressful moment, fooling the participants into believing that the situation is the source of the conflict rather than the occasion for its expression. In such a case,

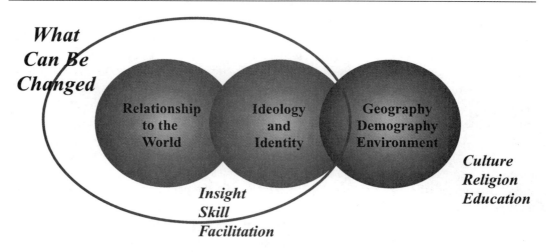

Figure 3–2 Value Conflicts

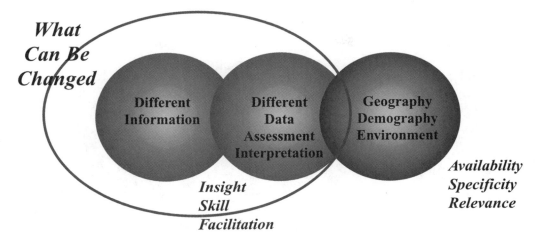

Figure 3–3 Information Conflicts

trying to deal with the conflict within the context of the situation will likely escalate the conflict, and so it is better to put the participants into a different environment or deal with the conflict at a later time and focus the dialogue on the issues, not the events.

Remember, conflict is primarily about behavior, not about people (although see the section below on identity-based conflict). In dealing with a conflict, the leader needs to be clued into the behavioral patterns and concerns and their impact on the parties' relationship, for the ultimate goal is to sustain this relationship. The leader is looking for accommodation and the ability to develop a working relationship that evinces the values and commitment necessary to do the work and continue to do it. In addition, the goal is to fix the problem, not affix blame. No conflict is unilaterally driven—there is enough fault to

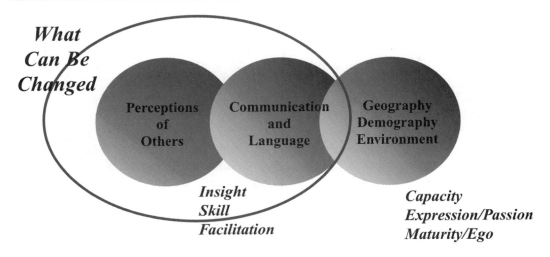

Figure 3–4 Interaction Conflicts

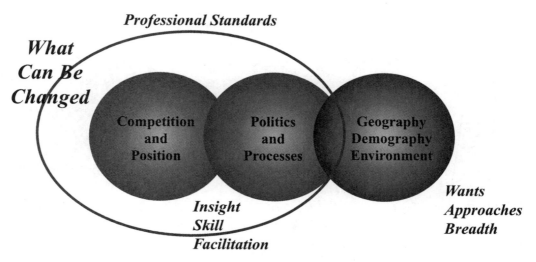

Figure 3–5 Interest Conflicts

go around. Wasting time on trying to affix blame delays long-term resolution of the conflict.

The resolution of a conflict depends on the achievement of some level of agreement about the parties' behavior or responses. Further, the agreement must be clearly articulated and must be understood by all the parties. In addition, at some point the parties must define their common ground in a joint meeting.

If a conflict is to be resolved, the parties must feel a sense of ownership over their own feelings and the agenda. The leader must ensure that they own their feelings and do not cast them on the shoulders of others and that they do not interpret what others mean without confirming that their interpretation is correct. The use of "I" approaches is critical to the dialogue. By making certain that each party's insights, feelings, and views are expressed from the party's own perspective and in his or her own language, the leader is able to keep both parties away from "us versus them" statements and "you" statements. The leader also can help maintain the focus and flow of the dialogue by making certain it stays within the limits of self-directed communication and personal ownership of the dialogue.

A flipchart or other visual tool can be used to get the conflict elements out in front of the parties in a two-dimensional way. The use of visual tools can overcome some of the obstacles likely to be raised by poorly

> **Key Point**
>
> *Facilitators must understand that the conflicts they attempt to resolve never belong to them. A conflict is owned by those who experience it, and transferring the locus of control is good neither for the parties nor the process.*

chosen language and place the ideas of all the parties before their eyes in a way that automatically creates equity. It also can help balance the dialogue and move the issues closer to real resolution by expanding the foundation of understanding between the parties.

Vagueness is to be constantly fought against. Although a certain amount of ambiguity is unavoidable as people sort out the issues, continuing vagueness obscures the issues and stops the dialogue. The leader must work to facilitate clarity around every issue of concern. By naming names, identifying events, describing situations, and illustrating behaviors, the leader seeks to get down to basics. The goal is to ensure that the real issues and processes are laid out on the table in clear enough terms that all the players can see them plainly.

Each party is looking for something, and unless this something is obtained or willingly given up for something else, the conflict will not end. First, each party must be able to articulate what he or she wants and what the other parties want in a way that all can understand and agree to. Second, each party must leave the conflict with a sense that he or she obtained something valuable, and each must feel good about what the other party got as well. In other words, the parties must view the resolution as equitable. This does not mean that what everyone gets is equal. It means that the resolution dispensed to each party is enough to satisfy that party, regardless of how important what was given may be to any of the other parties.

The above advice on how to manage conflict is not all-inclusive. For instance, leaders must take into account both situational and cultural factors when trying to facilitate the resolution of a conflict. The flexibility necessary to incorporate these factors is part of the conflict management skill set.

Team-Based Conflict Issues

Working together to provide health care services can be intense and difficult and can easily lead to conflict. To reduce the chance of unnecessary conflict, leaders must pay attention to relationship issues and create and keep an open and honest context for the work. Still, even in the best context, the behaviors and characteristics of people can lead to conflict.

Different personalities deal with conflict in different ways. Some folks are naturally generators of conflict, whereas others are skilled avoiders of it. Most of us fall somewhere in between these two extremes. Because different interests and personalities are present in the workplace, there is always ripe opportunity for conflict to emerge.

The leader of a health care organization should always be on the lookout for the potential for conflict. Because conflict eventually arises in any human environment, its potential is always present, at least to some degree. Further, if a conflict can be detected in its very early stages, it can be addressed soon enough to keep it from becoming critical and requiring extensive intervention. In general, the amount of effort needed to resolve a conflict is directly related to how early in the conflict's development the issues are dealt with.

Leaders must be aware of the main factors that lead to team-based conflict. Some of these are discussed below.

If team members believe that they are on the receiving end of *unfair or inequitable treatment,* they will descend down Maslow's ladder. Conflict and acting out inevitably will occur unless everyone is given an equal opportunity to provide input and have an impact. Another source of inequity is the tendency of people to use each other or the team for their own agendas or advancement. All team members must try to be just and fair in their dealings with each other to ensure the ground is even and everyone gets treated impartially.

Everyone does not need to know everything, but there must not be a *lack of essential information,* especially the information people need to do their work and to function and relate efficiently. In addition, team members must have a common understanding of the information and be able to see it within the correct context. It is common for people to think they have the information they need but discover upon further investigation that each has a different understanding of it, and so the team leader must make sure that everyone shares a common understanding. Also, team members need to be able to share their knowledge, insights, and experience in a way that can influence the team and what it does. Expressing what they know and think is critical to their own sense of value and place on the team and is likewise critical to the viability of the team.

Game playing always leads to conflict. The team leader must therefore be certain that the members are singing off the same song sheet. The rules that govern the team's activities should be clarified to and by the team members at the outset and often along the way. The members also need to be reminded that they will be held accountable for respecting the rules. Although any team must be able to accommodate different personalities, the interaction of team members must keep within certain boundaries. Processes that impede good interaction and communication between members ultimately lead to conflict.

Not acknowledging everyone's uniqueness can be a source of trouble. Every person approaches his or her work differently, has a different array of talents and skills, and has a different background and set of experiences. The team leader must not only recognize the differences between team members but must use them to advance the work of the team. For instance, some members are more reflective, and others are more active. Whereas the leader need never fear that the more active members will not make themselves heard—they are usually the first to initiate dialogue or action—the leader may have to ask the more reflective members for their views. Since the reflective members often have excellent insights and thoughtful opinions, they also must be involved in the team process to ensure the team's work is fully effective. Thus, the leader must recognize that the presence of personality and role differences can actually enhance the team's effectiveness, and that getting the full range of contributions from members will help avoid conflict, because no one will feel unjustly neglected.

Behavior based on *hidden agendas* is a prevalent source of team conflict and is extremely difficult to address. Almost every team has members who are not "on board" because they are pursuing their own agendas. They attempt to realize their goals by manipulating others and preventing others from attaining their objectives. They tend to see the world solely from their own position and treat others simply as a means of advancing their own interests. Whether they keep the team from growing or move the team in the direction of their choosing, they damage

> **Point To Ponder**
>
> *The team is the basic unit of work, not the individual. The individual must always be seen in the context of his or her relationship with others. Because work is the aggregation of the efforts of many people, for work to result in sustainable outcomes, these efforts must be coordinated and integrated. The task of any team leader is to synthesize the efforts of the team members and take advantage of the resulting synergy to achieve the team's goal efficiently and effectively.*

the integrity of the team and its sense of purpose. The team leader must try to detect these patterns of behavior early in the team process to correct them before they do serious harm. If members are allowed to pursue their own agendas with impunity or for a long period of time, they will reduce the team's effectiveness and eventually cause the team to descend into a state of chaos and conflict.

Lack of mutual appreciation among team members will impair team integrity. An old Zulu adage says, "I can only be me through your eyes." Who people are and the gifts that they bring are sacred and important. All team members should feel that they have value and are there because they have a unique contribution to make. They should know what it is they offer and be acknowledged for it by the other members. Each member should be aware of the character and role of any other member and understand how they advance and honor his or her own role. By clearly articulating the gifts that everyone brings to the table and the value of those gifts, the team leader keeps all the team members in mind of everyone's importance and thus diminishes the potential for conflict and breakdown.

> ### Key Point
>
> *Power is a sensitive issue in health care. For example, the word power is rarely used by health professionals, as if they do not really believe it operates in their relationships with each other. Of course, it always does. It is vital that the issues of power and authority be open for discussion, as they are critical elements in the interaction of team members at every level of the system.*

Power issues are a common source of conflict. How power is dispersed and used has a great influence on the occurrence and intensity of conflict within a team. In particular, conflict inevitably will occur if the expression of power is not seen as competent or balanced, or if the location of power is not seen as appropriate. A team operates like a community, and the team leader has the responsibility to maintain a sense of community among the members. The leader is always looking for breaks and potential problems in the relationship between members as a way of anticipating conflict and dealing with it before it develops into a major crisis requiring substantial time and resources.

Getting ahead of the conflicts that emerge is the best possible method for diffusing them and mitigating their consequences. The team leader should set up the team's structure and processes so as to make conflict processes a normal part of the interaction and relationship between members. The leader should not ignore conflict but instead implement strategies to expose the essential differences between members early enough to resolve the inevitable episodes of conflict as quickly as possible. By valuing and validating differences between team members and accommodating them, the leader will reduce the number of conflicts and at the same time decrease the chance that any of them will be crippling.

IDENTITY-BASED CONFLICT

Conflicts generally fall into two categories, interest-based conflicts and identity-based conflicts. Interest-based conflicts arise from circumstances or interactions and often can be resolved quickly. Identity-based conflicts go much deeper and last longer. Rothman (1997) suggests that identity-based conflicts are rooted in threats to people's need for dignity, recognition, safety, control, purpose, and efficacy. For these conflicts to be adequately addressed, their origin and their meaning to the opposed parties must be adequately appreciated. In general, identity-based conflicts

- reflect the parties' culture and beliefs
- involve questions of identity and sense of self
- arise out of the parties' commitment to their values
- are of long duration
- are the most difficult conflicts to resolve
- can be passed on from one generation to next

Their sources include

- values
- religion
- language
- heritage
- culture
- family
- community
- country

Each person has a unique background and set of life experiences and brings a personal as well as a cultural framework to any dialogue or deliberation with others. Further, it is because everyone is a unique individual that relationships and interactions exhibit a dynamic pattern and that identity-based conflicts are possible. It is the differences between people that create life's mosaic—its fabric. The richness of human experience is driven by the broad diversity that is characteristic of human life and that forms the foundation for human interaction. It is no surprise that, for conflict resolution activities to be successful, they must be based on an understanding of the ingrained differences between the parties and must encompass a respect for and appreciation of these differences.

Group Discussion

Look around the room at the other occupants and note down as many differences as you can in a few minutes. After listing all the differences on a flip chart, discuss how each might lead to a conflict. Also discuss how the resulting conflicts might affect relationships, interactions, and the work environment. Then identify how the different types of conflict are related to each other and consider the possibility that together they could result in an irresolvable state of conflict. Finally, discuss how the conflicts identified could escalate and describe the impact such escalation could have on patient care.

Conflict is a normal part of all human affairs, from marriage to politics. Recognizing this fact encourages us not to ignore conflict, downplay it, or leave it unaddressed. The best strategy is to accept that conflict is inevitable and acquire the skills and methods for safely and effectively dealing with it, including paying attention to what it means and where it is trying to move us.

Identity-based conflicts are very difficult to either define or resolve. Because they are rooted in historical, psychological, cultural, and experiential factors, their boundaries and content are hard to determine. Because they are deeply embedded in personal sentiments, the contending parties are less willing to compromise. Therefore, they demand a deep and creative engagement.

Giving the Parties a Voice

When confronted with an identity-based conflict between two or more parties, a leader must try to facilitate the resolution of the conflict. Acting as facilitator, the leader's first job is to give the parties a voice and to listen to their essential concerns and their perceptions of the conflict. They must be allowed to express where they are in the conflict and what their feelings are about the conflict. Note that their perceptions do not have to be correct, for the main goal is to find out what each party has experienced *from inside the experience*. The stated perceptions of each party constitute a personal expression of his or her experience of the conflict and are bound to be different from the stated perceptions of the other party. In some cases, the parties' perceptions are so different that an objective third person may wonder if each is describing the same situation.

> **Key Point**
>
> *Difference is a cause of conflict and, as a prerequisite of dialogue, part of the solution to conflict. In fact, both difference and dialogue are necessary for good and sustainable human interaction.*

Getting the parties to give expression to their perceptions of the conflict is an essential first step in understanding and resolving it. The way the perceptions are formulated should reflect the feelings and sentiments of those who have the perceptions. This stage, when the parties give voice to their sentiments and perceptions, is not the time for clarification and process. The facilitator needs to allow the expression of perceptions to be natural and unconstrained. The result is sometimes uncomfortable because the emotion can be intense and raw. Yet, intensity of feeling will indicate to the parties how critical the process is and just what the stakes are.

In order for there to be movement toward resolution, the facilitator must make sure that all of the issues and all facets of the

> **Point To Ponder**
>
> *Although conflict is normal, unresolved conflict is dysfunctional. Further, a particular conflict will remain unresolved if it remains unnamed or undiscussed.*

issues felt by the parties to be critical are laid out in detail, including issues related to dignity, recognition, value, and meaning. There is nothing more threatening to the process of resolution than a belief on the part of any party that his or her story was not told, the origin of the conflict has not been fully appreciated, and, as a result, the process is flawed.

Identity-based conflicts are rooted in the parties' need to protect their value and identity (Exhibit 3–2). They feel there is a threat to *who they are*—a threat to the very foundation of their being—and they often respond by going on the attack. For example, conflicts between nurses and physicians over practice are rooted in their notions of who they are as professionals and their sense that their value and even survival is threatened by the other professional group. Physicians feel that nurses jeopardize their independence as practitioners and their economic well-being, and nurses feel that physicians obstruct their ability to practice, grow, and thrive. In fact, each group views the other group as a major threat to its own interests, predisposing members of both groups to let their negative perceptions of the conflict inform every interaction they have on issues of practice and service.

Interest-based conflicts, if left unresolved long enough, can and often do become identity-based conflicts, but the latter, no matter what their origin, require strategies different from those used to resolve conflicts that are simply interest based. For instance, legalistic and negotiation-oriented strategies tend to alienate the parties to an identity-based conflict. These strategies limit the amount and types of dialogue that occur, preventing the parties from establishing the kind of relationship they need to deal with the issues affecting them. Using resolution strategies aimed at getting to an early agreement can poison the conversation and keep the parties from finding common ground. People are not willing to compromise those things that they feel are fundamental to their own identity and survival. Some issues are simply not subject to negotiation.

Time and Patience

In trying to resolve an identity-based conflict, it is a mistake to begin by pushing the parties to compromise, often the strategy of choice for interest-based conflicts. Another mistake is to try to get the parties to separate their feelings from the so-called facts of the conflict, for their feelings, especially their sense of identity, are at the root of the conflict. Using a strategy that threatens their identity will make the parties more suspicious of each other and of the conflict resolution process.

Exhibit 3–2 Identity Characteristics

• Needs	• Balance
• Self-image	• Clarity
• Insight	• Investment
• Knowledge	• Breadth
• Skills	• Ownership

The resolution of identity-based conflicts takes a great deal of time, especially the first stages of the process. However, these stages are the most crucial and warrant the extra time and patience. Naming and certifying issues, feelings, and positions clearly at the outset establishes a firm foundation upon which to construct a process that moves effectively to a successful outcome.

In a traditional negotiation process, the parties try, through compromise, to arrive at a place where they can essentially "split the difference." This process works best when the issues are clear, the goals are well defined, and the parties are reasonably clear on what the common ground looks like. Unfortunately, the underlying issues in an identity-based conflict are blurred, and the parties feel especially vulnerable because the stakes are seen as so consequential. The parties therefore are hesitant to compromise early in the process, and moving too quickly toward a resolution could threaten the process itself and prevent the parties from dealing with the underlying issues, in which case these issues would ultimately give rise to another episode of discord.

> ## Key Point
>
> *Identity-based conflicts take longer to resolve than interest-based conflicts. They arise out of people's identity—who people are as opposed to what they do—and often have substantial historic content. In an identity-based conflict, the two parties, in order to reach a resolution, must come to appreciate each other's value and respect each other's uniqueness—a very challenging task given the passionate attachment of each party to his or her own identity.*

Building Trust

Much of the early work in the resolution process is directed toward getting the parties to change the way they think about each other and agree on a process and method for interacting. The parties are essentially suspicious of each other. Their suspicion is itself a great source of conflict, and getting to a place where the rules of engagement are clear and can be used as the vehicle for dialogue increases the probability that the parties will be able to work out their differences.

In an interest-based conflict, the root issues are not always put on the table, and the negotiation strategies are typically as important as the issues. In contrast, in an identity-based conflict, posturing and positioning are generally ineffective, because the parties need to disclose their powerfully held sentiments and beliefs—those things that reveal who they are and what they do. To build a proper foundation for resolving the conflict, they must fully understand these sentiments and beliefs—their own and those of the other party—and identify whatever common ground exists.

Because of the high stakes involved in an identity-based conflict, the facilitator should move the parties toward negotiations slowly, after a trusting foundation has been established. In the initial stages of dialogue, the facilitator should encourage the parties to set practical goals, such as arriving at a common view of the conflict and agreeing to a description of the issues in a common language. By achieving these goals, the parties will be more inclined to accept that resolution of the conflict is a real possibility and will feel comfortable with the resolution process. In short, the parties must develop a sense of relationship with each other before moving further along toward resolution.

> ### Point To Ponder
>
> *Conflicts love to hide in ambiguity. If a conflict remains unclear or undefined, it also will remain elusive and hard to eradicate. The parties, only able to deal with the symptoms, almost certainly will allow the conflict to have an impact on all their joint activities, leading to negativity and uncertainty far beyond the boundaries of the conflict itself.*

The facilitator must realize that building a trusting atmosphere and getting the parties to recognize they each have a substantial stake in resolving the conflict are both essential steps. By showing the parties their relationship to the larger context, the facilitator helps them see where their common values lie and what a resolution equitable to everyone might be.

The facilitator is likely to find that one or both parties exhibit a currently prevailing pattern of behavior characterized by deviousness, secretiveness, manipulation, and a sense of "us against the world." This pattern provokes a response of unilateral defensiveness that is hard to break through. To fight against it, the facilitator must try to nurture cooperative inquiry, establish credibility, and engage in relationship building. A good part of the resolution process must be devoted to creating a *common identity* around the issues in a way that allows all the parties to feel that they are mutually contributing to the end of the conflict.

The parties must arrive at a place where they can honestly say what they value and believe. Getting them to this place may not be easy, as the parties may have strong emotional blocks preventing them from articulating what their issues really are. Sometimes the parties believe they are articulating the issues by stating how they feel, but in doing this they are focusing on the results of the issues, not the issues themselves. The facilitator must be able to get them to focus on what caused these feelings—the conflicts that lie at the heart of their emotions.

The long-term work involves helping the parties reconceptualize the conflict, perceive their relationship in a new way, change the language they use to describe the conflict, and even change the nature of the conflict altogether. The conflict may be rooted in a lack of clarity, and one or both parties may say things that are inconsistent with what they do. They both need to achieve a good understanding of their own motives and desires before attempting to move toward an end to the conflict. Otherwise, each will be unable to hear and understand where the other is coming from.

Finding Differences

As mentioned above, each person is a unique blend of differences, and their differences from each other are what make people exciting and intriguing to each other. We celebrate our differences and honor diversity in culture and personality. Yet, differences can become an impediment to understanding and relationship, and given enough time any human relationship will give rise to some level of conflict. When it does, those in the relationship must understand that it is not the conflict that is problematic but its nonresolution.

> **Group Discussion**
>
> In any organization, unresolved conflict eventually creates a culture of conflict, increasing the incidence of conflict at every level. After identifying personally experienced unresolved conflicts in the workplace, discuss the impact that each conflict had on relationships in the work group. In talking about this issue, consider the following questions: What kinds of factions formed? Did the one conflict lead to others? Did the group leader take any action to ensure that the conflict would be resolved? That it would not be resolved? What was the long-term impact of the unresolved conflict? Was the conflict ever resolved? How?

To figure out just what caused a conflict, the parties to the conflict must be able to frame the issue in a way that gives it focus. One method is for each party to ask, what do I want here? And to answer this question, each must be clear on how he or she stands on the differences between the two parties. Framing their notion of the conflict or of their position in relationship to it gives the parties a foundation upon which to take a position. To get there, they need to ask themselves some pretty specific questions.

Do the parties remember the period before the conflict existed? Looking at the before and after can help the parties give the conflict a time and a frame of reference, allowing them to identify its elements in a way that makes it real. Furthermore, the parties, in reviewing the period before the conflict, give the facilitator an opportunity to see how each perceives the beginning of the conflict and to detect any differences in their perceptions.

What antagonisms emerged? What did they look like? How did they feel? Here the focus is on perceptions of the moment of conflict. The issues of resentment, behavior change, and cultural and personality differences get expressed in the unique language of each party. Both parties begin to express their special insights about the feelings and animosities that emerged and grew as a result of their differences, and the individual flavor of the conflict starts to become clear. The parties now get a chance to express not only how they felt but why and what it meant to them at the time, allowing the circumstances to be reflected through the lens of personal experience. This process disciplines their insight and forces them to focus on the conditions and circumstances that give form to their sense of the conflict.

Who is to blame and what are they to be blamed for? Answering this question is a good way to get to the dynamics of the conflict. In almost every conflict, a strong element of blame lies at its heart. The parties need to get some idea of what the blame is, where it resides, and what form it takes. Not only is it important to uncover the blame, the facilitator must push each party to describe the content of the blame it points at the other party and explain why it is justified. The explanation is likely to make reference to stress, pain, or anguish experienced by the party doing the blaming and indicate how the other party was responsible for it.

These questions get at the fundamental antagonisms causing the conflict. The parties' perceptions and feelings need to be articulated at the beginning of the resolution process for two reasons. First, both parties must see and say where they are in relation to their notion of the conflict. Second, the facilitator must get some sense of where the parties are at the start of the resolution process. The agenda for building the process and achieving reconciliation is constructed at the very beginning of the process. By getting the parties to delineate the differences in their perceptions and positions, the facilitator gains information about the work yet to be undertaken.

To get this information, it is best to talk with each party independently. The facilitator should keep the meetings informal and focused on gathering information and helping the parties get ready for their work within the process. These meetings also offer a good opportunity to discuss the rules of engagement that will be used when all the parties are at the table. Note, however, that the rules of engagement must be finally deliberated and agreed to when both parties are present.

Who Wants What?

People in conflict generally know what it is they think they want. When individuals or groups are at the point of conflict, they generally have reached the stage of holding black-and-white positions—positions that are mutually exclusive and sit at some distance from each other.

To bring the positions closer, the facilitator must be steeped in the resolution process and look for every opportunity to foster congruence, strengthen trust, and improve the interface between the parties as their relationship begins to grow. As noted above, the parties to an identity-based conflict must establish a relationship rather than simply obtain a resolution of their issues. The facilitator helps them do this by knowing them as well as possible and being familiar enough with their issues and positions not to miss opportunities for bridging differences and constructing common ground, for such opportunities rarely are presented twice. The facilitator's knowledge is his or her main tool for advancing the process and moving the relationship through the tough times.

ARIA*

In his seminal work on identity-based conflicts, Rothman (1997) suggests a format for the resolution process. The stages of the format, which he calls ARIA (antagonism, resonance, invention, and action), are outlined below.

Antagonism

In the first stage, the facilitator pushes the parties to express their antagonism, which, besides helping the facilitator move the process along, helps the parties lay out their raw

---

*Source: Resolving Identity-Based Conflict, J. Rothman, Copyright © 1997, John Wiley & Sons. This material is used by permission of John Wiley & Sons, Inc.

emotions in plain view and, in so doing, diffuses them, thereby reducing the temperature of the conflict. Given the proper context, this initial expression of antagonism also pro-vides extra motivation to do something about the conflict and the negative feelings that it generates—to end the pain and dis-cord and move to a better place, where there is more peace and stability and opportunity.

In addition, it can reveal to the parties their own limitations and constraints. They are able to see how their own intensity of emotion polarizes their views and positions. Although unlikely at this point to be able to make substantial changes, they can at least get a picture of what their positions look like and how strongly they hold their views, possibly opening a window to understand-ing. Indeed, expressing their antagonism and hearing it reflected back in the language of the facilitator may surprise them and

> ## Key Point
>
> *Parties to a conflict must be allowed to express their feelings, even their passionate feelings. If not expressed, these feelings will become intensified and move deeply inward, poisoning every interaction and preventing a reso-lution from being achieved. Therefore, facilitators must create a safe space for the parties to get their feelings out.*

finally make them realize just how fixed, strident, or polarized they have become. After all, the flames of antagonism are fanned by a wide range of emotions that, regardless of their legitimacy, are strongly felt and often strongly expressed.

In a typical conflict, one or both parties blame the other side in order to strengthen their own position, at least in their own eyes. Blame serves to escalate the conflict and give it a justification. It creates an "us and them" position, locates the enemy, and defines the terms of opposition. It puts the other party at fault and provides a reason to be angry at and in conflict with the other party. The nat-ural tendency to place blame is best exem-plified by the common childhood claim "He hit me first."

Blame helps the parties avoid focusing on their own part in the conflict. By concen-trating on why it is the other party's fault, each party evades having to reflect on the role he or she has played. The parties never have to consider how they might have acted differently, experience the pain of admitting their own contribution to the conflict, or engage in the work of reaching a resolution. Indeed, blame suggests that a resolution to the conflict is not possible.

> ## Point To Ponder
>
> *Blame keeps the parties from owning their part of the conflict—from naming their own issues and identifying them as causes of the conflict—and thus keeps them from achieving a resolution. In pointing a finger, each party focuses exclusively on the other party's actions, whereas each should instead attempt to see clearly and admit to his or her role in the conflict dynamic.*

Blame helps keep the conflict external—safe and free of personal content. It puts the responsibility for resolving the conflict in the other party's court and suggests that if the other party would make certain changes or act differently, the issues and the conflict would simply disappear.

Blame never has any real value. The facilitator's best strategy is to pursue naming the feelings of each party and their intensities. Even when restating accusations of blame, the facilitator does not spend time in the blame. Discussing the blame that has been leveled merely helps the facilitator figure out (1) where the parties are in relation to each other and to the issues at the root of the conflict and (2) how to move the parties toward reconciliation.

Blame also generalizes feelings and perceptions and keeps the parties from being specific and reaching clarity. The facilitator's role is to get the parties to focus on the particulars and delineate their own positions.

Posturing and positioning commonly act as intensifiers of conflict. They support the culture of justification and rights and lead to rationalizations of the polarization that typically occurs in a conflict. The parties will give reasons for the polarization and construct a whole logic to support it. In other words, they circle the wagons and make the war their cause rather than the issue at the root of the war. They then devote more time and energy to conducting the war than they ever did in pursuing the underlying issue.

Group Discussion

Greg Shue, manager of a hospital department, was angry with the head of critical care. She had beat him out of a part of the budget he needed in order to make programmatic changes in his own department. He occasionally referred to her in derogatory terms and seemed unable to get past his anger, which was beginning to have a serious effect on the relationship between Greg and the other department head and on the entire organization. You are the conflict mediator in this case. How would you begin the conflict resolution process? What would you do to get Greg to own his anger? What would you do to induce Greg to move beyond his feelings and begin dealing with the real issues?

At this stage, the conflict has taken on a life of its own. Nothing the other party does with regard to the issue is right or appropriate. Further, because each party is acting out of his or her own identity, the other party not only does the wrong thing but becomes wrong. The next step is to describe the other party as bad and to conclude that he or she must be opposed. If the one party did not oppose the bad party, the former would be bad too, and in the same way. This would be untenable. Thus builds the polarization between the parties and the intensity of the conflict.

Also, as the characterization of each party by the other grows increasingly negative, the less necessary each feels it is to resolve the conflict. Who would want to resolve a conflict if it meant giving up a justifiable fight against what is bad, perhaps even evil? In the mind of each party, what needs to happen is for the other party to stop being bad. If that occurred, the conflict would automatically end.

The facilitator must realize that each party has a selective memory. Each vividly remembers events that led to the conflict and for which blame could be laid on the other party. On the other hand, each tends to forget contributing events for which he or she was responsible, not to mention dishonorable motives.

When the negatives run high, the parties' desire to resolve the underlying issue wanes. Their energy is instead devoted to building a culture of opposition and to placing themselves in the right. They act to strengthen their position and get it validated by prospective allies. Correspondingly little energy is devoted to pursuing strategies that might lead to a resolution of the conflict.

As time goes on, each party becomes increasingly critical and disapproving of the behaviors, practices, and even culture of the other party. Words and actions become opportunities for the one party to challenge, skewer, or demean the other and further validate continuation of the conflict.

Projection is commonly used by parties in a conflict to strengthen their positions. Projection involves attributing to others problematic behaviors we engage in or embarrassing characteristics we possess. It is universally understood as a defense mechanism for avoiding responsibility for such behaviors and characteristics. In a conflict, one party, in addition to viewing the other party as fundamentally different, might project, for example, unacceptable motives onto the other party and thus avoid confronting the fact that these are his or her own motives.

If this occurs, the facilitator's goal of getting the parties to see what they share in common becomes even harder. Each party resists admitting that the other could in any way be similar because doing so might involve having to acknowledge engaging in certain objectionable behaviors. Though daunting, the facilitator's task at the outset is to achieve as much clarity about the antagonism as possible, and his or her initial activities largely will be spent on getting the parties past this part of the conflict so that they can pursue resolution strategies.

Resonance

Resonance is the process of moving away from antagonism and toward the identification of common ground. Through "reflexive reframing," the parties begin to articulate their values and concerns and seek commonalities on which to build dialogue.

In the preceding phase, the focus of each party is on the behavior of the other. Each party's view is outward and other oriented. Reflexive reframing refocuses the gaze of the parties back to themselves so that they can clarify who they are and what they want before trying to fashion a resolution.

An identity-based conflict is likely to involve intangible and subjective issues. The facilitator might have a hard time believing the two parties are talking about the same concerns. In point of fact, they may not be. The two parties are likely to have different cultural and experiential backgrounds, have different perceptions of the conflict, and use different language to express their perceptions. The notion of objective truth is irrelevant because each party cannot help seeing the conflict through his or her own eyes and treating his or her own perceptions as true.

However, by expressing their deepest feelings and values, the two parties start to fashion a common frame of reference. Each begins to sense that the other shares certain sentiments and to develop a fuller picture of the other. By going deeper into their own experiences, the parties build the foundation for future dialogue. They discover that their initial views and positions—those expressed during the first stage—are inadequate and cannot be supported. The personal and "why" questions they ask help turn the conversation into a vehicle for learning about each other's different perspectives and values.

Group Discussion

The parties to a conflict each possess their own values and beliefs. If the conflict is identity based, their ownership of their values and beliefs and their sense of who they are will unavoidably impact their interaction with each other. Assume you are assigned the job of facilitating the end of an identity-based conflict between two people. How do you break through the identity issues to get the parties to talk with each other? What should you explore and settle with the parties separately before you bring them together? Break the discussion group into two and give each subgroup the role of acting as one party in an identity-based conflict (a conflict arising out of a difference in nationality, ethnicity, religion, or politics). List the elements of conflict as they come up during the ensuing dialogue.

Reflexes come in two varieties, the automatic reflex to external stimuli and the reflective response based on study and assessment. The latter type is characteristic of good conflict management. It requires the ability to step back and look at issues and concerns from a far enough distance to see the whole landscape related to the conflict. The goal of the facilitator is to get the parties to take the necessary step back. Ideally, they would see each other's pictures of the conflict, understand the circumstances and variables placing them in the conflict, and understand how all of that stands in relationship to everything else. Ultimately, the facilitator wants to create a double-loop experience for the parties. Once each has articulated his or her own experience and completed the circle of experience, the two parties would link their experiences in a way that exposes their similarities and intersections. Common elements and frames of reference begin to emerge as a result, and the relatedness of the elements become clear to the parties and form a foundation for further dialogue.

The two parties also need to see clearly that both have the same fears, uncertainties, meanings, and values and to recognize that they could find themselves saying the same things. When one party says, "I am concerned," "I am afraid," or "I am angry," the other should be able to admit honestly that he or she could easily utter the same statement. Furthermore, through the "I" form of the expression, the individual ownership of thoughts and feelings ultimately becomes mutual. It is precisely because of the deep ownership each has of his or her own insights and feelings that mutuality can begin to emerge without causing the threats of challenge, accusation, or alienation. It is hard to reject in another what you just affirmed in yourself.

Identity-based conflicts can exhibit elements of reaction. Each party's sense of self may actually be formed in opposition to the other party's sense of self. The parties' discernment of who they are not can sometimes be as important as their definition of who they are. For instance, they might see themselves as not having characteristics that they attribute to the other party, possibly just because they perceive the other party as having them. They are likely to view themselves, not just as possessing different interests, but as being fundamentally different. Religious, cultural, ethnic, national, and sexual differences often serve as the basis of identity-based conflicts. After all, there is nothing any of us can do about our sex, nationality, ethnicity, or religion and so these are seen as defining us.

> **Key Point**
>
> *Fear keeps people from disclosing how they really feel and focusing on resolving the issues at the root of a conflict. Therefore, early in the conflict resolution process, the facilitator must give the parties a strong sense of safety so that they can confront their anxieties and talk openly and honestly.*

In health care, discipline, role, function, and license can similarly act to divide people in fundamental ways and create a priori positions that are hard and sometimes impossible to get around. For example, "I am the doctor; the buck stops with me." Or "I am the nurse; I manage the processes of care." Or "I am the caregiver; I do the work of health care." Each of these statements is partially true, but by holding to them, the parties can become polarized and entrenched. Moving them from their positions is a challenging task, but it can be done by persuading them that no role is the most special, important, critical, powerful, or viable and that no person can do what needs to be done if the other parties fail to meet their responsibilities. The fact is that "I am because you are." That is, we are all interdependent, and indeed the clearer I am as to how I stand in relation to you, the clearer I am as to who I am and who I can become. It is essential that the parties understand the interdependence of their roles so that they can reach a sustainable resolution of their differences.

The parties to an identity-based conflict are faced with a fundamental choice: they can continue to maintain an isolated identity against the world or they can search for and uncover their common roots and frames of reference and find their mutuality. To get them to do the latter, the facilitator should help them move

- from blaming to articulating their sense of self
- from antagonism toward the other to identification with the other
- from the attribution of negatives to understanding
- from projection to ownership
- from anger to acceptance
- from fear to a sense of safety

As the parties move through these initial stages of the conflict resolution process, they clarify the conflict, obtain ownership of the process, and explain to each other what is most present in themselves, thereby deepening their self-understanding and establishing a foundation for the later stages.

Invention

During this stage, the parties begin to see some payoff for the work they have done. The focus is on inventing solutions that can take the parties to a place where they can live in peace and engagement.

Their main task is to look at solutions through a larger lens or use a greater frame of reference—in other words, to think outside the box. They should try to develop new ways of looking at the conflict and come up with new solutions. As noted, in identity-based conflicts, negotiating a compromise is fraught with difficulty, because the parties would view compromising as giving up something of who they are, not simply something they have, and would thus find it unacceptable.

Instead of seeking compromise, the facilitator must challenge the parties to apply a broader framework and see the situation in a new way. They both have a stake in the outcome and will stand to gain from a solution. They must, therefore, reconceptualize the conflict, which is the purpose of the invention process. This process is about developing whole new ways of seeing the issues and working through them. It demands a focus on the practical and the real, and by going through the process, the parties should be able to develop a different vision of their concerns and a different image of each other. In particular, they should recognize that they are interdependent and need each other and that the resolution of the conflict requires everyone to get on board.

The first step is to develop and agree on statements of objectives. These are derived from statements of the issues. They help the parties see and say what they want to get from the process, especially as relates to their fundamental needs for safety, security, value, dignity, and so on. They also will inform the more detailed discourse the parties will engage in regarding the steps and processes intended to move the parties to where they would like to be.

This step includes components that allow the parties to educate each other on what they need and to explain why. The education expands on what has already been shared but with a new focus on safety, security, values, and so on. Because the issues at the root of the conflict are identity issues, the parties must try to explain how what they are asking for advances or protects their identity.

Working out the details is critical. Watching negotiations, uninformed observers often feel that the haggling that occurs over the smallest detail is ingenuous and foolish. In an identity-based conflict, each detail has implications for the identities of the parties following the resolution, and thus each one counts.

Note that there is a significant difference between interests and needs. Interests generally play a central role in resource- or interest-based conflicts but a subsidiary role in identity-based conflicts, where needs are primary. Consequently, in an identity-based conflict, the most critical task is to get parties to express their needs, then to reach an understanding of their interests based on their needs. For example, as they see it, the nurses in a health care organization need to give care to patients unconstrained by financial considerations. On the other hand, the managers, as they see it, need to ensure the financial health of the organization. Both needs—the nurses' need to give good care and managers' need to ensure financial viability—relate to a common interest, ensuring the existence of enough financial resources to render good service to the public. If the two groups understand that because of their needs they share an interest, they are more likely to reach a resolution of their conflict.

Of course, achieving a resolution does not mean that the parties get everything they desire. At best, they will be able to negotiate a method for meeting their needs—a method that may involve working together, such as one of those described below.

Sometimes *differentiating between the parties* more clearly, that is, accentuating and enumerating their differences, can lead to a more suitable resolution for each. Although their needs may differ, clarifying them and seeking alternative ways to satisfy them through common action can help move the parties to a new place. For example, imagine a respiratory therapy union is seeking greater recognition for its members and a stronger role for its leaders, whereas the management wants a reduction in complaints and grievances instituted by the union. Both groups agree to apply a different method of problem solving, one in which the union leadership plays a more direct role. The result is less use of the grievance procedure. Here the different needs of the two groups provide a basis for resolving their conflict creatively.

> **Point To Ponder**
>
> *In trying to resolve an identity-based conflict, the facilitator should help the parties differentiate themselves and develop a clearer sense of who they are and what they bring to the table.*

A second technique involves *expanding the playing field* so the parties can each get more of the resources they need. For example, nurses may request more staffing, and management may want to save more money. The two groups may agree that if the nurses meet set productivity targets, management will use part of the savings to hire more nurses. By consenting to work together to expand the organization's resources, they each help meet their

---

Group Discussion

Nina Conners really did not want to settle the issues she had with Frank Kliener. They had been feuding for three years. Both she and Frank used their conflict as a way of getting more for their own departments and keeping their staff energized and competitive. However, the organization has been paying the price, and its goals are sometimes held hostage to the war between the two departments. Discuss how a mediator would begin to resolve this conflict. What are the apparent issues? What might be the real issue? How would the mediator structure the resolution process? As part of the exercise, create a resolution plan that contains steps for addressing the issues and resolving the conflict.

own needs and those of the other party. The result is a win-win resolution of their conflict. To reach a mutually beneficial resolution, the parties usually have to identify joint activities that move them past the issues that prevented them from ending their conflict in the past.

If the parties find that their needs are seemingly irreconcilable, the solution may lie in *offering compensation* for not meeting a certain need by bestowing something of equal value. If one party is asking for money that the other party cannot afford to give, it may agree to accept something it views as equally valuable, such as more vacation time. The two parties must engage in clear and creative dialogue to ensure that the substitute is truly viewed and explicitly accepted as equivalent; otherwise, the issue of just compensation will likely arise later and cause problems and further conflict.

The leader-facilitator must look for signs of enough movement and energy to take the parties to the next step—or provide the necessary energy. There is nothing like a small success now and again for *maintaining the momentum*. Once successes begin to occur, they serve to spur the process and move it in ways that nothing else could. The process, energized by the successes already achieved, begins to change the dynamic, the emotions, and the relationship of the two parties without any further intervention. Through good timing and careful pushing, the facilitator can get the parties to work on the more difficult issues in the midst of good momentum, increasing the chance that they will be finally settled.

The inventing stage is when the parties' interaction changes from being oppositional to being collaborative. It is an essential stage on the journey to a resolution, and the techniques of differentiation, expansion, compensation, and momentum all have the potential of increasing the probability that the parties will achieve an end to the conflict.

Action

The final stage is devoted to crafting a plan of action. There is nothing more disheartening than to get through the touchy issues and concerns, establish a strong commitment to pursue possible solutions, build an effective relationship, and then have the process fall apart because an action plan either could not be constructed or was not detailed enough to guide the parties to a final resolution.

As the process progresses toward action, the parties need to reaffirm where they have come from and where they believe they are in relation to their own needs and their interaction with each other. The mutual understanding that results will serve as the ground for the subsequent focus on action. In the action phase, the new questions are what to do, who is to do it, why is it being done, and how to do it.

The first step is to set the agenda for action. What are the priorities of the agreements reached? Where do the parties start? What are the items that must be translated into substantive work, enabling the agreed way of relating and behaving to be realized? These questions serve as the basis for the next level of critical dialogue. Here again patience and attention to detail are required from both parties and from the leader-facilitator.

Setting the agenda includes deciding the priority of actions, their timing, their criticalness, and what other actions must be done in preparation. It also includes reaching an agreement on who is to be accountable for the actions.

New kinds of structures and institutions may have to be constructed as vehicles for implementing the actions. If built early on, they provide a framework for implementing the actions and evaluating their progress. They also help ensure that the issues that are important to the parties are addressed as expected and that any problems or concerns that arise are defined precisely.

Once problems are defined, they need to be solved, which means building problem-solving mechanisms into the implementation process. Unaddressed problems have the potential to negatively impact the relationship between the parties and eliminate the progress made to date.

The parties need to clarify immediate and long-term goals and priorities based on the critical elements identified during the reflexive reframing process (which occurs in the first stage of ARIA). They also need to ensure that the principal, pivotal, and relational items are handled first during the implementation.

The facilitator must try not to upset the delicate balance achieved between the parties. The facilitator's tasks include determining the specific needs each party wants to satisfy as a result of the implementation process and devising an evaluation schedule so that progress can be assessed at critical points. Evaluating the process regularly will help keep the parties on board and ensure the process remains in line with their expectations.

Equally critical is the assignment of accountability for specific outcomes. Who does what should be a practical rather than a political issue, yet at this stage politics often take precedence in a way they never should, typically because the skills, talents, and roles of the participants have not been discussed in advance of the assignment. These must be ascertained before the point of assigning accountability if political machinations are to be kept at a minimum.

Content (goals) must always be placed before process (methods). Once the parties set their goals, however, they need to choose methods for achieving them. In thinking about methods, they need to anticipate potential impediments and select those methods that are most likely to succeed.

The parties should keep in mind that each is going to judge the other by his or her actions, because these actions are the visible evidence of that party's commitment to the agreement. They represent what the one party has done on the other's behalf. The parties'

> **Key Point**
>
> *Conflict resolution is a process with its own timing and techniques. It requires training and experience. Leaders should undertake to develop the necessary skills and practice using them until they are adept at bringing parties in conflict step by step through the process to a sustainable settlement of their differences.*

> **Point To Ponder**
>
> *A conflict resolution facilitator must keep the parties centered by reminding them what is at stake and which issues need to be addressed. The facilitator must also remind the parties of the expectations agreed to so that these can be reaffirmed or altered as the process moves forward.*

actions, therefore, require as much attention as any of the other components of the resolution process.

The leader-facilitator must always keep the parties focused on what is at stake and how important it is. The parties must have the sense that they are a part of an meaningful effort that is larger than their own contributions and that will lead them to a better place.

In any conflict resolution process, no matter whether the conflict is interest or identity based, the leader-facilitator must establish his or her neutrality at the outset. If that cannot be done, the leader-facilitator may consider relinquishing his or her role. A facilitator who is seen as too close to the issue or unable to act in a neutral manner will be more of a hindrance than a help.

The facilitator must be as committed to the process as to the parties. He or she has an important position of trust and is responsible for moving the dynamic in critical ways. If not careful and skillful, the leader-facilitator will cease to be credible to the parties and will lose their confidence, thereby crippling the process and ensuring that further problems will arise.

The facilitator must make it clear at the outset that he or she is working for the whole, not one side or the other, regardless of how he or she got there. Further, the parties must agree to the notion that the facilitator is neutral or the process simply will not progress. If one side or other is paying for the facilitator's services or the facilitator holds a specific role in the organization, accommodation may have to be made at the outset of the process to ensure that the parties trust and support the leader-facilitator equally.

Although identity-based conflicts are the most difficult of all conflicts to deal with, they can be resolved using the processes and mechanisms outlined here. Many of them are allowed to continue because leaders have no idea that these tools even exist and mistakenly try to employ approaches suitable only for interest-based conflicts.

In the current world of health care, the potential for conflict is greater than ever. The various disciplines and work groups are being forced to revise their relationships and their boundaries—or even establish them for the first time. Team-based and continuum-driven approaches to service place a great emphasis on who people are rather than simply what they do. Thus, a vital part of the leadership role in the new age of health care involves working through the differences between professionals and building mutuality as a basis for preventing unnecessary conflict and resolving unavoidable conflict when it arises.

INTEREST-BASED CONFLICT

In dealing with an interest-based conflict, a leader will act essentially as a mediator, a neutral third party who helps the parties resolve their issues and bring closure to the conflict. There is much more negotiation and give and take than in the resolution process for an identity-based conflict. Offers are made and countered as the parties try to work out an agreement consistent with their interests.

The mediator typically undertakes two kinds of intervention, contingent and noncontingent. The noncontingent interventions focus on the processes necessary to any mediation. The contingent interventions are implemented in response to specific circumstances arising from the process itself. Problems, emotions, issues, and other contingencies can individually or collectively have an impact on the mediation process (Figure 3–6), and the mediator occasionally will have to respond by adjusting the process accordingly.

Ten Steps To Resolving an Interest-Based Conflict

The resolution of an interest-based conflict typically includes 10 steps (Figure 3–7). Each step requires a different amount of time and a different approach. By keeping track of each stage of the process, the mediator is able to discipline the parties and keep the process moving steadily in the right direction.

Establishing the Initial Relationship

The mediator's first task is to establish credibility with the parties and introduce them to the process. A conflict resolution process has components and rules that the parties must understand and agree to if the process is to result in a resolution.

Developing Strategies To Guide the Process

Discussing approaches and processes as well as the rules of engagement with the parties up front is a good way to strengthen the relationship between all the participants. In addition, it will help the parties learn about the process and select those activities they determine will best assist them in moving effectively toward resolution.

Constructing the Initial Database

The mediator needs to become familiar with the parties and the issues as soon as possible. Thus, early in the process the mediator should ask the parties about their histories and experiences and also ask them for their insights in order to build a foundation for estab-

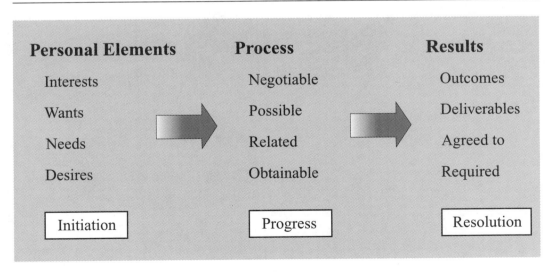

Figure 3–6 The Interest-Based Conflict Resolution Process

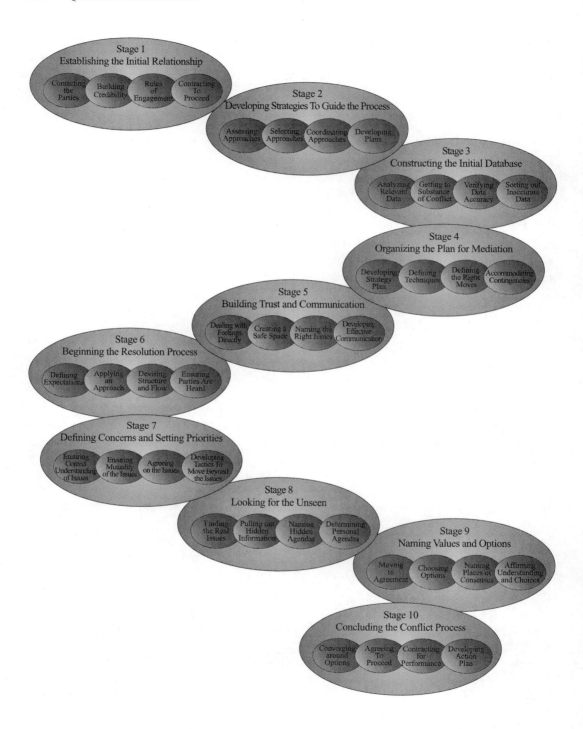

Figure 3–7 The 10 Stages of the Conflict Resolution Process

lishing priorities and deciding on an approach. Verifying the accuracy of the collected information and the central issues of concern is part of the data-gathering process. Following the gathering stage, the participants should spend time reflecting on the content of the conflict and its implications for the resolution approach and process. Here again they get to know each other better. In particular, the mediator obtains a view of the personal processes and behaviors of the parties within the context of the mediation process and can adjust the approach accordingly.

Organizing the Plan for Mediation

In this stage, the mediator considers the approach and structures to use for the mediation. The goal is to develop a plan of approach that fits the situation and the parties, accounting for the contingent factors discernible thus far. The mediator designs the non-contingent structures, considers process elements that could move the parties closer to agreement, and constructs a framework for guiding the process. The plan is simply a plan and is not cast in stone. The participants need to be flexible and adjust the process in response to the inevitable emergence of new information and unexpected factors.

Building Trust and Communication

It is essential to build trust between the parties and to strengthen the parties' trust in the mediator. The challenge is obvious—the parties have entered the mediation process precisely because they are in conflict and have negative feelings toward each other. The mediator's job is to get the parties at least to trust the process enough to get from it what it has to offer. Through exploring the emotional component of their perceptions of each other and of the process, the participants can lay a firm grounding for the subsequent work they will do.

Beginning the Resolution Process

The first stages of the conflict resolution process set up the parties for everything that is to follow. The mediator clearly lays out rules of engagement at the beginning, ensuring that the parties understand what to expect and how to proceed. These rules include guidelines for meeting together and for expressing feelings. The mediator also clarifies the areas of focus and the mechanisms used to proceed and apprises the parties of the opportunities they will have to be heard, have their issues considered, and be included in deliberations. Familiarizing everyone with the structure of the process is essential, for that will increase the participants' flexibility. Flexibility is especially important for the mediator, as he or she must be able respond appropriately to what emerges along the way and take advantage of any opportunity to bring the parties to agreement.

Defining Concerns and Setting Priorities

Here doing one's homework pays off. The mediator, having come to understand the beginning issues, gives the parties an opportunity to explain their individual perceptions and how they formed their related expectations. The mediator also gets agreement from the parties on their understanding of the issues. The participants discuss the substantive points and positions until they are clear to everyone, work out the flow of events, and express their expectations of the methods for dealing with the issues.

Looking for Hidden Information, Agendas, and Interests

The mediator is constantly focused on what the real issues are and on finding clues that could direct the parties toward sustainable solutions. During this stage, many issues, concerns, and problems are likely to emerge, and the mediator must be on the lookout for opportunities to get the parties to work them out. The seeds of solution are to be found in the parties' dialogue. The parties will be engaged in a great amount of detailed work, sometimes together and sometimes apart or one-on-one with the mediator.

Finding Potential Solutions and Determining Their Value to the Parties

As the parties move closer to an agreement, the mediator concentrates on getting them to understand where they appear to be in accord. The mediator's main task is to help the parties work out and state in detail any points of agreement between them, assess the applicability of potential solutions to the issues, determine their acceptability, and do whatever else is necessary to bring closure to the issues. As part of this process, the participants figure out the expected benefits and costs of meeting the obligations of the solutions.

Formalizing the Agreement

Once all the issues in the dispute have been dealt with and the parties understand what they have agreed to and find it acceptable, the mediator and the parties fashion an official agreement that is both clear and acceptable to the parties. Depending on the breadth and complexity of the agreement, different levels of documentation may be necessary. The parties must do whatever they can to make certain that they all have the same understanding of what they have agreed to. In this final stage, the mediator prepares the documentation that formalizes the agreement and forms the foundation for carrying out the solutions. The parties, once they are satisfied there is a mechanism for implementing the agreement, formally accept it.

Keeping the Process on Track

The conflict resolution process outlined above will of course be impacted by the issues, behaviors, personalities, and circumstances of the parties to the conflict. Some of these will be unanticipated and will move the process in directions not initially imagined by the mediator. However, the mediator, by paying attention to the dynamics of dialogue and remaining flexible, will be able to guide the process in a way that will ultimately get the parties to an agreement and/or an end to the conflict.

The mediator uses many techniques to get the parties unstuck and moving toward a workable consensus. Taking the parties aside and working with them individually (commonly called *caucusing*) helps each deal with the issues in a way that is impossible when they are all in the same room. Getting more information, expanding the options, introducing new considerations, moving horizontally on the issues, pressing the parties to consider other factors, and expanding the parties' perceptions, among other strategies, are all part of the mediator's tool chest.

The mediator is always attempting to move the parties toward a negotiated settlement by means of a joint problem-solving process in which the parties work out the solutions themselves. The mediator is not invested in any particular outcome. It is the parties who must be satisfied. They own the issues and the solutions. The mediator is simply providing them with tools and a structure within which the resolution can be more assuredly achieved. The mediator stays neutral, favoring neither party and moving both toward a state of mutual satisfaction.

The mediator is also constantly aware of the need to maintain a balance of power between the parties. In any dispute, issues of power are embedded in the process, and each party is tempted to pursue his or her own advantage to the exclusion of the other party's interests. Aware that jockeying over power is going on, the mediator does everything possible to make sure that the balance of power remains constant so that no party is disadvantaged as a result of the process. The mediator must not become an advocate for one party, nor act in a way that creates a perception of favoritism. The best strategy for dealing with issues of power is to be as public as possible about maintaining a balance, making it clear to the parties that this is a necessary feature of mediation.

> **Key Point**
>
> *Mediating any dispute involves helping the parties remain "unstuck," often a time-consuming task. It is all too easy for the parties to retreat to known territory, pushing for their own advantages and sustaining the polarization that has occurred. The best strategy is to stay focused on the larger picture and on the mutual benefits to be gained from a resolution.*

Conflicts come in all shapes and sizes and levels of complexity, but in any conflict it is the mediator's role to guide people through the process of problem solving and solution seeking who have been unable to get through this process by themselves. Although what this fact entails for the mediator's role is subject to debate, the mediator must recognize that the issues and their solutions belong to the parties. The mediator can bring his or her insights and skills, as well as sophisticated techniques and new concepts, to the process, yet the parties essentially own it. Whatever solutions are chosen will be chosen by the parties and implemented by them. This is not to deny that sometimes the parties might want the mediator to control more of the process or take over responsibilities that properly belong to them, either because they view the responsibilities as too difficult or see the mediator as better placed to handle them.

The mediator must keep in mind that the process lends itself to tricks and stratagems that can slyly or inexplicably change the character or context of the interaction between the parties with such subtlety that it happens unnoticed. To avoid such shifts from occurring, the mediator needs to remain constantly focused on the process and its dynamics, evaluating its viability and efficacy and working to ensure that it is unfolding as it should.

PEOPLE AND BEHAVIOR

In conflict situations, stress levels are high and not everyone is at his or her best. Further, because of the history of conflict and people's general attitude toward it, people in conflict are not disposed to engage in relationship building and problem resolving.

Parties to a conflict generally take the position that someone must win and someone must lose. The role of the mediator is to see that this outcome does not occur. It should be clear that only a mutually satisfying solution is likely to end the conflict permanently.

In the effort to "win," either party might try one or more tactics to unbalance the situation. The mediator needs to be on the lookout for these tactics and counter them through good techniques and a good process. In addition, the mediator needs to be aware of other factors that often influence the outcome of a conflict resolution process. Several of these are discussed below.

Communication Technique

The mediator must always be listening. And not just listening but listening actively, which means continually restating points in a way that is understandable to all the parties and gets the issues out in the open. Almost any conflict is rife with emotional energy, and the mediator must manage and diffuse as much of it as possible through being clear and understandable and by translating every nuance and every embedded message into a explicit assertion. The parties are more likely to come to an agreement if they fully comprehend all the issues and each other's positions.

The Meeting Setting and Schedule

The meeting place should be comfortable and not favor one of the two parties. The room should exhibit balance, the table should be round instead of rectangular, the seating arrangement should be comfortable and informal, and the lighting should be conducive to dialogue and therefore not bright or irritating. It is important to schedule the meetings at a time of the day when the parties are alert and invested instead of tired and worn out. By being sensitive to the possible influence of the environment on the resolution process, the mediator can ensure the meeting place is pleasing and congenial and supports the process rather than works against it.

Demeanor

Mediators come from all kinds of backgrounds and have all kinds of personalities. Personality is always a consideration in mediation, and there must be a good fit between the mediator and the parties. If there is not a good fit, the mediator will have difficulty moving the process forward, possibly to such an extent that the process comes to a dead halt. The mediator must exhibit confidence and competence and present him- or herself as someone the parties can depend on in the times of challenge. The mediator is responsible for the process and its culture and dynamics, and by showing a proper demeanor and gaining the respect of the parties, the mediator can do much to create a suitable culture and stimulate movement toward resolution.

Information Exchange

During a conflict resolution process, lots of information gets laid out. The mediator must facilitate the transmission of correct information. The more accurate the information exchanged between the parties, the more likely the process will move along smoothly. There is always a danger of having more information than is necessary for good decision making. Having lots of information is not the same as having the right information. The mediator tries to ensure the parties have the information they need and can differentiate between desired data and needed data (needed data are data they can use to fashion an agreement).

The Use of Experts

The mediator tries to provide the parties with access to whatever will help them resolve their conflict. Because no mediator could be an expert in all the elements and processes associated with every kind of conflict, others may need to be involved in the process. There are no rules limiting access to what or who is needed to resolve issues. Planning for and scheduling the use of experts or other resources and determining the focus of their use are among the critical responsibilities of the mediator.

CONCLUSION

Resolving conflicts is a fundamental part of managing human relationships. All relationships have the potential for conflict embedded deep within them, especially in our increasingly diverse health care system, where professionals with widely different backgrounds and roles are now required to work together. As they sort through their unique contributions, they will face many opportunities for conflict and are almost guaranteed to fall into disputes and disagreements. Health care leaders are responsible for supervising the relationships between the disciplines, and as the roles of the disciplines change and their relationships become more complex, the leaders will have the critical task of helping all who work in the health field to respond to the changes and build stronger, more positive relationships.

The kind of intense interdisciplinary interaction characteristic of continuum-based teams is new to health care. Historically, there were only a very few types of professionals, and each type performed a wide variety of tasks. With the advances in technology that have occurred, more types of professionals exist, but the activities of each type are more narrowly focused. As a consequence, more people will be negotiating the clinical practice landscape, and, to complicate matters, these people will have more divergent roles and views. Working through their differences to find common ground will be essential to creating a more aligned and integrated health care system. Leaders have an important role to play in bringing this kind of system into existence by assisting others in solving problems and resolving conflicts.

Dealing with conflict is a normal part of the leadership role as it currently exists, and therefore leaders must understand the basic elements and learn the essential skills of conflict management. Like any skills, these will require development. Leaders must recognize this and persevere in their learning efforts. The payoff is that these skills will serve any leader well in dealing with the increasingly complex set of relationships in the delivery of health services. To the extent that a leader develops the necessary skills and takes on the role of conflict resolution facilitator, he or she will strengthen the relationships between health professionals and, most importantly, increase the effectiveness of health care.

REFERENCE

Rothman, J. 1997. *Resolving identity-based conflict*. San Francisco: Jossey-Bass.

SUGGESTED READINGS

Costantino, C., and C. Merchant. 1998. *Designing conflict management systems*. San Francisco: Jossey-Bass.

Kalb, D. 1997. *When talk works*. San Francisco: Jossey-Bass.

Levine, S. 1998. *Getting to resolution*. San Francisco: Berrett-Koehler.

Slaikeu, K. 1995. *When push comes to shove*. San Francisco: Jossey-Bass.

Slaikeu, K., and R. Hasson. 1999. *Controlling the cost of conflict*. San Francisco: Jossey-Bass.

Zemke, R., C. Raines, and B. Filipczak. 2000. *Generations at work: Managing the clash of veterans, Boomers, Xers, and Nexters in your workplace*. Chicago: AMACOM.

Quiz Questions

Select the best answer for each of the following questions.

1. Conflict in everyday relationships is:
   a. to be avoided
   b. unacceptable
   c. normal
   d. destructive

2. Conflict resolution facilitators must recognize the value of:
   a. uniformity
   b. diversity
   c. anxiety
   d. humanity

3. Conflict is destructive only if it:
   a. is not resolved
   b. is accompanied by anger
   c. is secretive
   d. becomes physical

4. The perceived imbalance of power can lead to conflict. To mitigate its potential for mischief, power should be:
   a. viewed as a necessary evil
   b. placed in the hands of managers
   c. placed in the hands of staff
   d. distributed equitably across the organization

5. Two parties in conflict generally know:
   a. each other's position
   b. why they are angry
   c. what they want
   d. what they dislike

6. The difference between interest-based conflict and identity-based conflict is that:

a. interest-based conflict concerns how the parties view themselves
b. identity-based conflict concerns how the parties view themselves
c. identity-based conflict involves tangible issues
d. interest-based conflict is harder to resolve

7. The primary role of a conflict resolution facilitator is to:

a. bring the conflict to a sustainable end
b. establish a good resolution process
c. keep the parties moving through the process
d. help both parties get what they want

8. A conflict resolution facilitator must never:

a. take sides
b. stop the process
c. get angry
d. interject personal insights

9. To reach a successful completion of the 10-step conflict resolution process, the mediator should ensure that:

a. the interaction between the parties is friendly and their dialogue is courteous
b. the parties use effective techniques for communicating and exchanging information
c. the parties always meet with the mediator together, never one on one
d. the parties receive all the information the mediator is able to acquire

10. The attribution by each party of negative motives and qualities to the other party usually indicates that the parties:

a. hold fluid positions
b. have an accurate understanding of each other's positions
c. do not fully understand the issues at the root of the conflict
d. want to avoid dealing with the real issues

CHAPTER 4

Living Leadership:
Vulnerability, Risk Taking, and Stretching

Take comfort in the notion that we have never been in control!
—Anonymous

Evolved people respect differing views, understanding that life's
meaning is to be found everywhere. They are open, always learning and growing. An evolved person knows that there is only one
truth, but many different ways of seeing it.
—Lance Secretan

Chapter Objectives

At the completion of this chapter, the reader will be able to

- Understand vulnerability as a positive leadership trait.
- Identify four essential relationship skills that support vulnerable leadership.
- Discuss the process of complexity communication.
- Evaluate open communication as a means of improving leadership expertise.
- Critique vulnerable leadership as a moral imperative.

Leaders of postmillennium quantum organizations must be able to use resources effectively
in an environment in which control and direction are lacking. They must grow comfortable
with the idea that uncertainty is the norm and that they can never know everything there is to
know. They must be willing to take risks, recognize that their colleagues come from a wide
range of backgrounds, and realize that they will never obtain a complete picture, no matter
how good their communication with others. Finally, they must use new strategies based on
vulnerability principles if they are to succeed in designing a health care system that works.

In the Industrial Age, leaders were expected to be in control. Whether chief executive officers or case managers, they were viewed as being in charge and in possession of the information that consumers and employees wanted and needed. According to the classical theories of management, good leaders knew everything and could do everything better than anyone else. They held all of the information necessary for operating the organization and shared this information with the employees only when it was appropriate.

Now, things are much different. Information is currently available to the masses and in great quantities, minimizing any leader's potential for being in control of anything! Furthermore, all leaders have limitations—strengths and weaknesses—and as they move through the chaos of the transition into the Age of Technology, they typically experience feelings of defenselessness, helplessness, and inadequacy. The fact is, in order to act with vigor in this time of great uncertainty, they need to replace their old skills with new ones.

LEADERSHIP FITNESS IN THE NEW MILLENNIUM

The leadership fitness profile is very different from in the past, when the leadership role was basically one of command and control. In the new millennium, leaders find themselves in an environment of great uncertainty, and in order to navigate in this environment, they need to be comfortable with taking risks, being vulnerable, and stretching the boundaries of current thinking and current practices. They also need to be able to coach employees to develop the same performance characteristics. Engaging the staff to work collectively to interpret the events of change in a way that makes sense of them is essential for success.

Vulnerability, risk taking, and stretching are required for several reasons. First, the present is very different from the past, and the skills that will be needed in the coming age, the Age of Technology, are very different from those needed in the Industrial Age. Past practices of bureaucratic command and control cannot be assumed to be effective in a new environment in which the distribution of knowledge has been radically altered and the skills needed to manage the environment are undeveloped. The quantum leader, besides exemplifying the spirit of incompleteness, must shift from managing content to guiding process and outcome over and over again until order finally emerges.

In addition, the leaders of the various health care professions need to maintain a focus on creating a new framework for each profession, a framework that will allow them to understand and manage the future rather than sustain the past. As part of this process, they need to scrutinize the relationships between the professions, examine the specific services provided by each profession, and assess the value of these services in the marketplace. The services that add value will be retained and those that do not will be eliminated.

> **Point To Ponder**
>
> *The paradox of our time in history is that we have taller buildings, but shorter tempers; wider freeways, but narrower viewpoints.*
>
> —George Carlin

> ### Group Discussion
>
> Compare the behaviors of classical management and those of vulnerability leadership. Examine the practices of coaching, facilitating teams, building relationships, and empowering others in each model.

VULNERABILITY

In the Industrial Age, vulnerability in a leader was seen as a weakness. Indeed, the word *vulnerability* tends to conjure up the idea of susceptibility to physical or emotional injury or to corrupt influence. This type of vulnerability is very different from the type required of leaders in the Age of Technology. The essence of vulnerability, as the term is used in this book, is openness to others and to new ideas (Exhibit 4–1). It encompasses being able to

- examine long-held beliefs and change one's mind without feelings of inadequacy
- recognize personal limitations and strengths
- work from a clearly defined personal identity

Vulnerable leaders know and show their limits, whether these pertain to knowledge or abilities. Rather than work beyond their limits, they allow people with the right kind of aptitude to assume responsibility for particular tasks. According to their mindset, their role is to create the conditions that will allow employees to make their maximum contribution and simultaneously enjoy their work.

Leadership vulnerability is not about weakness or incompetence. Team members and colleagues do not want leaders to be weak, ailing, or whining. They look for strength and self-confidence, but the kind of self-confidence that permits someone to admit his or her limitations and not maintain a stance of immunity to anxiety, fatigue, or doubt. Leadership vulnerability is also about creating conditions that encourage safe and healthy dialogue as the way to do business.

In contrast, leaders who act out of a sense of invulnerability tend to be aloof, separate themselves from those they lead, and avoid making time for the meaningful discussion of

---

Exhibit 4–1 Leadership Vulnerability

Facilitators	Barriers
• Openness to new ideas	• Aloofness, arrogance
• Recognition of personal limitations	• Strong ego
• Feelings of adequacy	• Fear of losing control
• Self-awareness of strengths and weaknesses	• Fear of discovery
• Absence of ego	• Believed immunity to anxiety, fatigue, illness, and overwork
• Trust in others	

complex issues. Their purpose in behaving in this manner is to keep control over situations and to abstain from dialogue that might lead to the revision of their chosen courses of action. Charisma, too, is suspect. A leader who exhibits charisma is almost always partly covering up a lack of substance. Further, charisma tends to lead to arrogance if the leader is successful and to paranoia if not.

The traits and behaviors associated with invulnerability play a big role in protecting the leadership ego. Traditionally, leaders have feared not just losing control but also being found out. They have worried that others would discover that they are not what they seem to be, that they do not have all of the answers to all of the questions. Quantum leadership, on the other hand, is about the absence of ego. Quantum leaders seek exposure of their limitations as a means to improve organizational performance. According to Torbert (2000), vulnerability is paradoxically powerful. When power is exercised by a leader who remains vulnerable or open to transformation, the result will be voluntary transformation in others rather than mere external conformity and compliance (or resistance). In addition, there is no point in fearing discovery or losing control, because in reality no one ever is in control!

> **Key Point**
>
> *Quantum leadership is about the absence of ego, not its presence.*

Relationships in a quantum organization are based on three principles:

1. Power is a pluralist, not an elitist, commodity.
2. Diversity is valuable.
3. Personal boundaries must be clearly defined.

These principles provide the framework for developing new and more effective relationships.

POWER

The notion of power has both positive and negative connotations and often produces feelings of ambivalence. Further, because power is associated with the conflicting ideas of strength, influence, coercion, and dominance, it is difficult both to understand and to use. Yet, as we move into the Age of Technology, leaders must be able to comprehend the nature of power and make use of it in their relationships.

> **Point To Ponder**
>
> *Knowledge really is power. Intellect is a gift, but learning is hard work.*

First, quantum leaders consider the quantity of power to be infinite and thus conclude that sufficient power is generally available for all individuals to exert influence, mobilize resources, and meet their goals. They view power as located in each person, not centralized in an elite group, and they treat the legitimate exercise of power as a right that belongs to everyone.

In a traditional organization, power is concentrated at the top of the hierarchical pyramid, and work is compartmentalized and controlled from that central point. The organizational power structure always benefits some at the expense of others, and, if anything, revisions of the structure tend to enhance the power of those who have it. In other words, leaders seldom design themselves out of a position.

> ### Group Discussion
>
> Consider power from both an elitist perspective and a pluralist perspective. How is power perceived in your organization? In your department? Describe the power behaviors that occur in your organization as a whole and in your department. Identify at least two opportunities to shift power behaviors from elitist to pluralist.

In a quantum organization, the response to centralization is not decentralization but *uncentralization*. Uncentralization, unlike decentralization, does not attempt to preserve hierarchical workways by subdividing and parceling out the work while hanging onto central control through the use of more and more creative accounting systems. The new organizational structure is fluid and flexible, allowing easy rearrangement of work groups to meet point-of-service needs.

To be sure, there are still distinctions between organizations. In some, the style of leadership is looser and more collegial; in others, recommendations mostly go up and orders mostly come down. The intent, however, is the same—to minimize bureaucratic control and the concentration of power and to maximize involvement while still getting the work done.

The point is not to create "nobody in charge" systems. Yet, regardless of how the leadership power transition occurs, some leaders will experience real or perceived threats to their power, and their instinct for self-preservation may override their concern for organizational goals.

In many cases, employees who have high expectations will be quickly disillusioned by the leaders' perceived failure to meet their expectations. In fact, traditional employees will discourage leaders from becoming vulnerable. This means that leaders not only must change their own mindset but must create the

> ### Point To Ponder
>
> *What no Greek political theorist imagined or people's revolutionary accomplished—a devolution (or transfer) of real power to hundreds of thousands of people—is coming to pass as the social consequence of modern science and technology. We have our aristocracy, but it is increasingly an aristocracy of achievement. By common consent we no longer entrust the setting of styles to any one class, any one race, any one priesthood or courthouse gang—or even to the White House staff. . . . The complexity of organizations is diffusing the opportunity to lead and multiplying the requirements for leaders.*
>
> —Harlan Cleveland

conditions for employees to adapt to the new culture. As the necessary changes proceed, the resulting battles for survival are likely to cause organizational confusion and even chaos.

THE CYCLE OF VULNERABILITY

Learning to live and thrive in vulnerability is a lifelong journey. It is often a circuitous journey, reversing on itself and then moving forward. For the purposes of discussion, learning to live and thrive in vulnerability is presented as a cyclical process (Exhibit 4–2 and Figure 4–1). The six steps of this cycle are as follows:

1. becoming vulnerable
2. taking risks
3. stretching one's capacity
4. living the new reality
5. evaluating the results
6. cherishing the new knowledge gained

Becoming Vulnerable

The first step in the cycle involves recognizing the value of being vulnerable. You need only enroll in a computer class with a teenager to discover the value of vulnerability—the value of being open to receiving new ideas about how to use a computer. By admitting you are uncertain and not all-knowing, by being willing to put aside longstanding mental models, you open yourself to the possibility of incredible growth and rewards.

Frustration and fear typically fuel the search for certainty, a search that wastes significant time and effort. In any organization, situations and relationships are usually too complex to be predictable, and therefore a degree of uncertainty is avoidable. If fear of the unknown is allowed to rule, the result will be organizational inertia and continued reliance on past practices. Despite believing in the need for change or in the savings to be gained from a new technology, leaders will place too much emphasis on the failure of past innovations and will sit back and do nothing.

Employees as well as leaders long for certainty. Formerly, securing a position in an organization meant getting employment for a lifetime. This is no longer true. As organiza-

---

Exhibit 4–2 The Six Stages of the Cycle of Vulnerability

1. Become vulnerable and open to new ideas. Recognize and value uncertainty.
2. Choose to take risks that challenge the status quo.
3. Stretch organizational capacity by stimulating the latent potential of employees.
4. Live the new capacity.
5. Evaluate the outcomes.
6. Cherish the resulting new knowledge.

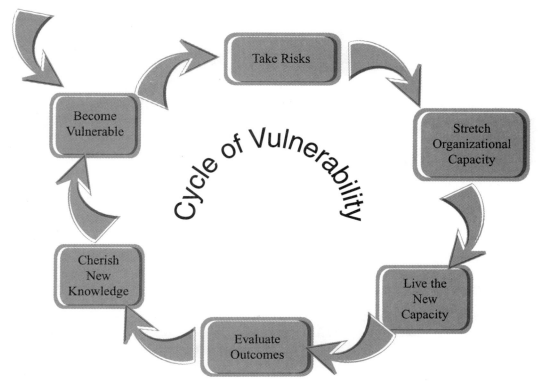

Figure 4–1 The Cycle of Vulnerability

tions face more challenges than ever before, employees face more uncertainty, particularly about the security of their jobs. As a consequence, they experience additional stress as well as feelings of isolation. In struggling to find a new vision, they become frustrated and often panic. What they should do instead is learn to tolerate and respect the discomfort of their uncertainty and thereby unleash their creativity in the interests of organizational change.

Quantum leaders need to give up the quest for certainty and discover the benefits of admitting fallibility. One benefit is that leaders can expend their efforts in designing the future rather than become petrified by feelings of panic and loss of control. After all, leaders never have possessed a crystal ball capable of predicting the future. Leadership judgment is called judgment because certainty is missing. Besides judgment, what leaders can use is creativity. To do this, though,

> **Point To Ponder**
>
> *Traveling naked into the land of uncertainty allows for another kind of learning, a learning that helps us forget what we know and discover what we need. It is this journey that leads to the discovery of what is needed to help us create the future.*
> —*Robert E. Quinn*

they need time for thinking, for designing the future. Unfortunately, many leaders deny they have any extra time. Most believe that they are working at their highest level of productivity and are unable to fit in additional work, especially if it is merely inventive headwork.

> **Key Point**
>
> *Leadership judgment is called judgment because certainty is missing.*

The reality is that their organizations will suffer severely unless they make the time to engage in creative thinking. In some cases, new employees will have the extra time and energy to explore possible innovations and reforms. More often, the necessary time can be found by examining current work from a value perspective and eliminating particular tasks that fail to add value (i.e., that fail to make a difference in patient care). The time formerly spent on these fruitless tasks can then be used to think creatively and work toward constructing a vision of the future.

Taking Risks

The second step requires leaders to begin to take risks. Much like vulnerability, risk taking is not viewed as a classical leadership behavior and is rarely welcomed or encouraged. Instead, it is seen as increasing the organization's exposure to unforeseen hazards and to the loss of net income.

Classical leadership behavior encompasses strategic planning and the purposeful review of ideas. With the recent advances in information technology, these processes are becoming increasingly outdated. New approaches, such as the "tinkering" described by Abrahamson (2000), a management professor at Columbia Business School, will become the norm.

Tinkering, in fact, is a good way to learn how to take risks, for it involves making small changes to reconfigure existing practices and business models rather than create new ones. A little tinkering and a lot of expertise allow small groups of providers to make changes with big goals in mind and to evaluate the changes efficiently. In addition, the providers' skills are stretched with little risk to the organization. Support for constant tinkering minimizes the chance that the organization will drift into inertia. Risk becomes the norm, change is internalized as essential for survival, and employees gain new experiences and develop new skills.

Embedded in tinkering processes is the expectation that leaders will routinely challenge the status quo—indeed, seriously challenge it, which means not asking questions out of idle curiosity but looking carefully at current dogma and raising issues that open the door to substantial improvements. For quantum leaders, examining the work of their organizations is not a meaningless exercise but is intended to guarantee accountability and make certain that all of the work is value producing. Asking the unaskable questions about structure, principles, and customs requires a comfortableness with vulnerability and an openness to and passion for new realities (Exhibit 4–3).

When leaders ask the unaskable, they are ostensibly inviting employees to mention the unmentionable, which the employees can perceive as very risky, especially when the leaders' body language says, "Do not raise difficult issues." Brusque or otherwise unwelcom-

Exhibit 4–3 Risk Taking

• Encourages creativity	• Requires resiliency
• Supports "tinkering"	• Is avoided by most leaders
• Requires continuous evaluation	• Is inconsistent with classical leadership
• Allows for mistakes	behaviors
• Requires vulnerability	

ing behavior must be replaced with genuine openness so that the employees feel safe and the inquiry into problems can be fruitful and lead to growth. Although decisions made under conditions of incomplete information sometimes fail to have a positive outcome, leaders must be willing to risk changing course if there are good reasons to do so. No one knows the future for certain, as shown by the many mispredictions perpetrated by supposed experts. (Perhaps none is more famous than the implicit prediction regarding the future course of movies that was contained in the question asked by Warner Brothers in 1927: Who the heck wants to hear actors talk?)

Group Discussion

Harlan Cleveland (1972) in *The Future Executive* notes that "planning cannot be done by a few leaders, or even by the brightest whiz-kids immured in a systems analysis unit or a planning staff. Real-life planning is the dynamic improvisation by the many on a general sense of direction. The sense of direction is announced by a few . . . but only after genuine consultation with those who will have to improvise on it." Do you agree with Cleveland? Review the current strategic planning processes in your organization, then challenge the status quo by modifying them. What is the rationale for your recommendations? List the advantages and disadvantages of the suggested revisions.

Some risky decisions have paid off well. Consider the cash register, which was introduced in the late 19th century by Patterson as a help in cash management and as a means of double-checking the honesty of sales clerks. Patterson took an incredible risk in challenging the status quo, and indeed at first everybody resented the product. Owners, for example, refused to have this "thief catcher" in their stores. Patterson had to use great leadership skills to convince others to accept his idea and motivate his sales force to sell the product. Today, of course, no store is without one.

The role of the leader is to inspire creativity and hard work and to challenge the past as prologue, recognizing that the past is past. The work of inspiration requires not just inspirational *phrases* but inspirational *behavior.* Risk-disposed leaders motivate others by showing what can be done, not merely by sermonizing about opportunities. They also need to exhibit candor and vulnerability, be able to identify value in marginally successful efforts, and be willing to allow others to take risks and experience success and failure.

Risk-disposed leaders develop a very high level of self-discipline that allows the processes of risk to evolve. A strong sense of commitment can be more valuable than intelligence, education, luck, or talent. Leaders adept at taking risks neither surrender nor overreact to crises or marginally successful efforts; they regroup and return. They take stock of the situation, often pulling back temporarily (but not too long) while they plan the next steps. They realize that sometimes it is best to put aside personal feelings and let bygones be bygones. Finally, they focus on the present and the future, both of which offer perils and possibilities, rather than on the past, about which nothing can be done.

Resiliency is the key. Leaders must be resilient in order to manage the uncertainty and inherent risks that are features of the leadership role. They must act with confidence, purpose, and enthusiasm rather than hesitation and self-doubt. To manage risks through resiliency, they must apply determination and energy, inspiring those around them at the same time.

Stretching One's Capacity

In the third step of the vulnerability cycle, the leader of an organization works to stretch the organization's capacity. In doing this, the leader looks for new and untapped potential. Typically, this potential lies mostly within the organization. For example, new employees as well as old employees in continuing education programs represent two main sources of serviceable potential.

In spite of the chaos and uncertainty in organizational operations, quantum leaders learn to mitigate and overcome their reluctance to implement new processes in the face of perceived dangers, including the threat of failure. This is not to say that the dangers are not real. Yet there are also serious dangers that arise when an organization fails to adapt to the changes in its environment or undergoes unmanaged change.

Risking serves to stretch the organization's capacity. Indeed, overcoming risks by making use of the potential of the members of the organization should become the new golden rule. Once everyone in the organization sees the emperor has no clothes, the best strategy is to put new ideas out into the open and begin to design new services and products once thought unattainable. By sharing the uncertainty, leaders can increase the level of trust in the organization and strengthen the social connections, thereby raising the levels of reciprocity, information flow, collective action, happiness, and wealth.

Kellner-Rogers (1999) states that a complex web of relationships and meaning-making characterizes all living systems, including organizations, gangs, families, and political movements. This web is not describable using neat organizational charts or flow diagrams. Even more importantly, it cannot be used to predict outcomes. The relationships that make up a living system display an incredible capacity for engaging in sophisticated, coordinated behaviors. These behaviors, however, are seldom the result of directive leadership, strategic plans, or engineered solutions but instead usually occur when the conditions that support risking and creative stretching are present. In short, they emerge to the degree that the members of the organization are open, vulnerable, and willing to take risks.

Capra (1982) has described the emergence of coordinated behaviors using the analogy of chemical combination. Sugar is made up of three atoms: oxygen, hydrogen, and carbon. Where is the sweetness? The sweetness is in the relationship between the atoms. It is not a quality of any of them individually but emerges in the molecule as a whole. Likewise, when vulnerability, risking, and stretching enrich the communal capacity of an organization, out of the relationships of the members tend to emerge behaviors that produce positive results, although not always.

Group Discussion

As described in the text, at the end of the 19th century, a common orchard was used to graze livestock by everyone in a small Midwestern village. Because the feed was free, everyone felt the temptation to add animals to their herd. Eventually, after a rapid increase in the total number of livestock, the grass became depleted, the trees died, the livestock starved, and the villagers went bankrupt. Obviously, new rules were needed. Who should create the new rules for use of the orchard? What strategies would you recommend to correct the situation and make the village prosperous again? How should the strategies be evaluated? What is the relevance of this case history to the role of leadership in the transition from the Industrial Age to the Information Age? Identify at least two scenarios in your organization that bear some resemblance to the case history and critique how the main issues were managed.

In fact, less than optimal results often lead to a new and better order, as shown by the following story. In a Midwestern village at the end of the 19th century, a common orchard was used by all of the villagers to feed their livestock. Over time the villagers, despite working diligently, went bankrupt and even faced starvation. What happened? Each villager thought, "The more livestock I have, the better off I will be. The feeding is free, so I will increase my herd as fast as I can." The number of livestock grazing in the orchard increased so rapidly, however, that the grass was soon depleted and the trees died. The livestock began to starve and the village faced destruction. The main problem was that the villagers all engaged in the same behavior without awareness of their interdependence and of the impact of their behavior on the village as a whole. It was by experiencing the dire outcome of their actions that the villagers were able to recognize their interdependence and gain the power to reverse the course of events.

Living the New Reality

The fourth step is living the new reality. Living the new reality is about trial and error, about learning what works and what does not work. Once a new path has been identified, the leader, along with the team members, supports the unfolding of additional capacity (new work processes or services). Ideas become reality by being applied by the organization on a trial basis. For the organizational leader, living the new reality involves

- allowing the new work processes (or services) to become integrated into the system
- determining the fit between the processes and the stakeholders (patients, employees, and the entire organization)
- accepting that unanticipated outcomes will occur, both positive and negative
- coaching others to sustain the new knowledge
- encouraging vulnerable behaviors
- leading the way to a state of mutual trust

During this phase of the cycle, the leader and team might easily lose sight of its purpose. The tendency is for them to become so anxious and pressured for success that they do not always examine the new processes carefully enough to determine the full range of their effects. The goal here is not to ensure the success of the new processes but to allow them to become integrated into the system in order to evaluate their goodness of fit (i.e., their advantages and disadvantages for the organization, the employees, and the patients).

The leader and the team must allow the new work processes to unfold, to live and breathe, rather than expect perfection immediately. The leader and the team must carefully examine the processes from all perspectives, looking for opportunities for improvement. Timely evaluations become the norm. What the leader and the team should not do is implement the new processes as if they were permanent and fully refined, hoping that no rework is necessary and that no additional costs will be incurred.

Evaluating the Results

In the fifth step, the results of implementing the new work processes or services are evaluated. Mechanistic principles of thought presuppose linear cause-and-effect relationships. Given the nature of health care organizations, such principles are inappropriate for evaluating work processes and must be replaced by nonlinear evaluation models for two reasons. First, the increasing complexity of work in the Age of Technology minimizes the number of simple cause-and-effect relationships. Second, living systems, especially systems that encompass human beings and their behavior, cannot be understood mechanistically.

Because of the complexity of organizations, the assessment of processes and outcomes requires the use of multiple indicators and a nonlinear evaluation model, such as the Performance Measurement Matrix. This model accommodates different data levels and data measures and traditional performance measures while taking into account the limitations of cost-benefit analysis. It examines nine categories of data that represent quality, productivity, and cost measures (Exhibit 4–4).

The Performance Measurement Matrix provides a framework for assessing the impact of selected indicators on organizational performance and can help minimize the tendency to make a decision on the basis of one positive indicator. In some situations, for instance, it might show that a course of action, despite increasing the organization's net income in the short term, will negatively impact all the other eight indicators, including customer and

Exhibit 4–4 Performance Measurement Matrix

	Quality Indicator	**Productivity**	**Cost**
Customer	Satisfaction	Service time/event	Unit cost of service/product
Employee	Satisfaction	Turnover	Cost of labor and benefits
Organization	Reputation	Net income margin	Administrative cost of overhead/ all costs

Source: Reprinted from K. Malloch, The Performance Measurement Matrix: A Framework To Optimize Decision Making, *Journal of Nursing Care Quality,* Vol. 13, no. 3, pp. 1–12, © 1999, Aspen Publishers, Inc.

employee satisfaction and the organization's reputation, in both the short and long term. The matrix can also be used to compare two or more options and their overall impact on the organization.

Group Discussion

Suppose your organization is exploring which of two possible employee retention programs to implement. One applies to all employees, whereas the other applies only to nurses, who have an especially low retention rate. The same amount of funding is available for each program. Select indicators for the nine dimensions of the Performance Measurement Matrix to evaluate each program, then identify the potential positive and negative effects of each on the organization. Which program offers the greatest benefit to the organization? Explore other scenarios in which the Performance Measurement Matrix could be applied.

Whether the matrix is used or not, the goal of this stage of the vulnerability cycle is to

- measure multiple process and outcome indicators
- evaluate the quality, productivity, and cost of the new work processes
- avoid cause-and-effect assumptions

Cherishing the New Knowledge Gained

The goal of the final step of the vulnerability cycle is to cherish and make use of the knowledge gained by going through the entire cycle. Each time a risk is taken, an outcome occurs—an outcome that may not have been anticipated. Consider the two following scenarios. In scenario A, an organization implemented a new work assignment process based on the recommendation of the staff employees. The project was more successful than anticipated. Not only were the original goals accomplished, but the professional behaviors of the employees improved and their job satisfaction levels increased (owing to their involve-

---

Group Discussion

The six steps in the cycle of vulnerability present leaders with different levels of challenge. Consider two recent projects that were implemented in your organization, one believed to be a success and the other not. Using the cycle of vulnerability, determine for each project at which stage the implementation processes were most successful and at which stage interventions would have been especially helpful.

---

ment). In scenario B, the management team selected a reputable work management system without input from the employees. The employees did not support the system, and the costs for additional education and monitoring were much greater than anticipated. Employee satisfaction declined. Both projects were well thought out, and positive results were anticipated in both scenarios. In scenario A, the new process was retained. In scenario B, the project was discontinued or modified in step 5 (evaluation), but the knowledge that the style of implementation used was ineffective will be retained and applied when future projects are developed.

At the end of the vulnerability cycle, the challenge is to identify what was valuable and what was problematic. Repeating positive efforts is as important as avoiding negative results. Although sometimes it is easy to see the value of implementing new processes or services, at other times it is difficult to discern anything more than that the implementation was not effective at this time and place. Nonetheless, leaders should always document both the positive and negative results and try to view the implementation as a lesson in the value of vulnerability.

Point To Ponder

Preparing an environment that will nourish creativity is, in itself, a creative activity. Spontaneity, dynamism, fun, humor, freedom from fear of failure, incentives, sympathetic values and culture, a soulspace, and celebration are just a few of the essential ingredients of a creative culture. Leaders who seek to liberate the soul through creativity must establish a sanctuary in which failure is not punished but valued as a learning experience.

—Lance Secretan

Coaching and mentoring employees in the development of vulnerable, risk-taking behaviors is the logical next step. To guide employees toward these behaviors, a leader must first establish a culture of trust. The leader and employees must then discuss the value of risk taking and its potential impact on organizational productivity and morale. The coaching process—in which leader and the employees learn together rather than alone—becomes transforming for everyone and for the organization as a whole. Guiding each other to become more vulnerable requires attention to both the content of the situation and the new relationships that emerge once the culture supports vulnerable behaviors.

> **Group Discussion**
>
> Imagine you are a leader coaching employees in the acquisition of vulnerability behaviors. Develop a coaching outline that (1) describes the components of the vulnerability cycle, (2) provides examples of the relationships that emerge in a vulnerability culture, and (3) presents three strategies to sustain vulnerability behaviors.

Quantum leaders must develop patience to wait for the vulnerability cycle process to emerge, learn to trust in the value of fostering a vulnerability culture, and maintain their confidence in the inevitability of progress. Mutual trust evolves when the leader and employees experience the positive realities of the vulnerability cycle and when employees are valued for their efforts as well as the results of their efforts.

In addition, leaders need to guide employees toward new behaviors rather than direct their work. Guiding is not about judging but about recognizing new behaviors when they occur and inviting the employees to offer feedback on their performance and perceptions of success. It is also about maintaining composure and showing tolerance, as vulnerable behaviors and risk taking are learned slowly and employees who have not yet acquired the necessary skills will be able to only partially finish new behaviors. Finally, it is about communicating well and developing and sustaining the kind of relationships that support new behaviors.

NEW RELATIONSHIPS

Although much attention has been given to the differences between the emerging Information Age (or Age of Technology) and the Industrial Age, the fact is that successful leaders in all periods of history have valued information and knowledge. Being timely and well informed has allowed leaders to craft effective solutions to problems and take full advantage of opportunities. Seldom do leaders rely on secondhand or outdated information. Instead, they develop networks of reliable sources to provide them with steady streams of current information. Indeed, their relationships with information sources in the organization and the community will take on ever greater significance as the availability of information increases.

Noted leadership expert Kouzes (2000) holds the view that, for leaders, social capital will be as important as intellectual capital, if not more important. After all, leadership is about relationships. Whom people know and what they can do for each other facilitates the work of the organization. This is not to say that brains or intellectual capital are not important, especially in the Information Age, but knowing is different from doing and does not necessarily translate into action. Making something happen requires having information *and* having good relationships. Furthermore, with the opening of the floodgates of new communication pathways, relationships are even more complex than previously. Removing the traditional hierarchies of communication brings new obligations, such as the need to value diversity and personal privacy and to respect boundary setting and self-disclosure (Figure 4–2).

Valuing Diversity

People differ in more than gender, race, and ethnic background. People grow up in different geographic locations, speak different languages, practice different religions, and belong to different generations. In addition, people think and act differently. Some think quickly, some slowly, some are analytic, others are creative, some are detail oriented, some prefer the big picture, some want facts, some depend on intuition, some are outgoing, some are reserved—and the list goes on. Given these differences, it is a wonder that we can relate to each other at all. Yet the diverse reality of our universe requires that we maximize our efforts to form relationships, despite the prejudices that unfortunately form because of our

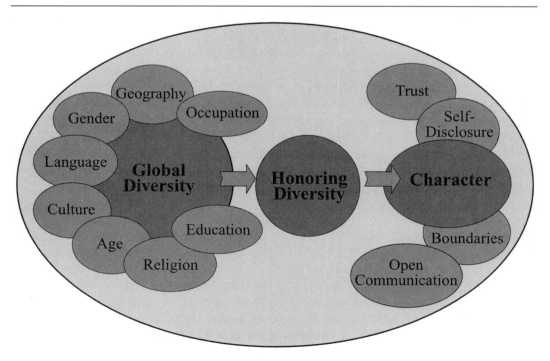

Figure 4–2 Relationships in the Information Age

differences. Labeling individuals who differ from us and profiling their behaviors may make it easier for us to function at times, but because they create irrational biases, they often prevent people from forming meaningful relationships or fracture the relationships that do get established.

Perhaps the greatest obstacle in the way of getting people to value diversity and develop new relationships is the common reluctance of individuals to accept change. Even when they are given a clear explanation of nonmechanistic processes, for example, and shown how these processes have led to success, many people will continue to adhere to mechanistic and linear approaches and remain convinced that these would have brought about still better results. In short, these people resist admitting that the good old days were not really all that good, not even as good as today or as the future could be. Furthermore, because of their reluctance to change, the challenge of guiding others on the journey into the next age is monumental, and leaders can become disheartened at the prospect of leaving behind those who, for whatever reason, have cold feet. Nonetheless, if they are to lead the journey, leaders cannot afford to spend the majority of their time trying to convince everyone that the world is in fact changing.

The beauty of diversity has yet to be truly discovered. Seeing differences as enhancements rather than deterrents is increasingly important in the Information Age, for attempts to filter out data can discourage creativity and obstruct an organization's creative potential. Keeping an open mind is necessary for gaining a richer, more complete understanding.

By contrast, in the Industrial Age, creative thought was discouraged and consensus was encouraged. "Be a team member" was the slogan. The former emphasis on harmony and accord should be abandoned; however, instead we need to embrace the idea that organizational success lies in transforming our notion of organization and accepting that the chaos of competition and the order of cooperation can and do coexist.

Diversity in Health Care

The health care leadership remains less diversified than the health care work force and the overall population (Weber 2000). Eighty-two percent of Americans describe themselves as white, 13 percent as black, 11 percent as Hispanic, 4 percent as Asian or Pacific Islander, and about 1 percent as American Indian, Eskimo, or Aleut. Health care organizations employ 11.5 million workers. Approximately 75 percent of the workers are white, 15 percent are black, 7 percent are Hispanic, and 3 percent are Asians or Native Americans. Of the 50,000 health care leaders, a remarkable 98 percent classify themselves as white. Given this mismatch in diversity, opportunities certainly exist for including more (and more widely varied) perspectives in leadership decision making, not only for purposes of fairness but also to better serve ethnically diverse communities by delivering care that respects cultural traditions. Health care organizations have a responsibility to understand and meet the needs of their communities by developing partnerships with representatives from all local cultures.

Opportunities for Change

When things go wrong, what usually goes wrong are relationships, not physical objects or processes, and these go wrong because of poor communication. Unfortunately, as a society we have very little idea how to get along with one another. Wars rage around the globe, the divorce rate is greater than 50 percent, and violent crime is rampant. The legal profession has been dubbed "the undertakers of relationships."

Fortunately, health care leaders are realizing the importance of establishing and maintaining productive relationships. Furthermore, although the Internet is a valuable new communication tool, there are reasons to worry about its dehumanizing effects. For example, it allows people to inhabit a virtual world and spend less time relating directly to others. Although technology is necessary for leading an organization, it is not sufficient. *Who you are* in your relationships with others may be just as important as *what you do* in the way of delivering technologically sophisticated care. Quality relationships are characterized by trust, the honoring of differences, clear personal boundaries, comfort with self-disclosure, and open communication—all of which confer a degree of vulnerability.

Privacy

The explosion of the Internet as a means of communication has made privacy into a hot political issue. Historically, privacy advocates have had difficulty building support for their position. Now, Internet users are becoming especially concerned about their privacy, largely because of the trails of e-commerce "cookie" crumbs that make it easy for companies to sift through these and sell the personal data they garner to other companies. Until laws are passed to force companies to inform consumers before they sell their personal data, the onus is on each individual Internet user to protect his or her privacy.

> **Point To Ponder**
>
> *Leaders have always been set on stage, in sight and view of the whole world. The Internet puts the leader under the electron microscope for all to see in the finest detail!*

Furthermore, whether out of boredom or curiosity, we are spying on one another like never before. Tiny wireless cameras are used not just for espionage but to detect shoplifting in department stores, and there is a world of Web sites aspiring to publish our dirty laundry and private thoughts. Although people in general need to be more open to ideas, to be more vulnerable, they also understandably want barriers around their private lives. For example, few people, if any, are willing to allow the rest of the world access to all of their personal, financial, and health information. Where the boundaries lie is unique to each person, and determining what to consider private and public in the Information Age requires careful reflection.

Unfortunately, it is not a simple process to identify what will be shared with whom and at what time. For one thing, individuals do not present appropriate component parts of themselves whenever these are desired. Instead, individuals are unified wholes. Mary Parker Follett, noted management expert, points out that "it is unrealistic and wasteful to organize work on the basis that a person can be abstracted from the totality of their being and put into the exercise of one particular skill, taught to perform it to a certain standard, and expect continuous performance at that level—and nothing else. One cannot disconnect themselves, leaving most of themselves at the work-gate and take in just that bit relevant to their job" (Graham 1995, p. 75).

The lack of clearly defined personal boundaries (personal firewalls) is a major cause of relationship problems. As privacy diminishes, the importance of personal boundaries increases. Personal boundaries are different for each individual, and creating effective boundaries requires a healthy sense of identity. Boundary violations often run rampant in organizations. Saying no is frowned upon. Yet excessive overtime, for instance, violates the employees' family boundaries. The best course of action is to respect assumed or articulated boundaries until permission is given to cross them.

Personal boundaries include physical, mental, and spiritual boundaries. In general, a person's physical boundaries extend beyond the person's skin to encompass a space surrounding his or her body. Hugging or standing too close is a violation for some and welcomed by others. A person's physical boundaries also pertain to his or her possessions, money, time, and energy. Touching personal belongings in someone's office may be viewed as acceptable or as a violation. Mental boundaries pertain to beliefs, emotions, and intuition. They are violated, for example, when people are told they do not have the right to feel and appropriately express their emotions. Spiritual boundaries pertain to people's self-esteem, their sense of identity, and their relationship with a higher power. Destructive criticizing, yelling, and uttering abusive words are violations of spiritual boundaries.

Group Discussion

Create a list of expectations regarding your physical boundaries, emotional boundaries, and spiritual boundaries. For example, would you consider your physical boundaries to be violated if someone stood very close while talking to you? Touched you on the arm? Ask a colleague to create a similar list and then share your expectations with each other.

Traditionally, boundaries and boundary violations in health care have been assessed from a patient-provider perspective. The point is that the patient is especially vulnerable by virtue of illness or injury and is dependent on the provider for help, whereas the provider has access to sensitive information about the patient and may uncover medical problems that the patient normally would share only with intimate friends. Given the imbalance of power, the provider has very clear responsibility to delineate and maintain appropriate boundaries.

The power imbalance between managers and employees creates similar expectations. In any relationship between a manager and an employee, both are responsible for delineating their personal boundaries, a task that is an essential step in creating an effective working relationship. Lack of boundaries blurs the purpose of the relationship, creating an ambiguous situation in which harm to either person may result. In addition, uncertainty is unnecessarily increased, to the detriment of the relationship and the entire organization. For far too long, command-and-control leaders have unwittingly violated the personal boundaries of employees without their consent—not with malicious intent but to ensure that the work of the organization was completed in a timely manner. The challenge for leaders today is to avoid dwelling on the rights and wrongs of past practices but instead to move forward and create the conditions in which personal boundaries will be acknowledged and respected.

Self-Disclosure

No relationship can develop fully until the participants expose something of their deeper selves to each other. Revealing oneself to others—one's thoughts, feelings, and intentions—is about telling one's story. Self-disclosure leads to greater understanding, trust, compassion, and commonality—in short, to a better relationship.

> ### Point To Ponder
>
> *Make your ego porous. Will is of little importance, complaining is nothing, fame is nothing.*
> *Openness, patience, receptivity, solitude are everything.*
> —*Rainer Maria Rilke*

The idea that self-disclosure is valuable is often difficult to embrace, especially in a business context, for it runs contrary to classical management theory. In traditional organizations, people who stand around talking about matters unrelated to work are seen as wasting time. The obsession with efficiency is an obstacle to appreciating the value of strengthening relationships through casual conversation.

Self-disclosure is based on trust, on having total confidence in the integrity, ability, and good character of the other person. In other words, the person making the personal disclosures must believe the other person reliably follows through on commitments, has the competence to carry out his or her responsibilities, is emotionally balanced, and consistently chooses the "right" action.

Relationship Skills

In establishing relationships with employees and helping them develop a vulnerable and open style of behaving on the job, leaders must not assume that the employees have well-honed relationship skills. In fact, many employees, like many leaders, have less than adequate skills. Relationship skills, unfortunately, are not necessarily learned by growing up in a family. Many adults, because of how they were raised, have developed patterns of behavior that obstruct learning and accountability (e.g., conflict avoidance and assuming a victim attitude). In addition, many have failed to acquire the skills needed to cope with change, deal with personality differences, and communicate effectively.

Rather than becoming Information Age aliens, quantum leaders learn when to spend time building relationships and when to focus on tasks. In a healthy organization, the distinction between performing tasks and building relationships becomes blurred. For one thing, the latter can be used to develop the relationship skills needed to incorporate vulnerability and open communication into the organization's work and grow its capacity. Developing these skills takes time as well as a strong commitment on the part of the leaders. In addition, leaders can enhance the effectiveness of these skills by using the principles of complexity communication.

COMPLEXITY COMMUNICATION

In sharp contrast to traditional hierarchical organizational structures, the new organizational structures will be virtually flat, with a minimum of mid-level layers between executive management and staff. Using information networks, organizational staff in different divisions will be able to communicate and collaborate with each other in a moment's time.

In many organizations, the entire focus is on sending information, which is only one-third of the communicative interaction. The assumption is that the receiver will understand what the sender intended. This assumption is often wrong, and the full exchange should include the sending of information by one person, its reception by one or more people, and, finally, a confirmation of their understanding.

Complexity communication is presented as an integrated process for improving the effectiveness of communication (Figure 4–3). It requires sensitivity to the myriad interrelationships and interdependencies that are characteristic of a quantum organization. It is based on three behaviors: critical listening, critical questioning, and critical thinking. The term *critical* here should not be taken as having a negative connotation; it is intended to have roughly the same meaning as *analytical.*

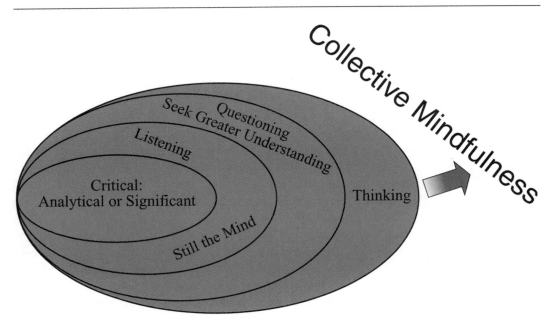

Figure 4–3 Complexity Communication Leads to Collective Mindfulness

Critical Listening

In a conversation, each listener has the responsibility to get the message, but often listeners are too busy thinking about what they want to say to listen carefully enough. People often understand only half of what is said to them. Being vulnerable requires expert listening skills—skills that most people obviously cannot claim.

The greatest challenge for listeners is to "still the mind," to stop the self-talk and mental rehearsing of what they intend to say when it is their turn. Stilling the mind is also about dismissing mental models, at least temporarily. Its consequences include allowing listeners enough time to formulate enduring and just solutions, as well as minimizing the tendency to seek quick fixes.

> **Point To Ponder**
>
> *Rest assured, no matter how bad it looks, I will not judge you until I have heard your side. Once a leader puts expedience above fairness, his reputation and integrity crumble away like something rotten.*
>
> *—Elizabeth I*

Our deeply held internal images of how the world works have a powerful impact on how we listen and react to information. Putting aside our perceptions of power, money, gender, culture, physical appearance, and so on, is simply impossible. Nevertheless, leaders who listen with an open mind and create the conditions for employees to do the same will see better outcomes from their decision making.

Another challenge is to deal with information overload. Some individuals want to tell everything they know, or at least provide more information than the listener needs, which puts a strain on the listener. The listener must then listen even more carefully to discriminate between what is worth retaining and what is not. Managing information is not an easy task, but it is essential for effective and efficient communication.

Critical Questioning

Lawyers are schooled to never ask a question that they do not know the answer to. Vulnerable leadership requires the opposite. The purpose of critical questioning, or asking for significant information, is to check individual perceptions of an issue or situation and render it more manageable. Leaders in the Information Age need to ask new types of questions, including questions about progress, value, and satisfaction. Asking for clarification is also a good way to minimize misinterpretation.

The wise leader never leaves a meeting without going through a checkout procedure. This procedure involves asking the participants questions such as the following: How do you think the meeting went? Did we accomplish what you thought should be accomplished? What was accomplished?

Asking questions about the value of work done will help ensure that all of the work planned or completed will in fact make a difference. Examples include these: What difference will this work make? To whom will it make a difference? At what cost?

Questions about the skills and roles of employees are also important. Do the skills of the employees match the needs of the marketplace? Is there a need to eliminate or add job duties? Is the organization and the community better off because of the services or products provided?

> **Group Discussion**
>
> Staffing is the largest expense for most health care organizations. One reason is that the uncertainty of patient care needs requires a health care organization to have sufficient staff on hand to cover upward swings in care delivery, including emergency situations. Use the principles of vulnerability and complexity communication to create an effective and efficient staffing system that incorporates staffing by ratios and/or patient acuity. Discuss the advantages and disadvantages of the system. How can you be sure that the right care provider is with the right patient at the right time? Is the highest quality care provided at the lowest cost?

In asking questions like the above, leaders attempt to learn more about those being queried and their perspective on issues related to their work and the organization. In the fast-paced world of health care, leaders run the risk of overgeneralizing from past experiences, and asking lots of questions can help prevent this mistake in reasoning. Unfortunately, listening is not always easy for leaders.

One of the keys to critical questioning is to refrain from offering advice or commentary to the person being questioned. Most leaders feel comfortable providing guidance to others, and they readily give advice. Critical questioning requires something more—the gift of an ear. Asking questions will garner the questioner more information if the respondent is allowed to express pertinent opinions. Examples of questions that leaders might ask are contained in Exhibit 4–5.

Receivers of information, or listeners, need a safe space to ask clarifying questions of the senders. In other words, the open exchange of information depends on the existence of a safe forum. If the sender of a message feels threatened by the receiver's asking of questions about the message, the resulting hostility will make for a quick end to the questions and a breakdown in communication. If the receiver feels unsafe asking questions about the message, the resulting silence could easily be misinterpreted as agreement and understanding. When leaders misconstrue the absence of questions as acceptance and understanding of their messages, they commit a grave error.

For some leaders, the challenge is different. Those who are steeped in the classic command-and-control leadership culture rarely ask questions to gain information. In their view, they are expected to be experts on all matters related to their role and are reluctant to ask for information for fear of exposure. Although their concern about looking less than

Exhibit 4–5 Examples of Critical Questions

- Can you tell me what your understanding of this situation is?
- Why is this important to you? To others? To the organization?
- Is the situation you are describing related to a technical issue, a systems issue, or a people-related issue?
- What do you need to know to make a decision on this issue?
- Do you think others have made false assumptions about this situation?
- Who else cares about this issue as much as you do?
- This sounds very rational. What do people feel about it?
- This sounds very emotional. What do people think about it?
- What are the choices in the situation?
- Can you propose a solution?

competent is generally unfounded, they still are not able to listen very well or feel comfortable asking for advice from others. In the new age, their main challenge will be to allow themselves to become more vulnerable and hence more open to input from others.

Critical Thinking

The ability to think critically has long been recognized as a necessary management skill. What is different in complexity communication is the sequence of events. The process begins with critical listening, followed by critical questioning and then critical thinking. It does not make sense to engage in analysis before listening and asking questions to clarify content so that all of the vital data can be considered. Further, complexity communication is a team process, and it involves the participants' assimilating information and then reaching a logical conclusion as a team, not individually.

Critical thinking encompasses

- analyzing the use of language
- explicating assumptions
- formulating problems
- weighing evidence
- evaluating conclusions
- discriminating between arguments
- justifying claims
- clarifying values

Critical thinking is helpful for seeking deeper meaning, validating perceptions, and setting priorities. The proper attitude for engaging in critical thinking is a mix of reflective skepticism and tolerance for ambiguity. Openness is essential for examining evidence. Too often, people proclaim they are thinking critically when in fact they have prejudged the issues, and their discussion supports preconceived notions rather than explores the range of available options. Managing the complexity communication process requires a more critical or analytical style of thought and communication.

For many leaders and employees, engaging in dialogue runs counter to the prevailing culture within their organizations—a culture that instead fosters internal competition and sets hierarchical limitations on who can contribute to the decision-making process. These leaders and employees find it especially difficult to recognize and practice openness and self-disclosure, learn to suspend judgment, and promote collaboration as a way of increasing collective intelligence. In complexity communication, it is normal to view disagreement as an essential aspect of dialogue and to avoid suppressing differences merely for the sake of preserving the peace. Although intensely painful at times, learning the necessary skills and engaging in complexity communication dialogue have a value that can hardly be overstated.

Developing dialogue skills and communicating with others based on the belief that every person is of value but has a limited view represents an overwhelming challenge. In this type of communication, careful listening is integrated with questioning for clarification and then analyzing the messages using critical thinking skills. Many leaders are quickly able to develop the three distinct skills of listening, questioning, and thinking but have difficulty with the sequencing of the skill application. Leaders commonly think or make a decision first (often before all of the information is presented), request information and clarification second, and then listen as the final step—the fire-aim-ready approach. In spite of the fast-paced work environment, which hinders contemplative communication practices, quantum leaders recognize the benefits of complexity communication and coach others to use the associated skills to mediate the internal competition and reinforce new and more effective behaviors.

COLLECTIVE MINDFULNESS

Complexity communication skills are especially important in health care, where the potential for catastrophic outcomes, should employees fail to perform, can be significant. Given the critical nature of the services they provide, health care organizations often develop what is known as the power of collective mindfulness, a phenomenon described by Sutcliffe and Weick (1999). Collective mindfulness is the capacity of groups and individuals to be keenly aware of significant details, notice errors in the making, and have the shared expertise and freedom to act on what they notice.

Consider the case of a patient who is experiencing cardiac arrest. A team of nurses, respiratory therapists, and physicians quickly assembles, prompted by a prearranged code call. Within minutes the patient's heart rate is stabilized, respiratory function is restored, and the team disperses. Those unfamiliar with emergency departments might think the actions of the health professionals had been tightly scripted and well rehearsed. Rather, the professionals all knew their particular role, had experienced similar situations in the past, and had only to listen to what was happening, ask for additional necessary information, and think through and integrate past experiences with the current event in order to perform the rescue.

To be effective in potentially catastrophic situations, health professionals depend on not just their mastery of standardized routines, but complexity communication at its best. They listen intently and with full presence, question only for clarification, and intervene as a finely tuned unit.

> ### Group Discussion
>
> Select two teams, one composed of experienced employees and the other composed of newer employees. Consider an emergency situation in which a patient is experiencing chest pain. Compare the two teams with regard to their working relationships, communication skills, and ability to prioritize and make decisions. Create a plan to develop the skills of the less effective team.

Collective mindfulness is not limited to clinical situations. It is evident in many types of situations in which there are complex interpersonal relationships. Consider health care staffing. Health care leaders are continually challenged to deliver reliable services in the face of fluctuating conditions, such as shortages of qualified employees and reductions in reimbursement. Quantum leaders create a culture that allows employees to be flexible (but in orderly ways) and to focus energy and expertise where and when they are needed. They can then use the employees to assist in dealing with the difficulties that arise by creating strategies that address the appropriate issues.

Hidden within the spirit of collective mindfulness is the essence of vulnerability—being open, searching for new solutions, taking risks, trying new strategies, retaining what works and discarding what does not work. What emerges is a delicate balance of processes that encourage continuous learning and improvement while at the same time promoting order and reliable performance, a very powerful combination.

STRATEGIES FOR CULTIVATING LEADERSHIP VULNERABILITY

In this section two strategies for fostering vulnerable or open leadership are proposed: open communication and syndication. Both strategies have inherent risks and require leaders to stretch current thinking. Although many other strategies support open leadership, these two are designed to begin the process of changing mental models and moving to practices that fit with the work of the quantum organization.

Open Communication

Some leaders have confused dialoguing with behind-the-scenes consensus building and decision making. Making decisions before all of the information is considered leads to poor outcomes and decreases trust in the integrity of the decision-making process. Although, according to the classic management model, conducting business in informal settings such as the dining room and the golf course may have some merit, recent advances in information technology have brought both challenges and opportunities to the way business is conducted. In particular, by aiding in the removal of secrecy and increasing the ease of dia-loguing, they support the open communication model.

The open communication model is based on the same principles as open meeting laws (Exhibit 4–6). The idea behind these laws, which have traditionally applied to meetings of public bodies, is that publicizing meetings and conducting them openly maximizes public access to governmental processes. All 50 states have enacted some type of legisla-tion providing the public with a statutory right to openness in government. The laws require meetings of public bodies to be conducted openly and notices and agendas for such meetings to be provided to the public. Open meetings expose the conduct of the business of government to the scrutiny of the public and prevent decision making in secret, thereby ensuring that appointed members of boards and commissions truly serve as representatives of the broader community and that the actions taken are in the best interests of the community.

The open communication model applies the principles of open meeting laws to organ-izations based on the belief that the work of any organization belongs to all of its mem-bers and that encouraging open communication will enhance organizational effectiveness and capacity. The following seven principles, if followed, will increase the incidence of open dialogue, improve trust among employees, and decrease bureaucratic processes. These principles focus on the manner in which members communicate and make deci-sions, and their overall goal is to increase the fairness of decision-making processes and prevent them from being influenced by off-the-record communication between decision makers and others.

Exhibit 4–6 Basic Principles of Open Meeting Laws

1. A meeting is considered to be a gathering that can occur not only in person but also through technological devices.
2. All meetings of a public body shall be open meetings, and all persons so desiring shall be permitted to attend and listen to the deliberations and proceedings.
3. An "open call to the public" is permitted but not required. The purpose of an open call is to allow members of the public to address the public body on matters not listed on the agenda.
4. Executive sessions will be used to seek legal advice and review confidential records. No votes are taken in executive session.
5. Appropriate notice of each meeting will be given (usually not later than 24 hours before the meeting), and the agenda and meeting location will be posted.
6. For each meeting, there will be written minutes or a recording that will include an accu-rate description of all actions proposed, discussed, or taken and the names of members who propose each motion.
7. The minutes or a recording of any meeting, except an executive session, must be open to public inspection no later than three working days after the meeting.

Source: Data from http://www.sec.state.vt.us.

1. *The business of the organization shall be conducted during open meetings, which are defined as gatherings of people physically, telephonically, or electronically.* This principle requires that issues brought before a committee be discussed in the presence of all members of the committee. It is not appropriate to discuss any topic without involving all the parties. Ex parte communication considers only one side of a situation and as such violates the first principle of open communication. E-mail communication, telephone conversations, and casual dialogue at social gatherings about committee meeting topics are not allowed. The intent is to eliminate selective collaboration and prevoting on issues prior to the actual meeting. Decision making that is inclusive from the start results in decisions that, because everyone is highly invested in them, are more likely to succeed.

2. *The date and time of each meeting, its location, and its agenda shall be posted.* The publicizing of this information allows unofficial but interested members to learn the issues to be covered in the meeting and to discuss them with other members ahead of time. It also helps eliminate the chance that decisions will be made in secret. In the meeting itself, only issues identified as being on the official agenda will be discussed, which means that no surprise or unanticipated issues will be dealt with. Although posting meeting information may be cumbersome at times, it minimizes the chances of reactive decision making.

3. *Every meeting shall be open to all persons desiring to attend and listen to the deliberations and proceedings.* The intent of this principle is to remove even the appearance of secrecy. It is based on the belief that the satisfaction felt by employees, along with their job performance, is highly correlated with their involvement in the making of decisions that directly pertain to their work.

4. *Every meeting shall include a "call to the attendees" to allow members of the organization or the community a defined allotment of time in which to address the official members on matters discussed.* Although dialogue on the issues is restricted to official members of a committee, other attendees should be afforded an opportunity to react to what the official members say. Allotting a specified amount of time for comments keeps the meeting from running past its scheduled end. In addition, the official members are not required to respond but are requested to consider the additional information when making decisions.

5. *Executive sessions shall be used for the purpose of seeking expert advice or reviewing information defined by law as confidential but not for the taking of votes.* Some types of information, such as performance evaluations and salary and wage data, are protected. In executive sessions, issues involving confidential information are discussed, but no voting or decision making occurs.

6. *Each meeting is documented by written minutes or a recording that includes an accurate description of all actions proposed, discussed, or taken and the names of the members who voted for each motion.* Documenting the work of a committee fully prevents decision makers from hiding behind the cloak of the summative vote count. It also forces decision makers to own their opinions and makes them accountable to the membership at large. Minutes serve as an historical record of the decision-making process.

7. *The written minutes or the recording of any meeting except an executive session must be open to inspection no later than three working days after the meeting.* Making sure that a record of discussion in the meeting is available to all interested parties in a timely manner again helps lift the shroud of secrecy.

Interestingly, the two most common violations of open meeting laws are discussion of agenda items without the full board or committee present (ex parte) and inappropriate use of the executive session. The same violations should be expected during implementation of the open communication model, because collaboration and prevoting on issues have been a traditional practice in organizations, as has the use of executive sessions for dealing with matters of organizationwide concern.

Syndication

The second strategy for cultivating leadership vulnerability is organizational syndication, which is basically a way of structuring business to tap latent potential. Based on the recognition that information is now widely available, syndication uses resources outside of an organization to benefit the organization.

Organizations, according to Dee Hock (1999), are extremely good at some things, are very good at many things, but are not good at everything. In fact, organizations are pathetic at some things! Although much organizational work is believed not to be amenable to syndication, significant work elements might be, especially those at which organizations are pathetic.

Syndication, which originated in the entertainment world, is expanding to define the structure of e-business. It involves the sale of the same good to many customers, who then integrate it with other offerings and redistribute it, similar to the way television programs or news stories are managed.

Syndication is a radical new way of structuring business (Table 4–1). It requires leaders to rethink their strategies, to reshape their organizations, to change the way they interact with customers and partner with other entities, and to pioneer new models for collecting revenues and earning profits. Integrating syndication into an organization is similar to creating a "chaordic" organization, as defined by Dee Hock (1999). Hock is credited with devising a new concept of organizations based on the belief that chaos and order, competition and cooperation, can be harmoniously blended. He conceived of a global system for the electronic exchange of value, and the result was VISA International, which is owned by 22,000 member banks that both compete with each other for 750 million customers and honor each other's transactions across borders and currencies.

Chaordic organizations present an unambiguous challenge to the traditions of independent organizations by bringing into existence an interconnected, international reality once believed impossible. They also offer courage to those considering syndication for selected services or products. At the moment, the chaordic model is mainly a learning aid, however, and cannot be quickly imprinted on existing organizations.

Syndication is based on the realization that needed expertise is often found not inside an organization but beyond its boundaries. In a syndication network, the roles of originator of content, syndicator or packager of content for distribution, and distributor of content to

Table 4–1 Business in the Syndicated World

	Traditional Business	Syndication
Structure of relationships	Linear supply and demand	Loose, weblike networks
Corporate role	Fixed	Continually shifting
Value added	Dominated by physical distribution	Dominated by information manipulation
Strategic focus	Control scarce resources	Leverage abundance
Role of corporate capabilities	Sources of advantage	Products to sell
Role of outsourcing	Gain efficiency	Assemble virtual corporation

Source: Reprinted by permission of *Harvard Business Review*, p. 90. From "Syndication: The Emerging Model for Business in the Internet Era," by Kevin Werbach, May–June 2000. Copyright 2000 by the Harvard Business School Publishing Corporation, all rights reserved.

customers are quite different from the traditional roles of content developer and distributor of content to employees.

In a syndication network, the content originator has greater responsibility and accountability than in traditional organizations. In some situations, leaders have established collaborative initiatives that can be moved to the syndication level. Health centers for indigents, school health education and treatment clinics, hospice centers, and training programs developed through cooperation between communities and financiers are candidates for syndica-

> **Group Discussion**
>
> A group of health care organizations has decided to apply the syndication model to its employee development program. Imagine you are on the team creating the product to be syndicated. Using the principles of syndication, your team has been assigned the work of content originators. Describe the content origination process and continue model development with the creation of packaging and distribution plans for the education program. What are the advantages and disadvantages of syndication as a way of developing and implementing programs? Who would support or oppose the syndication model? What performance measures could be used to evaluate it?

tion. Because of their need for standardization of services (to ensure quality), operational cost savings, and conservation of capital, each could be syndicated to create a greater network without substantial duplication of effort. The role of the originator is to assess and consolidate the work of many products into a single product desired communitywide.

The second key role, that of syndicator, encompasses packaging the content and managing the relationships between originators and distributors. The syndicator's goals include achieving consistency of products and services, uncovering user expectations, and supporting the established relationship between product users and the syndication processes. Time-limited agreements would support state-of-the-art products and services that provide appropriate quality at the lowest cost, because failure to meet the standards would cause users to turn to other syndicators.

Finally, the distributor is responsible for delivering the goods from originators to users. As the virtual world develops, many more information services and education programs are likely to be distributed through the Internet.

It is no longer cost-effective for every organization to provide every service. Not only is it costly, but individual organizations lack the necessary concentration of expertise. The syndication model offers opportunities for current providers of services to generate revenue through a shared process as designated originators. Designated originators provide the content of their expertise to the product and become co-owners of the syndication model. If syndication became common in health care, those organizations with significant expertise could earn income as a result of contributing to the origination process, whereas those with limited expertise could have access to standardized, state-of-the-art products for a reasonable cost.

IS THERE A CHOICE?

Are leaders obligated to develop a vulnerable leadership style? Do they need to replace closed leadership behavior with open leadership behavior? The obvious response is yes, there is no choice, the value of vulnerability is too conspicuous to deny. The move into the Information Age requires different skills and knowledge than those required in the Industrial Age.

However, some leaders will have difficulty making the transition. Some, for example, might support the concept of open leadership, but because of the perceived threat in admitting to a lack of answers or information, they might be resistant to living the new behaviors. They also will have great difficulty in creating a culture supportive of open leadership, for their failure to walk the talk of vulnerability will hurt employee morale and lower the level of trust within the organization.

Thus, the best strategy for leaders right now is to critically assess their personal status and their ability to assimilate vulnerable behaviors and integrate them into their performance. Acquiring the skills needed to implement the open leadership model is a long-term process that requires understanding, commitment, and persistence. Ethically, developing open leadership skills is the right thing to do. Not only that, but as successful behaviors emerge, leaders will see some of the benefits to be gained from changing to a better model for the times.

CONCLUSION

Currently, it is nearly impossible for a single person to know more than 10 percent of what there is to know about a particular topic. This is most disconcerting to leaders who have worked and studied diligently to know as much as they can. Unfortunately for these leaders, it is even apparent to their colleagues that they do not have all the answers. In addition, they have no chance of catching up, as information continues to accumulate too rapidly. The good news is that everyone is in the same situation; no one ever has all of the answers.

Consequently, the new challenge for leaders is to become comfortable managing the information that is available—to become competent as information access finders and relationship makers. Furthermore, as this chapter points out, the best approach to leadership these days is to understand that the high speed of change, among other factors, makes total control impossible and to therefore accept that vulnerability and open communication are required. In addition, throughout the journey of learning to become openly vulnerable, leaders necessarily will become competent in managing uncertainty, encouraging risk, valuing diversity, and communicating with others based on principles of complexity and respect for privacy and personal boundaries. Increasing vulnerability increases leadership excellence, but no leader will be able to achieve this desirable result without significant commitment and effort.

REFERENCES

Abrahamson, E. 2000. Change without pain. *Harvard Business Review,* July–August, 75–79.

Capra, F. 1982. *The turning point: Science, society and the rising culture.* New York: Simon and Schuster.

Cleveland, H. 1972. *The future executive: A guide for tomorrow's managers.* New York: Harper & Row.

Graham, P., ed. 1995. *Mary Parker Follett—Prophet of management: A celebration of writings from the 1920s.* Boston: Harvard Business School Press.

Hock, D. 1999. *Birth of the chaordic age.* San Francisco: Berrett-Kohler.

Kellner-Rogers, M. 1999. Changing the way we change: Lessons from complexity. *The Inner Edge* 1, no. 6: 18–22.

Kouzes, J.M. 2000. Link me to your leader. *Business2.com,* October 10, 292–295.

Sutcliffe, K.M., and K.E. Weick. 1999. The reduction of medical error through systemic mindfulness. In *Enhancing patient safety and reducing errors in health care* (conference proceedings).

Torbert, W.R. 2000. Exercising vulnerable power. *The Inner Edge* 3, no. 4: 19–22.

Weber, D. 2000. The lack of diversity at the top. *Health Forum Journal,* September.

SUGGESTED READINGS

Axelrod, D. 2000. *Elizabeth I. CEO: Strategic lessons from the leader who built an empire.* Paramus, NJ: Prentice Hall.

Krass, P. ed. 1998. *The book of leadership wisdom: Classic writings by legendary business leaders*. New York: Wiley.

Malloch, K. 1999. The performance measurement matrix: A framework to optimize decision making. *Journal of Nursing Quality* 13, no. 3: 1–12.

Werbach, K. 2000. Syndication: The emerging model for business in the Internet era. *Harvard Business Review,* May–June, 85–93.

Youngblood, M.D. 1997. *Life at the edge of chaos: Creating the quantum organization*. Dallas, TX: Perceval Publishing.

Quiz Questions

Select the best answer for each of the following questions.

1. Vulnerability is an essential leadership trait for the quantum leader. Its major effect is to:
   a. expose the leader's weaknesses to others in the organization
   b. improve the leader's ability to manage information
   c. reduce the leader's authority and control
   d. improve the leader's ability to uncover multiple perspectives on an issue

2. Uncertainty in organizations results in a wide range of reactions from leaders. Most leaders in quantum organizations believe that uncertainty is:
   a. normal
   b. the cause of errors
   c. a deterrent to creativity
   d. surmountable

3. Nonlinear evaluation of work is the norm for quantum health care organizations. The nonlinear evaluation of a work process looks at:
   a. the cause-and-effect relationships of the process
   b. outcomes that occur repeatedly
   c. multiple outcomes
   d. multiple process participants and multiple outcomes

4. The recognition that uncertainty and chaos are present in all organizations is changing the nature of strategic planning. Which one of the following tactics can be used to increase the utility of the planning process?
   a. decreasing the time frame under consideration
   b. tinkering
   c. adding team members with different perspectives
   d. increasing the attention given to specific measurable goals and objectives

5. Complexity communication leads to several important results, one of which is:

a. an increased focus on the sending of information
b. collective mindfulness
c. greater participation of team members
d. more risk taking

6. New strategies are needed for leaders to provide health care in an environment that is unpredictable and changing rapidly. The strategy of open communication is designed to:

a. prevent hasty decisions
b. increase team member participation in meetings
c. increase trust in the decision-making process
d. eliminate confidential information

7. A leader's understanding of his or her own personal boundaries, privacy needs, and self-disclosure limits is an important new tool in the leader's toolbox, for it allows the leader to:

a. set limits with employees
b. share feelings and expectations in a meaningful way
c. develop a clear sense of his or her own identity as a precursor to relationship building
d. avoid conflict and support team processes

8. A leader's relationships or social connections have increased in importance as a means to:

a. facilitate the work of the organization
b. increase the leader's visibility
c. interpret information
d. manage conflict

9. Privacy is a continuing concern for health care leaders. It is best controlled by:

a. government agencies
b. each individual
c. eliminating communication on the Internet
d. developing coded communication

10. Syndication is a new way of using health care resources creatively and cost effectively. One of its main disadvantages is that it:

a. is expensive
b. requires an increased number of employees
c. has not been used extensively in the health care field
d. results in the sharing of information

CHAPTER 5

Healing Brokenness: Error as Opportunity

It is often the best people that make the worst mistakes—error is not the monopoly of an unfortunate few. We cannot change the human condition, but we can change the conditions under which humans work.

—James T. Reason

Chapter Objectives

At the completion of this chapter, the reader will be able to

- Describe the concept of error as an opportunity to improve health care outcomes.
- Describe the advantages and disadvantages of mandatory reporting and disclosure of errors.
- Compare the advantages and disadvantages of managing error solely from a systems perspective with managing error from an individual perspective.
- Describe the advantages and disadvantages of remediation and discipline as interventions for minimizing error.
- Show how health care leadership errors can be transformed into practices supportive of the quantum organization.

Given the complexity of the health care system as well as the chaos caused by work force shortages and reimbursement limitations, it is not surprising that health professionals continue to commit significant medical errors and that health care leaders frequently feel challenged beyond their ability to cope. As a result, health care leaders and professionals are generally fearful of making the wrong decision or doing the wrong thing. Yet, the potential for errors or breakdowns in the care of patients is always present. Breakdowns can be caused by poor health care provider performance, the unavailability of essential resources, and systemic problems. In the best case scenario, good systems design and proper staffing will serve to minimize errors and crises. Health care leaders have the ultimate responsibility for making decisions that create safe clinical practice conditions and for responding to public pressure to improve medical care and reduce errors. This chapter presents new perspectives on both clinical and leadership error and describes opportunities for reducing the incidence of error in current systems.

ERROR IN GENERAL

The reality is that if human beings are involved, mistakes will occur sooner or later. Big mistakes, little mistakes, mistakes of consequence with adverse outcomes, and mistakes of little consequence occur every day. To be sure, not every error results in harm. Further, errors have many sources, from human incompetence to systemic problems. Near misses are also of concern. Although a near miss, by its nature, does not result in full-scale harm, the surrounding events offer a rich source of data to be studied as a means of avoiding similar situations in the future. Discussing near misses allows an organization to assess specific products or procedures and develop recommendations for improvement.

Given the inevitability of error, reacting to mistakes punitively is unlikely to minimize their occurrence, even though our culture leads us to expect the assignment of blame, correction of the situation, and, in most cases, punishment of those who made the mistakes. Punishment and blame are also meted out to those who come in second. For example, when there is a loser in a competition, even the competition between health care organizations for market share, people tend to seek a scapegoat, someone to blame for the lack of success. Winning is everything in our society, and coming in second place or losing a competition is not viewed as acceptable.

> ### Point To Ponder
>
> *Consider what would have happened if you had allowed shame and embarrassment to overwhelm you when you fell as a baby while trying to learn how to walk. You would still be crawling!*

Our drive to be the best, to have the most, and to be in control has led to substantial achievements, but it does not always bring about the best outcome for an organization and in some cases results in failure. When the outcome is less than optimal, the leaders and employees are held accountable, despite the fact that few leaders and employees, if any, ever achieve perfect success.

The constant attaching of blame to individuals has created a climate of shame and guilt and has decreased the candid reporting and discussion of mistakes. Unfortunately, the main approach to error, not only in health care but in society at large, is to punish supposed offenders. Given that punishment usually has the effect of quashing the human spirit, it is curious that leaders, or anyone else, continue to view mistakes as failures rather than as opportunities for improvement. In some cases, leaders use punishment for the purpose of retaining and reinforcing their power within the organization. In some cases, they simply believe that it is the right thing to do and to do anything less would tarnish their reputation for effectiveness. Whatever the rationale, punishment of error makers not only fails to produce the desired result (the elimination of error), but the negative impact of the punishment dissuades the employees from doing more than the minimum, as they fear making more mistakes and suffering additional punishment. In short, the mistakes themselves become less of a problem than the societal response to the mistakes.

Error as Foolishness

In attempting to gain an understanding of behaviors related to error, it is helpful to reflect on our cultural roots and values. According to the view of many cultures, humanity begins in a state of perfection, but the journey of life is filled with temptation and distractions. Understandably, humans eventually partake of the tree of knowledge of good and evil (Kaye 2000).

Consider the two spiritual traditions of Judeo-Christianity and Buddhism. Both espouse the view that human nature is fundamentally perfect but that people soon stray from their natural state of perfection and make mistakes. They become distracted and tempted by many things, especially worldly goods. Not surprisingly, people follow their desires, lose their awareness of perfection, ignore their inner voice of wisdom, and give in to temptation. Sometimes a person will risk everything for one more possession—another automobile, boat, computer, or vacation—and will thereby negate his or her sense of personal wholeness.

Although not everyone is an adherent of a particular spiritual tradition, looking at errors from the perspective of such traditions can help people understand the phenomenon of error in a more positive way, a way that humanizes the error factor. By recognizing that mistakes are expressions of inescapable foolishness rather than malice, people can let them go, avoid taking them personally, and prevent them from casting a shadow over a lifetime career. Further, when people accept their fallibility and view their own mistakes in this way, they will be more likely to respond to the mistakes of others with understanding rather than anger or resentment.

> **Point To Ponder**
>
> *Being foolish does not mean that one is inherently good or evil—just foolish!*

Leaders, like other people, find it a challenge to overcome the human tendency to hold a grudge when someone makes an error believed to be unnecessary. Yet leaders must learn to forgive others when mistakes are made and begin to coach others to learn from the mistakes. When leaders move beyond resentment, they encourage employees to expect to be treated with understanding and kindness. It is unhealthy when employees are in constant fear of mistreatment as the result of errors.

By perceiving errors as foolishness rather than failures, leaders open the door to a new approach to managing errors. Rather than punishing those who commit errors, they treat errors as opportunities for improvement (Exhibit 5–1 lists appropriate questions to ask when an error has occurred). One good example of the way errors can lead to positive out-

Exhibit 5–1 Asking Better Questions

Do Ask	Do Not Ask
• Why do you think this error occurred? • Is there a way to avoid this from occurring again in the future? • What can the team learn from this situation?	• Why did this happen? • What did you do wrong? • Who is responsible for this error?

comes is the invention of Post-its, in which the disaster of a newly created glue that did not work as planned was turned into a great success—the creation of easily removable stick-on notes. As this example shows, mistakes may bring good fortune, and learning to trust

> **Group Discussion**
>
> Reflect on a recent error that resulted in serious harm in your organization. How was the situation managed? Did the questions asked focus on identifying someone to blame, like these: What is wrong here? Who was responsible for this? Or were they questions that would allow the organization and the provider to learn more about the situation and be better positioned to avoid recurrences of the error? Better questions for investigating an error include these: Why is this error occurring again and again? Am I missing a lesson here? How can I turn this situation into an opportunity for growth and learning for myself and the team?

the potential of mistakes to create new opportunities is the only way to move from the toxicity of a blameful culture to the productivity of an accountability culture.

Recognizing and Recovering from Error

Nearly every spiritual tradition includes avenues to recognize and recover from error. The intent of each tradition is to learn from mistakes, to identify actions that will decrease the chance of repeating the same mistakes, and to improve performance as a result. For organizations to survive and thrive, they must develop traditions that support employees in recognizing errors and rectifying their effects. This includes allowing employees to take responsibility for the impact of their actions, as well as maintaining openness in the workplace, which is critical for reporting and discussing errors and using them as opportunities for improvement (Exhibit 5–2).

Exhibit 5–2 Recovering from Error

• Recognize the lack of provider or leader preparation to manage errors as opportunities. • Develop strategies to cope with the sense of failure, disappointment, and remorse that often follows errors.	• Create a coaching script for leaders to address serious errors. The process of dealing with a serious error includes: – identifying critical events – identifying opportunities for individual improvement – identifying opportunities for system improvement – following up on these steps by implementing changes

Coaching employees through the error recovery process ranges from simple one-time dialogue sessions to long-term counseling and frequent reassurance. A mistake that results in significant harm or in the filing of a lawsuit has the potential to destroy the career of an otherwise exceptionally competent health care provider. If the person has a hard time coping with the sense of failure, disappointment, and remorse, he or she also will have a hard time learning how to prevent a recurrence of the mistake. Getting stuck in personal grief or remorse or assigning blame to others will not prevent a repeat performance. In fact, by focusing on the negative emotions felt, the person will be distracted from taking measures to solve the problem that led to the mistake. On the other hand, by focusing on what others could or should have done, the person may allay his or her feelings of remorse but may begin to feel powerless or even victimized. The ideal strategy is to accept as much responsibility for the mistake as is warranted and then go on to explore measures for changing the system in a way that reduces the chance of repeating the mistake.

> **Key Point**
>
> *When you make a mistake, stop, center, and apologize. Reaffirm your respect for the other person or people (those you have offended) and reaffirm your positive intentions. Do your best to learn from the situation.*
> *—Carol Pearson*

Given the need for openness, effective coping strategies, and support for moving on, the work of the leader is clear. If mistakes are to be treated as opportunities for improvement, health care leaders must meet the challenge and create new structures and processes that support dialogue about errors and ongoing follow up. The overall strategy includes

- acknowledging the sense of remorse or failure a person who committed an error might feel
- seeking clarification from and providing social support to that person
- attempting to discover the sources of the problem
- taking concrete actions to prevent future repetitions

In addition, health care leaders must create or strengthen support structures for those in litigation, because all too often these individuals are subtly ostracized by the health care team.

ERRORS IN HEALTH CARE SERVICE

Health Care Providers and Error

No provider ever intends to make an error or harm a patient. Health care is about helping others to manage their health, relieving pain and distress, restoring functionality, or assisting in a peaceful death. Health care providers feel a sense of satisfaction and accomplishment when a patient experiences relief, a patient's functionality is improved, or a terminally ill patient dies tranquilly. They feel the opposite—discontent and guilt—when their care results in unanticipated bad outcomes. In such a situation, the essence of their healing work has not been realized. Learning to understand the role of the human error factor is one of the greatest challenges for providers.

> **Key Point**
>
> *The systems by which health care is delivered and financed must be designed to ensure that care is safe, effective, efficient, equitable, and tailored to each individual's specific needs and circumstances.*
>
> *—Institute of Medicine*

Expecting Perfection

Health care, by its very nature, is uncertain and imperfect. The variability in perceptions and in the interpretations of clinical data by both patients and providers means that many decisions are partially accidental. Further, medicine is inherently experimental, in that each patient has a unique set of characteristics (e.g., age, weight, metabolism, existing conditions, and behavior patterns). Regardless of the number of participants in a clinical trial, when a drug is given to a particular patient, it may or may not act according to the established standards. There is never total assurance in health care, and when the uncertainty of care is denied, when perfection is expected, care providers become the scapegoats (Exhibit 5–3). Although the mind may understand and tolerate error, the human heart is most unforgiving when things do not go well.

> **Point To Ponder**
>
> *All healers will make mistakes that hurt, and we need healthier ways to respond. The responsibility accepted by a healer is awesome because patients give caregivers enormous power and authority. It takes considerable spiritual maturity to accept patient trust and understand that mistakes happen.*
>
> *—David Hilfilker*

Additional complexity has been introduced by the advent of managed care programs, which were implemented in an effort to control escalating health care costs. These pro-

Exhibit 5–3 Two Strategies for Handling Errors

Expecting Perfection	**Honoring Excellence**
• Is unrealistic but is considered the proper attitude	• Takes into account the trial-and-error nature of health care
• Creates unrealistic expectations	• Supports the evolution to best practices
• Fails to consider the wide variability in patient situations	• Supports continual improvement processes
• Positions providers as scapegoats for lack of success	• Respects the nature of human interactions

grams unfortunately have produced immense pressures for organizations, specifically pressures for perfection at the lowest possible cost. The efforts of managed care programs to control access to services, standardize practices, and monitor quality have not been as successful as anticipated. Although early evidence of greater access in conjunction with reduced cost raised the hopes of many payers, providers, and patients, the longer term outcomes have indicated that the benefits of cost reduction were being achieved at the expense of access to services and patient satisfaction.

The most alarming outcome of managed care models has been the distancing of clinical decision making from the point of service. This distancing and the requirement that services be authorized solely on the basis of established standards created additional difficulties for the delivery of appropriate and timely care. Furthermore, the delays in treatment that were caused often resulted in negative patient outcomes. When decision makers do not have day-to-day contact with patients, they can confuse what produces dissatisfaction with what is truly erroneous. The health professionals providing the care—those closest to the patients—were expected to practice within the established norms regardless of their goodness of fit with the specific patient clinical situations. This approach, unconditional adherence to standards, simply does not lead to good care overall.

Honoring Excellence

In many cases, leaders work diligently to preserve the status quo, and they avoid tinkering with current processes for fear of making mistakes. When mistakes do occur, leaders usually act to rectify the situation immediately and return to the status quo ante. Unfortunately, their fear of disrupting existing routines discourages creativity and motivates employees to refrain from rocking the boat as well. In other words, their drive to sustain the *perceived perfect present* quashes their own spirit and the spirit of the employees, obstructing the investigation of potential improvements. Indeed, the fear of failure or retribution that employees feel causes them to essentially "retire on the job" and reduces their productivity. The reality is that trial and error are necessary for improvements to be discovered and implemented.

When things do not go as planned, the best response is to look for the message in the error and use the information received to chart a change in course (see Exhibit 5–3). It is through the continual remodeling of care that best practices or templates for excellence are uncovered. When leaders think that perfection has already been achieved, they will view modifications as inappropriate and a waste of time, thereby hindering the emergence of true excellence.

Point To Ponder

Expecting perfection eliminates the possibility of excellence.

Learning to appreciate errors as a catalyst for change and improvement opens the door to unexpected opportunities. Errors allow leaders to look at things differently and even revise their plans in light of their new perspective. Quantum leaders examine mistakes or misfires carefully and work to minimize or eliminate feelings of shame and embarrassment—the traditional response to mistakes. Growing from our experiences requires a mindset that recognizes human fallibility and uncertainty. Our expectations should not be based on perfectionism.

Further, an important organizational dynamic emerges when leaders acknowledge that being right all the time is not even a possibility. If leaders are not highly invested in always being right, they will find their employees appreciate their attitude and are more likely to approach them with new ideas.

Public Reaction to Error

Significant attention has been given recently to medical errors. The Institute of Medicine (IOM) report on errors, entitled *To Err Is Human* (Kohn et al. 2000), elevated not only the health care community's awareness of this issue but also the public's awareness, for the reported statistics have implications for every single American. The report raised new issues, proposed solutions, and challenged health professionals and the public at large to work to reduce medical errors by at least 50 percent in the next five years. Exhibit 5–4 lists four strategies identified by the IOM as potentially effective for managing medical errors and minimizing their incidence.

Exhibit 5–4 To Err Is Human: IOM Goals

- Establish a national focus to create leadership, research, tools, and protocols to enhance the knowledge base about safety.
- Identify and learn from errors through immediate and strong mandatory reporting efforts as well as encouragement of voluntary efforts to ensure the system continues to be made safer for patients.
- Raise standards and expectations for improvements in safety through the actions of oversight organizations, group purchasers, and professional groups.
- Create safety systems inside health care organizations through the implementation of safe practices at the delivery level.

Source: Reprinted with permission from *To Err Is Human: Building a Safer Health System.* Copyright 1999 by the National Academy of Sciences. Courtesy of the National Academy Press, Washington, D.C.

As regards these strategies, the recommendation to implement mandatory reporting is consistent with the idea that errors are opportunities for improvement, as is the recommendation to establish a national resource for error research, including research into standards and best practices. Putting these recommendations into effect will require the commitment of leaders and their trust that the open approach will work in the long term.

Second, the report leaves it unclear where the accountability for error management truly rests. The report recommends both internal and external oversight mechanisms. Management of errors internally—in fact, nearest the point of service (or the point of error)—offers the best opportunity for continuing improvement, especially if there is a national repository of data on safety and supporting practices. External control reinforces the blame approach to error management.

Third, mandatory reporting may be a blessing for the public but could be seen as a curse by care providers. Although the consumers must be given information to assist them in choosing providers and services, not all errors provide pertinent information or help in making such decisions. More specific approaches that support error as opportunity are needed, although negligence must of course be reported.

Mandatory Error Reporting

The reporting of every minor incident to a state or national board does not necessarily enhance the protection of the public. Mandatory reporting serves to inform the public of errors but can obstruct their use as opportunities for improvement. Because of the threat represented by reporting to a public body, care providers may be unwilling to declare their errors, particularly minor ones. Further, minor incidents in which patients are not placed

> **Group Discussion**
>
> A colleague in nursing reports the following incident to you: "I recently gave a patient the wrong medication. The patient was not affected, and I did not write an incident report because I did not want it noted in my personnel file or reported to the state board of nursing. This type of mistake happens often, because most facilities are understaffed." How would you handle this situation? Do you agree with the nurse? What changes could be made to the system to support the reporting of this type of error and create opportunities to learn from the commission of errors?

at risk of harm and the care providers' competence is not put into question usually can be handled inside the organization. Most health care leaders believe that if there are mechanisms in place to take corrective action, remediate deficits, and detect patterns of behavior, no additional benefit is gained from the mandatory reporting of minor incidents. In fact, punishing a provider for a minor error adds to the bureaucratic burden and results in costs to the organization. The approach favored here, of using errors as opportunities for improvement, can best be supported by informing the public of significant errors and care provider negligence but withholding information about minor errors so that these can be brought out into the open within the organization and be used as vehicles for improvement.

Disclosure

Not only is mandatory reporting a complicating factor in error management, so too is the expectation of disclosure. Morally, disclosure is the right thing to do. The ethics manual of the American College of Physicians states that physicians should disclose to patients information about procedural or judgment errors made during care if such information is material to the patients' well-being. The ethics manual notes that errors do not necessarily constitute improper, negligent, or unethical behavior, but failure to disclose them may.

The disclosure of errors provides the chance to recognize brokenness. In addition, depending on the circumstances, the person who commits an error may have an obligation to apologize for it or offer reparation. Although professional codes do not clearly state when an apology or reparation is expected, care providers in every discipline, not just physicians, may find themselves in a situation where some sort of acknowledgment of error is morally required. Other ethical issues arise with respect to disclosure. For example, care providers have argued that nondisclosure may be appropriate if the harm from disclosure exceeds the harm from nondisclosure, or if the error is inconsequential and disclosure does not empower the patient.

The disclosure of an error raises certain practical issues, especially the timing of the disclosure but also where and how to make it, whom to make it to, and what to expect as a consequence. However noble and right it is to disclose errors, the current litigious culture makes it nearly impossible for care providers to willingly divulge their mistakes, a problem not addressed in the IOM report. Their fear of malpractice suits and their resulting tendency to remain silent about errors could easily keep care providers from moving beyond the status quo of error management. In addition, the malpractice system is unlikely to change in the near future, and alternative methods of dispute resolution are unlikely to be instituted. On the other hand, changes in how errors are dealt with should not wait until the legal system is corrected.

> **Point To Ponder**
>
> *Safety is a cultural matter, and unless you create a cultural environment in which it becomes safe to talk about errors and near misses, you cannot get to work on the root causes of error.*
> —Donald Berwick

For one thing, care providers could be better trained in how to disclose errors and how to maintain a relationship with a patient after an injury caused by a medical error. Not only are leaders challenged to create a culture that supports disclosure, but in many cases they will need to provide educational processes for developing postdisclosure management skills. The acquiring of the skills necessary to handle disclosure appropriately requires incredible effort from every member of the health care team and patience for the expertise to emerge. Following is a set of guidelines for discussing errors (Wu et al. 1997):

- Treat the situation as bad news.
- Begin by saying that you regret that you have made a mistake.
- Describe what happened and the decisions made.
- Describe the course of events using nontechnical language.
- State the nature of the mistake.
- Describe the corrective action and any consequences.
- Express personal regret and apology.
- Listen to them—accept, empathize, and answer questions.

Care Provider Disenfranchisement

In addition to the fear of litigation, barriers to the disclosure of medical errors include shame, emotional upset, early denial, grief, and dread of the patient's reaction. It is painfully obvious that medical errors harm not only the patient but also the care provider. Feelings of guilt and worry about potential job loss and professional isolation are all too common. When a serious error occurs, the fear of repercussion demoralizes even the most competent care provider. The frustration and demoralization that follows the making of an error negatively impacts productivity and future practice not only for the person committing the error but for other providers in the practice environment. These providers may feel relief that they did not commit the error but will realize that it is all too probable that they will commit errors in the future and be faced with similar emotional upset.

OPPORTUNITIES FOR HEALTH CARE SERVICE

Once errors are perceived as opportunities, they can be managed using several new approaches. These new approaches, including modified interventions for addressing errors, are consistent with a new mental model of error that is more positive and reinforces the quest for excellence rather than perfection.

System versus Individual Errors

Identifying and understanding the source of an error or set of errors is an essential first step in identifying breakdowns and opportunities for improvement (Exhibit 5–5). Unfortunately, the information needed to achieve this step is commonly lacking, partially because those responsible for the errors are reluctant to volunteer what they know. An incomplete analysis of the situation stalls the process and can lead to inappropriate recommendations. The quality of the information surrounding an error affects the quality and sustainability of the follow-up interventions. Once all of the information is collected, the source of error can be localized, and the interactions between the individual and the system and their role in causing the less than desirable outcome can be examined.

Much rhetoric has been devoted to system-related causes of medical errors, partly as a result of the significant publicity generated by the recent IOM (2001) report on patient

Exhibit 5–5 Key Concepts

- **Adverse event:** An injury caused by medical management rather than by the underlying disease or condition of the patient.
- **Accident:** An event that involves damage to a defined system that disrupts the ongoing or future output of that system (Kohn et al. 2000).
- **Breakdown:** Situations that unfold in undesirable ways as the result of team members' performance, the unavailability of essential resources, and system problems (Benner et al. 1999).
- **Error:** The failure of a planned action to be completed as intended (error of execution) or the use of a wrong plan to achieve an aim (error of planning) (Kohn et al. 2000).
- **Mistake:** An error in action, opinion, or judgment caused by poor reasoning, carelessness, or insufficient knowledge.
- **Safety:** Freedom from accidental injury.

safety and medical errors. The media, policy makers, health care providers, and the public have all expressed concern and urged that something be done, and consequently health care leaders are expected to pay special attention to the system-related problems.

Although the IOM report emphasized the importance of system-related factors for reducing the incidence of errors, such as safety systems, job design, and medication administration, the solution does not lie in an either/or approach (Exhibit 5–6).

Although the problem is not one of bad people working in health care but of good people working in bad systems, those bad systems are created by people—people who have the capacity to fix them. Further, the systems approach used by itself has the disadvantage that it

- decreases attention to particular aspects of care, especially in the area of relationships
- flattens out beneficial variations in practice
- promotes a false and distorting vision of medicine as solely technical
- weakens the moral commitment of professionals (Benner 2000)

In other words, including both system-related factors and individual behavior in error analysis is important if leaders are to develop new approaches to error management that are effective and sustainable.

> **Key Point**
>
> *When an error occurs, do not react immediately. Take a deep breath and share your feelings. Learn to ask questions to gain as much information as possible about the error. Avoid the tendency to criticize.*

Further, neither assigning blame by itself nor locating the source of error by itself is likely to minimize the incidence of mistakes. Although each approach may have advantages in the short term, neither will lead to positive outcomes for the system or the individuals in the long term. For one thing, neither the organization nor the individual has total control over the events surrounding an error. Second, employing a sys-

Exhibit 5–6 Comparison of Individual and System Accountability

Individual	**System**
• Professional/legal mandates	• Human factors research
• Emphasizes individual factors	• Emphasizes structure and organizational factors
• Emphasizes individual expertise, thoroughness, and accountability	• Emphasizes standards, automation, and redundancy
• Views individual as locus of responsibility for errors	• Views the system as locus of responsibility for errors
• Aims to assign blame and/or extract compensation	• Aims to decrease guilt and increase honesty in reporting

tems approach by itself is liable to create new patient care risks by minimizing the significance of the individual customization of care and of professionalism, stifling innovation, discounting the relational aspects of practice, mitigating the power of personal responsibility, and spreading responsibility too thinly. Conversely, the individual responsibility model separates care providers from the community.

Remediation versus Discipline

The way in which the accountability of health professionals is defined by state licensing boards tends to push leaders toward instituting disciplinary action against error makers. However, the overall effectiveness of disciplining for improving practice or minimizing errors has not been substantiated. Further, state licensing boards have different reporting requirements. Some states, for instance, require only the reporting of significant errors that resulted in harm, whereas others require the reporting of all errors, including minor ones. The value of reporting minor errors with low risk for harm does not appear to be worth the trauma caused to the care providers.

For these reasons, the strategy of using remediation first and discipline as a last resort deserves consideration (Exhibit 5–7). For one thing, remediation (counseling and guidance provided in a timely manner) serves to protect the care provider's dignity and minimizes shame. In addition, remediation is consistent with the treatment of errors as opportunities for learning new, more effective behaviors.

This strategy also makes the system and the individual both accountable for addressing errors. The person who committed the error is expected to participate in the analysis of the error and identify alternative approaches that will reduce the chance of a recurrence. The other members of the team or work group also review the error and contribute to the list of recommendations. These individuals thereby gain insights that will help them avoid similar errors. In other words, all the members learn not only from their mistakes but from the mistakes of others, which is invaluable both for the individual members, the team, and the organization as a whole.

Finally, the strategy puts the leader of the organization in the position to manage errors without additional reporting to an outside agency. This is an advantage, as the leader is best

Exhibit 5–7 Remediation Guidelines

Consider remediation when
- the potential risk of physical, emotional, or financial harm to the client due to the incident is very low
- the incident is a singular event with no pattern of poor practice
- the employee exhibits a conscientious approach to and accountability for his or her practice
- the employee appears to have knowledge and skill to practice safely

suited to manage minor errors and work with the providers to ensure that these errors are not repeated. Although not traditionally labeled remediators, most leaders are skilled in remediation techniques, especially the giving of feedback. By discussing the situation in private first, by being specific and focusing on the facts, and by following up to increase the chances of success, the leader can reduce minor errors without causing the providers to feel unnecessary shame and guilt.

> **Point To Ponder**
>
> *Learn from the mistakes of others; you can't live long enough to make them all yourself.*
>
> —Anonymous

Errors that carry a significant risk of physical, emotional, or financial harm or errors that show a pattern of recurrence require greater scrutiny and management. The leader should still refrain from using discipline until the system-related and individual issues are evaluated and a pattern of incompetence and/or negligence has been identified. The goal, in the "error as opportunity" approach, is always to learn from errors by focusing on the relationship between the individual and the system and by implementing appropriate revisions in the work processes. Discipline should be the intervention of last resort.

HEALTH CARE LEADERSHIP: ERRORS AND OPPORTUNITIES

Everyone acknowledges that learning comes not only from the successful performance of an activity or practice, but also from mistakes—from breakdowns or situations that did not go well. But most people are reluctant to reveal their failures, especially at work in front of others. And this in itself is an error! The reluctance to talk about mistakes means the whole team risks losing vital pieces of information that can be derived from looking at the mistakes carefully. Even worse, the likelihood that others will repeat the same mistakes increases dramatically.

Clinical errors do not occur in isolation. As noted in the IOM report, an organization's system—its structures and processes—has a large impact on the incidence of errors. Indeed, the system not only is the most important influence on the type and number of errors that are committed but also provides the greatest opportunity for improvement. It is through understanding the errors of the past that leaders can redesign the future to support the practices that will minimize system breakdowns and individual mistakes.

Unfortunately, the recognition of errors is not a simple or obvious process. Habitual routines often obviate the need to recognize errors, and it is true that changing what has become established involves some short-term costs. Habitual routines are familiar, comfortable, and usually temporarily successful. However, long-term survival must be the focus. The desire of most leaders to experience stability in their work life makes it difficult for them to admit that the system is not working as well as it could be and that it needs to be revised. Quantum leaders realize that routine practices, standard operating procedures, and traditional protocols seldom meet organizational needs for any extended length of time. Constant tinkering with processes is always necessary to ensure continuous goodness of fit with the environment.

Traditional leaders have tended to put a premium on "being right." They have wanted to be seen as a competent, comprehensive resource and thereby win the respect of the employees. Nowadays, in contrast, leaders and their teams must learn to become comfortable quickly acknowledging the existence of outdated processes, suboptimal choices, and leadership mistakes and to move on regardless of the investment. They must identify current practices that are not working or have become obstacles to providing health care services and then tinker with them so that they function better. In most cases, these practices should not be looked on as errors but rather as outdated. They simply no longer fit the organization's needs and currently fail to result in the desired outcomes, no matter how effective they were in the past.

The remainder of the chapter consists of a discussion of five leadership errors, associated opportunities for change, and specific strategies for supporting the desired improvements. The purpose here is not to criticize or negate the work of leaders but rather to focus on common problems and stretch creative thinking to support our journey into the Information Age, where error is opportunity. The five errors are as follows:

1. failure to shift to value-based health care services
2. failure to own health care products
3. fragmented leadership
4. dehumanization of health care providers
5. demanding the impossible

Error 1: Failure To Shift to Value-Based Health Care Services

Dramatic changes in health care have occurred over the last 30 years, most notably in the area of reimbursement. Unfortunately, few if any health care structures have changed to the extent needed to ensure the delivery of high-quality health care services.

Financial resources have become the focus of clinical decision making. Financial officers work diligently to maximize reimbursement and reduce expenses while care providers do their best to deliver the comprehensive care expected by consumers. Many health care leaders continue to believe that good financial performance will support clinical quality in the same way as in the past. The role of finance has become so important, in fact, that in many organizations the chief financial officer has a line position and controls processes and operations, whereas the medical director holds a staff position and offers input and suggestions but is impotent to control patient care services. Such changes in authority and decision making, although perhaps not reflected in the organizational chart, are otherwise explicitly recognized.

For many health care providers, these role changes interfere with the real work of the organization, and they view health care leadership these days as more like *dealership*. Health plan contract negotiations are based almost solely on actuarial data and the expectation that patients will use the least amount of services available. Further, although recognizing that both productivity and a healthy financial base are essential for survival, care providers find it disconcerting these are to be achieved at the expense of patient care quality. In short, health care organizations have failed to adapt the health care system to the changing supply-and-demand factors and marketplace values, and this failure is the source of the incredible chaos being experienced by leaders, care providers, payers, and the public.

Prior to the advent of prospective payment systems, the issue of value was only a minor one. Expenses were covered by payers interested in increasing the access to health care services. Leaders worked to expand the types and numbers of services they offered in order to keep their organizations competitive. In this model, there is no accountability and no control. Not surprisingly, resources ran out, and the public rebelled against escalating health care expenditures. The imperative for leaders continues to be to reconnect the system with the marketplace and reestablish a balance between service (the providing of assistance), quality, and cost.

The separation of marketplace value and clinical outcomes was tolerable when no connection was expected in the marketplace. Consumers received the services provided, and the payers reimbursed providers as billed. Health care value in the retrospective payment system was determined by the provider, not by the patient. It is important to note that provider behavior was not intended to diminish the importance of fiscal issues. There was simply no demand for real fiscal accountability. Providers were expected to provide the best of everything. They delivered as many health care services as possible. Functional, role, and clinical issues were of central concern, not financial issues. In fact, discussion of financial issues by care providers was considered inappropriate and was discouraged.

Opportunity 1: Practice within the Marketplace

As they begin the journey of shifting organizational work to support marketplace values, leaders need to keep in mind how health care got to its current state of chaos. The main causal factor is the current imbalance between the types and amount of services being provided and the dollars available for their purchase. In fact, the lack of dollars has created serious instability in the marketplace. In many organizations, changes are being implemented to shift the focus back to the provision of health care services within the marketplace parameters. Unfortunately, not all organizations have begun the work of transformation, and some have yet to identify the revisions that are called for.

Every health care leader must critically assess the services his or her organization provides to ensure that they are consistent with the organization's mission. Fixing marketplace errors requires a shift from managing for profit to managing for the organizational mission of delivering value-based health care. The process of fitting care to the available dollars cannot begin without an understanding of the value that is being bartered. Reducing or controlling services without a clear notion of the value each discipline contributes to clinical outcomes is like taking a shot in the dark. At best, it is an example of irresponsible leadership.

What Is Value?

It is not uncommon for leaders to be unsure of the real value of the services provided by health care providers in their organizations. Some providers are not sure of this themselves! There must be evidence that shows that resources are being used efficiently to bring about clear improvements in patient conditions, increase the ability of the patients to manage their own health, and add to the patients' knowledge of their conditions and/or healthy behaviors. This is quite different from providing services as defined in a standards manual.

Determining the value of health care services is an integral part of quantum leadership. This value, which is defined by means of an equation containing the three elements of cost, quality, and service, is never simply a matter of dollars (Malloch and Porter-O'Grady 1999). Instead, its calculation takes into account what is actually gained and what are the real costs. The exact equation is expressed thus: health care value = resources (funds and labor and supplies) + quality (appropriateness of interventions) + service (satisfaction and effective relationships).

Finding the value of a health care service requires health care leaders and care providers to ask the following questions:

- What is the actual service provided?
- How do organizational processes support this service?
- What are the interactions between these processes?
- What impact does the service have on the patients and the community?

The answers to these questions guide leaders and health care providers toward wise choices—toward clinical decisions that are the most cost effective and result in the highest quality care being provided at the lowest cost. The challenge for leaders is to reframe the health care quality issue as a value question. Again, value is defined as the result of an interactive process involving cost, quality, and service. The cost of health care in the marketplace is determined by both the available resources and reimbursement; the quality of the service is determined by the outcome of the service (i.e., how delivery of the service changes the patient's state of health); and service, which is the rendering of assistance, is partly a function of the time and manner of provision.

Within this framework, the marketplace phenomenon becomes apparent. The value equation is out of balance in that too much care is being provided given the level of available dollars—or too few resources are being applied to health care. The greatest opportunity or leverage point for changing the value equation begins with the element of service, not the cost or quality. If there are limited resources, questions arise such as this: Should the response to every sign or symptom be some type of intervention, particularly if it results in minimal or no improvement in the patient's clinical condition? What an incredibly difficult challenge it is for providers and leaders to deal with the issue of rationing, especially those schooled in the philosophy that increased access to health care is always in the public's interest. Indeed, rationing of health care services has traditionally been seen as incongruent with the American spirit. Of course, the reality is that it has occurred throughout history; it is just more obvious when the issue moves beyond the closed ranks of health professionals to the community at large.

The Metrics of Value-Based Health Care

To determine the value of health care, leaders and providers are faced with deciding what should be measured. What are the metrics of success? What constitutes value for the consumer? How are all of the metrics interrelated? Current financial management is concerned with statistics such as net income margin, net present value, return on equity, return on investment, and return on assets. These metrics are unfamiliar to clinicians and are very different from the metrics they see as vital, such as responsiveness to treatment, level of pain management, and wound healing.

Traditionally, the financial mindset has focused on return on investment for dollars spent. This measure has limited applicability in health care. In a return-on-investment analysis, the cost-benefit ratio shows the worth of spending dollars to make dollars. If the benefits of a health care program or service can be priced in dollars, then a cost-benefit analysis is appropriate, and the alternative that leads to the greatest dollar benefits for the cost has a good claim to be chosen. However, many health care decisions and services involve far more than simply generating income. In fact, health care dollars are often spent on a clinical problem to improve the outcomes of patient care, and ascribing a monetary value to a health outcome is a complex if not impossible task. Another issue is that cost-benefit analysis is not sensitive to health care objectives, including the psychological benefits of improved health, the psychological and physiological benefits of clean air and water, and so on.

> **Point To Ponder**
>
> *Business must be run for a profit . . . else it will die. But when anyone tries to run a business solely for a profit, . . . then the business must die, for it no longer has a reason for existence.*
>
> *—Henry Ford*

Increasingly, health care leaders are switching to cost-effectiveness analysis (Buerhaus 1998). Instead of measuring benefits and costs in dollars, a cost-effectiveness analysis uses units such as years of life saved to measure health outcomes and dollars to measure the cost of the treatment. Although a cost-effectiveness analysis cannot determine whether a single program's benefits outweigh its costs, it can be used to compare alternative programs.

It is nearly impossible to draw conclusions about services on the basis of a single metric. Multiple influencing factors must be considered in reaching decisions on allocating resources. Health care leaders are best advised to develop a matrix of metrics in which multiple essential indicators are considered in the evaluation of resource use. Cost-effectiveness should be measured in the aggregate from the multiple perspectives of quality, productivity, and cost and from the patient, care provider, and organization levels. Blending the cultures of finance and health care is challenging at best, but it can be made somewhat more manageable if everyone understands the common ground shared by finance and health professionals—they are all dependent on their checkbooks and their health, neither of which is able to exist effectively without the other!

Giving up Non–Valued-Added Services

Most health care providers assume that every service provided is an essential service, and that there are no opportunities for changing service patterns. They believe that if a service did not make a difference to the health of patients—did not add value in terms of increased well-being—they would not be providing it. Yet most providers have not examined each service to determine whether it really does affect the clinical conditions of patients, enhance the patients' understanding of their conditions, or increase their ability to manage their own health. In many cases, services are provided to conform to standards but without improving patient outcomes.

Consider a patient who suffers from chronic uncontrolled diabetes. The patient is regularly hospitalized for stabilization and treatment. During each hospitalization, the patient receives diabetic education and attends two information sessions, in accordance with the established standard of care. Despite the instruction, the patient and family have never been able to commit to the required dietary changes, nor do they plan to make any changes. In this case, the diabetic education has failed to make a difference in terms of clinical stability, knowledge of the disease, or ability to manage the patient's health; consequently, it is a non–value-added service. Given the overwhelming workload of the providers, the service should be provided to this patient in an abbreviated form or possibly not at all. The patient medical record should reflect the reality of the situation, namely, that continuing education was considered but not implemented because of the lack of expected clinical effect.

When services that fail to add value are discovered, the leader must support the team in eliminating them, a daunting task at best. Fear of the unknown often overrides the need to change, feeding organizational inertia and reinforcing assumptions that the current way is the right and only way to do the work. Limited resources and concern about short-term costs can further impede progress. The leader's challenge is to create a culture in which all members are expected to continually seek better and more efficient ways of providing services and eliminate practices that are no longer effective.

Group Discussion

Consider the impact of an organizationwide policy that required the elimination of two policies for every new policy created. Would the outcome be the creation of more or fewer policies? Would the value of health care increase or decrease as a result of such an all-embracing organizational policy? Who might oppose the policy and who might favor it?

Once the leader is able to identify what actual services are delivered, what outcomes they produce, and what their costs are, the dialogue with managed care organizations (MCOs) changes dramatically. If the MCO negotiators want to decrease premiums, the leader can now translate the reduction into a decrease in services. Conversely, the leader can request premium increases to match improvements in patient outcomes. No longer will it be expected that the services will remain the same despite a reduction in available dollars. Further, the amount of negotiating power will be determined by the value produced rather than the number of individuals around the table or their negotiating tenacity. Decisions should be made from a consumer value perspective.

Team-Based Health Care

In order for health care services and leadership practices to receive the kind of critical examination that is needed, the leader and the other team members must undergo a renewal of team spirit and show a willingness to challenge the status quo and expose the sacred cows of health care. No provider should decide alone what to do for patients. Engaging in dialogue with each other is the only way providers can ensure that their value-based goals are achieved. In addition, dialogue between providers minimizes the potential for system breakdown and error. As collaboration increases, the team becomes more competent in frontline quality management and system repair. It then is able not only to monitor service value but to act as the agent in monitoring and managing system breakdowns. The quantum leader must create the context in which the necessary communication skills are both valued and expected.

Regardless of past practices, every decision made by a provider should take into account the choices and decisions of others. In practice, providers seldom act as a team in implementing interventions and evaluating care, and each provider delivers the kind of care that those within the provider's discipline believe is best (as indicated by the discipline's established practice standards). To combat unilateral decision making and ensure a good fit between decisions made along the continuum of care, providers and patients must exhibit a strong pattern of communication and interaction.

Error 2: Failure To Own Health Care Products

The increasing involvement of external agencies in determining appropriate health care services sounds an alarm for even the most inexperienced health care leader. Regardless of perceived past failures of health care organizations to manage internal processes, the return of health care oversight and management to the point of service is needed to minimize bureaucracy and support the shift toward using errors as opportunities for improvement rather than punishment.

Perhaps the chaos of the transition from a retrospective payment system to a fixed payment system has blurred the expectations of all stakeholders. The expectation for health care systems is that processes are in place to ensure that services are both effective and provided within the marketplace parameters. The oversight of staffing, scheduling, pain management, advance directives, and so on, by external agencies interferes with the performance and accountability of the internal leadership, yet the public call for organizations to meet the core responsibilities of error management, safe staffing, and pain management reinforces the notion that health care leaders have not previously been held sufficiently accountable.

Besides dealing with unclear expectations and uncertainty, health care leaders face intense financial pressures that distort the order of their stewardship obligations, which should be service first, survival second, and profit third. They also often are placed in ethical dilemmas in which the right decision is hard to determine, let alone carry out. As evidence of this, fraud and abuse stories have become all too common in the press. It seems that the prevalence of such stories is partly explained by the fact that leaders are in the position of desperately searching for financial revenues and sometimes choose questionable methods. Of course, not only is fraud, when uncovered, detrimental to the reputation of the organization, but the intense scrutiny that follows its discovery creates an atmosphere of mistrust between care providers, payers, and the government. Yet, although fraud is a criminal matter that must be addressed in the court system, there are many issues that are better managed internally. The challenge for leaders is to determine which issues are best managed internally and which issues must be managed externally.

Opportunity 2: Moving from External Oversight to Internal Accountability

There is a pronounced need for less external regulation and more professional accountability within organizations. The locus of accountability for clinical quality lies within each profession, and the content is defined by its standards. The accountability for an organization's systems, structures, and processes rests with the leaders, and the content is defined by the organization's mission, vision, and values. The control or oversight of the organization's services and leadership rests with the governing board, for its members understand the needs and expectations of the community being served much better than any external accrediting agency could. It should not be necessary for business and government agencies to force or direct care providers and organizations to address issues such as the high incidence of medical errors or perform their essential duties as providers of health care.

Living Accountability

Accountability-based health care is an essential foundation for the "error as opportunity" approach recommended in this chapter. To ensure accountability for system processes, expectations for performance must be clearly defined for and shared by all members of the organization, and performance that meets the stated expectations must be recognized and rewarded routinely. In addition, incompetence or failure to live the expected behaviors must be dealt with in a timely manner. All too often, leaders ignore incompetence because they want to avoid confrontation. Hoping that the problem will simply disappear is unrealistic and damaging to the morale of the organization, for it has the effect of lowering the performance standards. Quantum leaders are competent not only at managing incompetence but also at coaching other team members in managing incompetence. They know that managing incompetence is strongly associated with improved organizational performance and increased employee morale as well as decreased errors.

Political Competence

Developing political skills is essential for all members of the quantum organization. In the past, health care leaders have played a role in devising and implementing health-related policies at the local, state, and national levels, but as organizations increase the extent of their team-based activities, political competence will be a requirement for all employees involved in providing services.

> ### Key Point
>
> *Political competence is the dual capacity to accurately assess the impact of public policies on performance of one's area of responsibility and secondly the ability to influence public policy making.*
>
> *—Beaufort Longest*

Political competence is defined by Longest (1998) as the dual capacity to accurately assess the impact of public policies on one's area of responsibility and to influence public policy making at both the state and local levels. For each health care service offered by an organization, the organization's leaders must understand the service and try to determine the expected impact of public policies and the policies of accrediting organizations and health plans on the service. Further, each member of the organization must understand the internal policies that apply to the provision of services and know when to communicate concerns to the organization's leaders, when to use positional power to exert influence on policy makers, and when to remove or mitigate barriers to care to ensure that the services are provided.

Group Discussion

Health care providers are under pressure to discharge patients according to protocols and guidelines. When patients fall outside the guidelines, it is the providers who must advocate for lengthier stays with insurance companies and who, when their requests are denied, are put in the untenable position of discharging patients under unsafe conditions. As leader of the surgical unit, you believe patients are often being discharged prematurely, especially patients who are unsteady and not voiding well. In this situation, what is your obligation as leader? What information should you be communicating, and when and to whom should you be communicating it? What changes in practice are recommended? What rationale for these changes is likely to garner the most support?

Politically competent health care providers are also able to assist regulators and legislators in creating solutions and to describe the clinical and economic value of health care services to patients, purchasers, and policy analysts. Organizational policies and procedures are designed to incorporate professional standards, define expectations, and enhance service quality. When policies exist that are inconsistent with standards, contradict expectations, or impede service quality, politically competent providers can communicate the issues of concern and facilitate the revision of the policies.

Error 3: Fragmented Leadership

Traditional health care organizations rely on clinical professionals to deliver the services defined by the mission, and they rely on management professionals to make the service processes more efficient and effective. Given that the clinical and management professions have different knowledge bases and values, clinicians and managers are sometimes at odds with each other. However, their differences have become increasingly problematic for the delivery of health care services as the environment has been affected by burdensome new payer constraints, increasing competition for a larger share of diminishing resources, and a lack of qualified health care workers. Indeed, the internal competition between clinicians and managers has negatively affected productivity and, more importantly, discouraged innovation.

Because of the ongoing financial pressure and competition experienced by health care organizations, patient care often loses out to financial priorities. In fact, left with few opportunities for reducing expenses, health care leaders often end up searching for ways of managing the demand for health care services rather than managing expenses.

Most health care leaders are experts on health care infrastructure and marketplace principles. Very few are experts on clinical care and marketplace principles. As a result, many organizations are struggling because their leaders do not have clinical competence and are making decisions solely from a financial perspective. No longer can health care organizations afford leaders incapable of integrating patient care needs and financial survival.

Opportunity 3: Holographic Leadership

The strategy of minimizing competition between financial and clinical priorities and increasing collaboration demands a new model of health care leadership. Leaders in quan-

---

Group Discussion

Imagine a health care organization in which the leaders were competent in both clinical and management disciplines. Speculate on how the organization would be structured. What roles would be added or eliminated? Would the patient care outcomes likely be different? In what way? Would job satisfaction be affected? Summarize the advantages and disadvantages of this model.

---

tum health care organizations need to be competent and knowledgeable in both health care and marketplace management. The position of chief executive or patient care administrator should be occupied by someone who has advanced clinical training (e.g., a physician, nurse, social worker, or physical therapist) and has expertise in the management of these clinical services. The chief executive's knowledge base should include an understanding of how services are provided, what their outcomes are, how to estimate costs, and how to determine the availability of reimbursement. A background in the business end of health care is not by itself sufficient for leading a 21st-century health care organization, and neither is experience as a clinical provider.

> ### Point To Ponder
>
> *In business, the measure of success is the bottom line, a matter of dollars. This, however, is not the purpose of leadership, for achieving that bottom line measurement requires many skills as well as a commitment of character.*
> — *Alan Axelrod*

As the health care environment changes, so too does the set of critical leadership competencies. The new competencies reflect an integrated or holographic perspective on the health care experience that encompasses the technical, relational, and intentional aspects of patient care. The quantum health care leader must have a clear understanding of the procedural work of providers and must possess the skills to connect providers to the service and system infrastructure in such a way as to ensure value-based care is delivered within the limits of the available resources. Health care provided without a specific intention or without effective relationships between providers is fragmented care, and fragmented care is no longer acceptable or affordable.

Necessarily, all operational or line positions in health care require knowledge, skills, and abilities that jointly reflect a holographic health care perspective. Operational positions are held by health care employees accountable for ensuring that the value equation is balanced. Staff positions are those positions that support the work of the organization but do not require clinical competence. In many ways, this model should suit those who were in traditional staff positions but were pushed into operational roles without being given adequate

Group Discussion

Some leaders focus on processes alone, others on outcomes alone, still others on both processes and outcomes. What are the consequences for the organization when the leader is process oriented? When the leader is outcome oriented? When the leader is both process and outcome oriented? Compare the differing effects of the three approaches. What are the advantages and disadvantages of each? Which approach fits best with holographic leadership?

training. Such professionals (e.g., finance officers) are now expected to do what they do best without the additional burden of making decisions in areas in which they lack expertise. Experts in planning, human resources, and finance are ideally suited for staff or consultant positions, and together they can participate as team members in a shared leadership team model.

Leaders at the beginning of the new millennium must determine the most effective and efficient processes to achieve the three goals of high-quality patient care, organizational viability, and respectable profits. Given that health care economists focus on the supply and demand for services, reimbursement mechanisms, productivity, the impact of technology, work force issues, market dynamics, and health-related public policy, it is incumbent upon care providers to provide a clear description of the health care services and their outcomes, the time and skill level requirements for each service, and the cost of providing each service so that the economists can analyze the aforementioned factors and their relationships accurately.

Error 4: Dehumanization of Health Care Providers

The financial pressure experienced by health care organizations not only has impacted the type and number of services afforded patients but also has altered the way organizational leaders are managing health care providers. In some cases, the providers perceive their treatment as uncaring and ruthless and see themselves as pawns. As evidence, providers can point to regular rounds of staff reductions, staffing by ratios, elimination of continuing education programs, and the use of hiring bonuses.

Work Force Reductions

The elimination of leadership and care provider positions with little or no warning has seriously marred the morale of the health care work force. Competent leaders and care providers are finding it increasingly difficult to rebound and find new employment. Regardless of how the termination is handled, they find it nearly impossible to live with the notion that "it's not personal, it's business" when their livelihood has been dramatically altered.

The hidden costs that result from the disruption of relationships in the workplace have yet to be measured. One hidden cost is the loss of departing employees' knowledge of the job and the other workers and the organization. Another is the reduction in needed competence and experience, which, if severe enough, can lead to a phenomenon known as *failure to rescue* (described below). Further, because length of employment usually determines who gets let go, newly hired employees with up-to-date skills and knowledge are eliminated in favor of employees who have minimal or outdated competencies.

To understand the harm that can occur from work force reductions, consider the critical surveillance role played by nurses. Indeed, their vigilance is essential to rescuing many patients who have experienced a complication. In such a situation, nurses must first recognize that a complication has occurred or is impending, then they must intervene rapidly to ensure the patient's survival. When nurse staffing levels are reduced, the ability of the nurses on the floor to recognize a potential or an actual problem is compromised, sometimes to the extent that they fail to save a patient who might otherwise have survived.

Another common effect of decreasing the number of competent registered nurses is the implementation of mandatory overtime. In fact, more than 70 percent of hospitals in the United States have formal mandatory overtime requirements. Making health care providers put in extra hours can push them beyond their physical limits and reduce their ability to perform competently. Tired and overworked care providers are poorly suited for the level of clinical surveillance required for quality patient care.

Finally, in addition to reductions in the absolute number of nurses employed, licensed personnel are being replaced with unlicensed care providers, thereby diluting the skill mix. As a cost-saving measure, the shift to employing fewer licensed care providers has not been particularly successful. Not only do the overall number of hours of care increase when the licensed hours are decreased, but the level of surveillance also declines dramatically. There is no substitute for having a reasonable number of highly trained nurses provide care to the patients.

Staffing by Ratios

Staffing levels are closely tied to the incidence of medical errors. The potential of inappropriate staffing to cause an increase in the number of medical errors is generally recognized but not always taken into account in an organization's decision making. The reality is that there is little evidence to use in determining the necessary level of staffing to ensure that the quality of patient care is maintained, organizational goals are met, and the providers' working conditions are acceptable. Studies intended to assess the effects of different ratios of patients to registered nurses are numerous and conflicting. Thus, historical averages of hours of care provided for each patient are typically used as the basis of daily staffing.

The problem is that this technique wrongly assumes that the needs of all patients are essentially the same and, more importantly, that the skills of nurses are comparable. Instead, patient needs vary widely, as do levels of nursing competence. Indeed, if an historically based ratio is used, such as four patients to one nurse, the chance that there will be a match between patient care needs and on-the-job personnel is low. For example, on some days the correct ratio for meeting patient needs adequately might be three to one, whereas on other days it might be five to one. Frustration increases for both patients and providers when there is no adjustment in staffing, up or down, to meet the identified needs.

Evidence-based staffing confronts leaders with two challenges. First, although providers often dislike ratio staffing, they have difficulty when assignment ratios vary among colleagues. For example, nurses expect to be given reasonable workloads, but even when patient acuity is lower than average, they still resist accepting an assignment with a higher than average patient-nurse ratio. Getting nurses to understand and accept assignments based on workload instead of numbers is a challenge for leaders—and an opportunity.

The second challenge is to determine which health care interventions contribute to meeting patient care needs and how effective they are. The main problem is that the nature and types of interventions vary widely from organization to organization and from provider to provider. Valid and reliable information that demonstrates the value of each provider's contribution is sorely needed because it will improve the dialogue between care providers and leaders and help them find meaningful solutions to managing the workload.

Developmental Freeze

Equally demoralizing for providers is the inconsistency of leadership support for continuing education aimed at giving them skills they need to function effectively in the changing marketplace. Elimination of funding for continuing education programs, both internal and external, commonly occurs when resources become strained. The strategy of requiring employees to attend seminars on vacation time at personal expense and limiting out-of-state travel reimbursement sends a strong negative message as to the value of continuous learning to the organization.

In addition, these restrictions increase the probability of failure-to-rescue incidents and other crises. The unavoidable breakdowns that occur in providing patient care and in the organization's systems require quick responses to prevent the breakdowns from developing into full-blown catastrophes. Most educational programs focus on giving providers the knowledge and skills they require to meet current standards of practice, but few offer learning opportunities that would allow providers to develop the proper skills for responding to imminent breakdowns. As the environment changes, so will the skills and interventions needed to manage developing crises, and continuous learning is a requisite for gaining the competence to address the kind of breakdowns that are likely to occur in the present.

Hiring Bonuses

In desperation, leaders sometimes use economic enticements to recruit needed health care providers. The practice of offering sign-on bonuses is based on two assumptions—that individuals usually will act in ways that they think will make them better off, and that they generally believe that *better off* means more money. The reality is that each person has his or her own preference map and that dangling cash before health care providers does not always induce the desired behaviors. Besides money, providers want respect, involvement in decision making, and good relationships with colleagues, among other things. The bonus model, by treating providers as shallow and materialistic, has the effect of disparaging them. Some providers, of course, will respond to the enticement of a financial bonus in given situations, but most are motivated by a combination of social, emotional, and material needs, not just led by the dollar.

Sign-on bonuses also send the wrong message to existing staff, especially long-time employees, who will likely feel resentment because they have not gotten bonuses for their loyalty. Sign-on bonuses therefore tend to reduce employee morale and create a revolving door, which can seriously impact patient care. Further, there is no way the sign-on bonuses can neutralize the cost of turnover, which is between $5,000 and $50,000 per nurse. The assumption of sign-on bonuses is that health care providers are for sale to the highest bidder and are willing to go across the street for dollars. They thus cause competition among health care organizations as well.

Opportunity 4: Revaluing Health Care Providers as Vital Capital

The health care marketplace can hardly support guarantees of lifetime employment for anyone. Yet there are other options besides discarding employees whenever the marketplace demands change. In fact, some of these options, by respecting the dignity of the individual and encouraging creativity and innovation, are more likely to improve an organization's long-term performance than cyclical episodes of mass layoffs. The challenge for leaders is to make hiring and firing decisions from a broad perspective that takes into account multiple performance indicators, not merely the monthly cash flow or short-term costs. In particular, these decisions should be based on a full consideration of the effects of staff reductions and restructuring on patient care outcomes and on the ability of care providers to provide health care services efficiently and effectively.

Given the increasing documentation that experienced and credential employees have a positive impact on patient outcomes, other approaches to managing the work force are indicated. The first step is to shift to a type of evidence-based decision making that considers not only financial indicators but also the intellectual capital profile of the employees. The second step is to look at both short- and long-term effects of resource decisions. (Exhibit 5–8 contains a list of studies that show impact of staffing on patient outcomes and health care provider satisfaction.)

Evidence-Based Staffing

Effective staffing is a matter not just of numbers but of mix. It requires developing new and creative strategies to manage the combination of predictable and unpredictable workloads and the availability and supply of experienced and competent health care providers. Given that at least 80 percent of the health care workload is predictable and repeatable, one challenge is to develop a work force suitable for this portion of the workload. Core staffing must be able to meet the identified range of care needs on a shift-by-shift and day-to-day basis. The second challenge is to handle the remaining 20 percent of the workload—the unpredictable portion. Because the services needed are unpredictable, it is futile to attempt to plan for and manage this portion. People generally do not call ahead and schedule trauma, deliveries, and medical emergencies with any sensitivity to the time of day or the availability of care providers! The goal, therefore, is to build enough flexibility into the

---

Exhibit 5–8 Nurse Staffing and Patient Outcomes: Selected References

Aiken, L.H., et al. 1996. Downsizing the hospital nursing workforce. *Health Affairs* 15, no. 4: 88–92.

Behner, K.G., et al. 1990. Nursing resource management: Analyzing the relationship between costs and quality in staffing decisions. *Health Care Management Review* 15, no. 4: 63–71.

Blegen, M., et al. 1998. Nurse staffing and patient outcomes. *Nursing Research* 47, no. 1: 43–50.

Bolton, L.B., et al. 2001. A response to California's mandated nursing ratios. *Journal of Nursing Scholarship* 33: 179–184.

U.S. Department of Health and Human Services. Nurse staffing and patient outcomes in hospitals. Available at http://www.hrsa.gov/dn/staffstudy.htm.

Kovner, C. and P.J. Gergen. 1998. Nurse staffing levels and adverse events following surgery in U.S. hospitals. *Image: Journal of Nursing Scholarship* 30: 315–321.

Oermann, M.H., and D. Huber. 1999. Patient outcomes: A measure of nursing's value. *American Journal of Nursing* 99, no. 9: 40–47.

Shullanberger, G. 2000. Nurse staffing decisions: An integrative review of the literature. *Nursing Economics* 18, no. 3: 124–148.

Group Discussion

In many organizations, when staff reductions are needed, those with least seniority are eliminated rather than those with greater seniority. Seldom is consideration given to the specific skills and credentials of those who are let go. Review the following research data and create a plan to manage the next round of staff reductions in your organization.

- Compared with other health care providers, certified nurses report fewer adverse events, have higher patient satisfaction ratings, and are more effective communicators and collaborators with other providers.
- An extra hour of nursing care is related to fewer urinary tract infections, a decrease in pneumonia, and a decrease in the probability of postoperative blood clots.
- As the number of medical residents, registered nurses, registered pharmacists, medical technologists, and total hospital personnel per occupied bed increases, mortality rates decrease.

Should the plan take into account employee longevity? If so, how? What effects on patient outcomes should the new model be expected to have? Who will support the new model and who will oppose it?

staffing to ensure appropriate care providers will be on hand to respond quickly to an unscheduled event. Meeting these two challenges requires two very different philosophies regarding staff availability and compensation.

To regain the respect and support of employees, leaders must learn to manage employees continuously and in real time rather than implement regular rounds of layoffs. On the other hand, employees have a corresponding obligation to ensure that their skills and abilities are appropriate to the needs of the organization. When there is a gap between the organization's needs and what the employees are able to offer, change is indicated. How this change is managed is crucial for the organization. First, the leaders and employees must enter into a dialogue to reach a clear understanding of the organization's responsibility to support employee skill enhancement and the employees' responsibility to obtain the desired skills. Regardless, group layoffs that come as a "surprise" serve no useful purpose in the long term. Early collaborative dialogue between employees and leaders on how to respond to changing needs will lead to a more stable work force and greater employee satisfaction.

Staffing for Patient Needs

Attempts to devise accepted national standards for nurse-to-patient ratios have yet to produce meaningful recommendations, and with good reason: facility case mix indices, reimbursement plans, and available support services vary widely. Further, the standards would set average numbers for meeting patient care needs, and these needs, by virtue of their unpredictability, cannot be met by using average numbers for daily staffing. In most organizations, daily patient needs vary at least 20 percent above and below the average, and it is possible that at no time do the actual needs exactly equal the average. In fact, using average numbers in planning the daily staffing discounts the range of nursing activities that are needed to respond to different case mixes.

Revising the nurse-to-patient ratio daily is essential for minimizing discrepancies between patient needs and provider capacities. In some organizations, valid and reliable patient classification systems have been used to determine patient care needs on a shift-by-shift basis. The information gathered becomes the basis for daily staffing and long-term scheduling. Once a representative sample of patient care needs that reflects the full range of needs is determined, the average nurse-to-patient ratios can be calculated. These ratios serve as standards, although they can become problematic when used for shift-to-shift staffing, because they are not sensitive to fluctuations in patient needs, technology, and procedures required.

In determining daily patient care needs and the proper number and mix of providers, leaders need to consider the dynamic interaction of the economic factors, technology, and labor availability. The greatest hope for developing valid standards lies in understanding the interrelationships of nurse-to-patient ratios and patient needs (acuity).

Shared Accountability for Learning

Health care providers have an interest in continuing to acquire more knowledge and develop new skills throughout their career life, and the organizations that employ them share this interest. In fact, investing in their employees is a way for organizations to invest in the future, and therefore it makes sense for any organization to create programs that recognize the continuing education efforts of its providers. The providers, on the other hand, should be willing to make a commitment to continue working for the organization as a quid pro quo. It is not unreasonable for an organization to expect a promise of five years of employment in return for tuition support for a higher education degree. Similarly, if an organization compensates an employee for attending a conference or pays the registration fees, the employee should be expected to share new information with the health care team. The terms of any agreement must be determined prior to the investment.

In cases where employees pay for their own continuing education *and* show improvement in their performance because of their educational efforts, they can rightly expect the organization to recognize their increased ability through some form of compensation, such as an increase in salary. Employees should not suppose the organization will reward educational efforts that fail to affect their performance.

Error 5: Demanding the Impossible

Health care provider assignments are increasingly complex and sometimes overwhelming. Indeed, doable assignments are the exception rather than the norm. Providers, nurses in particular, frequently are demoralized by being asked to do more than they are capable of, and for many the gap between what is being requested and what is possible has grown wider.

The limitations and inflexibility of current staffing and scheduling systems, coupled with the pressure to minimize costs, have prevented leaders from adequately supporting providers who have been given arduous assignments. At best, these providers receive encouragement and sympathy; at worst, they are berated for their inability to manage the workload. Although not the intent of leaders, the result is that employees feel abandoned and mistreated, they seek assistance outside of the organization, and the relationship between the employees and leaders becomes increasingly adversarial.

It is disconcerting for the profession and the community at large to observe providers who believe themselves abandoned by the leaders of the organizations they work for. Exhortations to do one's best are no longer able to counter the professional discouragement felt by providers. As a result, some providers have become openly critical of the health professions, discouraging others from joining or even leaving themselves for another.

Opportunity 5: Managing the Needs-Resources Gap as a Team

Even using the most reliable and valid patient classification systems, leaders are rarely able to match actual patient care needs and staff resources, including hours of staff time. Because some gap between needs and resources is almost inevitable, the challenge for leaders is to create effective systems for managing the gap.

Providers and consumers must engage in a dialogue to identify more precisely clinical care needs, desired outcomes of services, and available resources. In addition, if they discover a gap between needs and resources, they must reevaluate these. Attempting to provide all services regardless of the available resources, as has been the practice in the past, is irresponsible.

Much of the difficulty in identifying and managing the needs-resources gap stems from the failure of society to decide whether health care is a right or privilege. Until society reaches a verdict on this issue, confusion will reign. As clearly as can be determined, health care is a cross between a right and a privilege—a right when you fit the parameters of the government, a privilege when there is limited access and nonemergency services are involved.

Several strategies offer help in minimizing the gap between health care needs and staff resources. These include the following:

- Ensure that the system used to estimate patient care needs is valid and reliable.
- Eliminate non–valued-added services. After carefully examining all services to determine how they impact outcomes, eliminate those that generally fail to have a positive effect.
- Delay noncritical functions until staff resources are available. Some interventions, in order to be effective, depend on the delivery of services at precise times. Other interventions are not time sensitive and can be delayed without compromising the overall treatment. Most medications cannot be delayed, but daily treatments can be moved to the next shift.
- Reexamine previous efforts to call in additional care providers, and move staff from unit to unit to uncover opportunities for putting personnel to better use.

Currently, the responsibility of managing the needs-resources gap is placed on individual providers, increasing their feelings of abandonment. Further, providers are often expected to administer decisions made elsewhere and on the basis of economic factors—

decisions that frequently put patients and families at risk. The above strategies can be used by individual providers to the best of their ability. The most common strategy is to eliminate or delay services, and each provider uses his or her own personal criteria in deciding whether to employ it, as open discussion of the associated issues has been discouraged. Failure of providers to manage their assignments is generally looked upon as a sign of incompetence rather than a sign of system overload. The challenge faced by health care leaders is to shift management of the needs-resources gap from the individual to the health care team—and ultimately to the community, if need be. Accountability for managing the gap must be elevated to the collective level so that health care providers, health care leaders, and the community can work together to find solutions.

Group Discussion

Consider a situation in which a unit is short two nurses. Using the principles of variance management, develop a plan to address the gap. Answer the following questions: When should the discussion about the gap occur? Who should be present? Identify the strategies that will be used (e.g., eliminate nonemergency-related work, request nurses to work overtime, stop admissions). How will the actions taken be documented? What future discussion will occur to avoid the same situation or to prepare for managing a similar situation?

CONCLUSION

It is not errors that are the problem but how we respond to errors when we forget that errors are natural—natural as long as there is any shred of humanness present. By keeping in mind that errors are natural, we will be more likely to recognize that errors, besides causing inconvenience or hardship, offer opportunities for improvement. Unfortunately, most leaders view errors as solely harmful and believe it is their responsibility to discipline those who commit them. They therefore look for someone to blame and possibly punish. Herein lies the problem. The punitive approach to error management encourages secrecy and discourages analysis of the situation and development of strategies to avoid repeat errors.

Any changes to the current system have the potential to threaten the established power base of leaders. The structure of power and the organizational culture often bias the perspectives of those who benefit from the existing system. Alterations in the organization's structure and the roles of its members may increase the power of some members and reduce the power of others. Some will resist reward systems or metrics that diminish their status and authority within the organization. Nevertheless, shifting from a culture of blame to an open culture in which error is perceived as an opportunity for improvement will require leaders to reconsider how power is perceived and used in the organization. Punitive power will become passé and intolerable, while the power of dialogue will emerge as the propulsive force driving the organization toward success.

Managing errors as opportunities and improving our services without debasing our values and subverting our commitment to public safety remain important challenges. The presentation of the five leadership errors discussed in this chapter is intended to heighten the readers' awareness that many long-held practices may no longer be effective. The opportunities discussed are just a few of the many available to creative health care leaders—opportunities waiting only for discovery and testing. One of the opportunities that is currently prevalent, the opportunity to reframe the work of health care using a value-based model, can only serve to enhance a system in which partnerships between patients, families, and providers work to empower the patients to manage their own health.

Finally, even when things are going wrong and mistakes abound, trust in your journey and look for the lesson to be learned. Find the gift in the goof!

REFERENCES

Benner, P., et al. 1999. *Clinical wisdom and interventions in critical care: A thinking-in-action approach.* Philadelphia: Saunders.

Benner, P. Error in medicine: A complex sorrow. Presented at conference, University of California-Berkley, March 11–12, 2000.

Buerhaus, P. 1998. Milton Weinstein's insights on the development, use, and methodologic problems in cost-effectiveness analysis. *Image: Journal of Nursing Scholarship* 30: 223–227.

Institute of Medicine. 2001. *Informing the future: Critical issues in health.* Washington, DC: National Academy of Sciences.

Kaye, L. 2000. The spiritual roots of mistakes. *The Inner Edge* 3, no. 2: 5–7.

Kohn, L.T., J.M. Corrigan, and M.S. Donaldson, eds. 2000. *To err is human: Building a safer health system.* Washington, DC: National Academy Press.

Longest, B. 1998. Managerial competence at senior levels of integrated delivery systems. *Journal of Healthcare Management* 43: 115–135.

Malloch, K., and T. Porter-O'Grady. 1999. Partnership economics: Nursing's challenge in a quantum age. *Nursing Economics* 17: 299–307.

Wu, A.W., et al. 1997. To tell the truth: Ethical and practical issues in disclosing medical mistakes to patients. *Journal of General Internal Medicine* 12: 770–775.

SUGGESTED READINGS

Committee on Quality Health Care in America, Institute of Medicine. 2001. *Crossing the quality chasm: A new health system for the 21st century.* Washington, DC: National Academy Press.

Fagin, C.M. 2001. *When care becomes a burden: Diminishing access to adequate nursing.* New York: Milbank Memorial Fund.

Reason, J. 2000. Human error: Models and management. *British Medical Journal* 320: 768–770.

Rosner, F., et al. 2000. Disclosure and prevention of medical errors. *Archives in Internal Medicine* 160: 2089–2092.

Silber, J.H., et al. 1992. Hospital and patient characteristics associated with death after surgery: A study of adverse occurrence and failure to rescue. *Medical Care* 30: 615–629.

Quiz Questions

Select the best answer for each of the following questions.

1. Marketplace value incorporates the essential factors affecting health care. Which of these factors is not included in the marketplace value equation?

a. available reimbursement
b. time and type of provider
c. return on investment
d. appropriateness of clinical service

2. Errors in health care are inevitable. Given the nature of the interactions between providers, patients, technology, and the environment, errors should be:

a. expected and tolerated
b. managed by the team
c. viewed as opportunities for learning and improvement
d. eliminated at all costs

3. Disclosure and mandatory reporting of errors are both recommended as strategies for managing errors in health care. Why are these two behaviors incompatible?

a. Mandatory reporting removes the safety from disclosure and makes providers unwilling to admit to their errors.
b. Disclosure of errors implies failure.
c. Malpractice cases do not allow disclosure of errors.
d. The goal of mandatory reporting of errors is to establish blame, whereas the goal of disclosing errors is to generate an open dialogue.

4. To shift from external regulation to internal accountability, an organization will require:

a. an increase in the number of committees
b. elimination of licensing requirements
c. the commitment of the leadership to monitor and manage the meeting of health care standards
d. support from the Joint Commission on Accreditation of Healthcare Organizations

5. Cost-effectiveness analysis has been proposed as more appropriate than cost-benefit analysis for evaluating health care services. Its advantages include the fact that it:
a. takes into account health outcomes and the cost of treatment
b. takes into account the cost of treatment and the cost of health outcomes
c. takes into account the cost of the service and the savings achieved
d. uses units such as years of life saved instead of dollars to measure health outcomes

6. Providers have not been able to manage the gap (variance) between patient needs and health care resources effectively because:
a. it is difficult to determine the actual variance
b. the interventions selected by an individual provider to manage the variance are not known to the others on the health care team
c. the individual provider feels abandoned by the system
d. ownership of the problem and the solution rest with the health care team

7. Staffing by ratio (the ratio of patients to providers) requires:
a. sufficient funding
b. a valid and reliable baseline of patient care needs
c. historical trend data to support the ratio
d. approval of the legislature

8. Holographic leadership and fragmented leadership differ:
a. philosophically
b. in the skills required of leaders
c. in the leaders' scope of responsibilities
d. in the degree of financial expertise required of leaders

9. The process of recovering from the negative consequences of committing a medical error has not been discussed openly in the past, most likely because:
a. the emphasis of health care education and practice is on doing things right
b. the threat of lawsuits forces providers to keep silent about the errors they commit
c. most providers do not need guidance in learning to live with errors
d. most providers receive help confidentially

10. Managed care is believed to increase the incidence of error. If this is true, the reason probably is that managed care:
a. removes clinical decision making from the point of service
b. leads to a lack of funding to support quality care
c. encourages the use of noncredentialed providers
d. is more productive and leads to more patients being treated

CHAPTER 6

Emotional Competence:
A Vital Leadership Skill

> The illiterate of the 21st century will not be those who cannot read
> and write, but those who cannot learn, unlearn, and relearn.
> —*Alvin Toffler*

Chapter Objectives

At the completion of this chapter, the reader will be able to

- Explain why the leaders of health care organizations need to attain emotional competence.
- Identify the theoretical underpinnings of the claim that emotional competence is an essential leadership skill.
- Explain the role of self-awareness, compassion, passionate optimism, and impulse control in the development of emotional competence.
- Describe the stages of acquiring emotional competence for the individual and for the team.
- Discuss the challenges of measuring and documenting the organizational impact of emotional competence.

To support the work of the organization, leaders must have not only technical management skills but also skills in managing emotions, theirs as well as those of other individuals in the organization. Emotionally competent leadership exhibits a high regard for colleagues and subordinates, an understanding of basic motivations, as well as basic justice, a willingness to take responsibility, a willingness to correct faulty situations, and a willingness to take positive, quick, and aggressive action when indicated. This chapter examines the philosophical shift in leadership theory necessary for emotional competence to become a recognized essential leadership skill. It also presents behaviors demonstrating leadership emotional competence, including self-awareness, compassion, passionate optimism, and impulse control, and describes five stages of emotional competence acquisition for individuals and teams. Finally, it explores the emotional risks of leadership and the challenges of measuring the impact of emotional competence on organizational performance.

Quantum leaders recognize that they have no more control over organizational outcomes than police officers have over the movement of a large crowd. The officers may be able to herd the crowd in a certain direction for a period of time, but their control over the crowd is only temporary and cursory. As noted in prior chapters, leaders can no longer rely on command-and-control leadership methods and are being challenged to shift to behaviors that support team building and shared decision making and allow all team members to gain an understanding of the work.

Leaders must replace traditional leadership methods with coaching, mentoring, and facilitating. To do this, they must gain an understanding of the emotions and attitudes of all members of the organization and communicate this understanding to everyone else. Only when all members have an appreciation for each other's emotions and share an understanding of the goals of the organization can the real work be accomplished. In short, integrating emotional competence into the leadership model will substantially impact the quality of the work processes and their outcomes.

Managing the feeling side of the organization requires emotional competence. For leaders, emotional competence encompasses the abilities to identify, understand, use, and regulate the emotions that arise during the course of their work. Emotions in organizations are similar to emotions experienced in all walks of life and are seldom definitive of the workplace or personal life. Although it is difficult to separate emotions by setting, this chapter attempts to focus on the typical emotional experience in the workplace and the behaviors that organizational leaders tend to employ.

UNDERPINNINGS OF EMOTIONAL COMPETENCE

The worldview of the quantum leader differs significantly from the traditional Newtonian worldview, and leadership theory for quantum organizations takes into account the realities of dissipative (transforming or chaotic) systems. In these systems, there is spontaneous formation of structures that exchange energy and matter with their environment. Given that health care organizations experience continuous and complex interactions during the formation of the new structures, competence in managing the feeling side of work becomes essential. Following is a description of some quantum organization characteristics that reflect the emotional realities of human systems.

Holism

Quantum organizations are holistic rather than fragmented, which means they recognize the connectedness between work processes and individuals. Holism, as an organizational value, supports the organization's integration with the world besides being inconsistent with organizational structures made up of distinct departments and processes.

Intrinsic Motivation

A quantum organization operates on the principle that human beings, by their very nature, are internally motivated. In other words, the leaders of a quantum organization use a Theory Y style of management and fully recognize the creativity, capability, and motivation of all members of the organization. Further, the leaders do not structure the organization hierarchically, with chains of command encompassing many levels of superiors and subordinates, nor do they believe that the members are inherently lazy and uncreative and always in need of specific directions to be productive. They believe instead that, for members to show initiative, ownership, and high productivity, the only requisites are positive support and a context for performance. Quantum leaders also think that collective wisdom is most likely to emerge when all members are treated as if they are internally motivated to act in the organization's best interests. The idea is that individuals who are valued and encouraged to thrive will make up a synergistic cooperative that itself thrives.

Emergent Leadership

According to quantum leadership theory, organizational leadership emerges from the combined active engagement of all members of the organization. Thus, as the engagement of individuals in the work of the organization increases, the leadership also increases. In this view, leadership is not attached to individuals but rather occurs in the space between individuals. It is not something done by one person (the leader) to many others (the followers), nor is it a role reserved for the people at the top of the organization.

> **Key Point**
>
> *Leadership occurs in the space between individuals working together. It is an emergent property of their relationships and not the management or direction of work by individuals placed in superior positions.*

The model of leadership as emergent differs importantly from the dyadic model of leadership, which is based on hierarchical (superior-subordinate) relationships (Allen 2000). In this latter model, leadership is treated as a solution to particular organizational problems, specifically problems of performance. An organization that employs the dyadic model tends to be equilibrium seeking and structure preserving, taking certainty and stability as important goals but not expecting control to be complete, as the managers know that some degree of change is either unpredictable or uncontrollable, and that change in structure results in energy loss. High levels of performance only occur when a leader of superior capability defines and directs the work to be done.

Treating leadership as emergent fits well with the belief that individuals are intrinsically motivated, creative, and capable, and it also fits well with dissipative models of leadership, which are discussed next.

Dissipative Leadership

Whereas the traditional dyadic model of leadership considers disruption as an anomaly that should be eliminated as soon as possible, the dissipative model views change and the disruption it brings as necessary for survival and growth (Barker 1998). Because of the complex nature of today's society, simplistic problem-solving models based on linear command and control are no longer adequate tools for managing change. Administrative or leadership theory must be revised, therefore, to reflect the current nature of organizations as complex, dynamic, dissipative systems. Change is not merely a problem to be solved, change is.

The dissipative model of leadership rightly treats change as normal. It also favors transferring leadership responsibilities to a group process in which no specific person is in charge but every person is assumed to occupy a leadership role to some degree. It views leadership as a dynamic, community-building process rather than a means for achieving organizational goals—as a process of change where the ethics (rules of conduct) of individuals are integrated into the mores (customs accepted without question) of a community. Further, in this model, leadership becomes a form of participative democracy in which the actions of individuals are motivated by their own wants and needs and directed toward a perceived collective good. The focus is on the intrinsic and foundational values of individuals and the group rather than on causes and effects; leadership, in this view, is the emergent property of relationships, not the management of work by individuals placed in superior positions.

INTEGRATED LEADERSHIP

The new leadership model makes emotional competence an even more important skill, especially for leaders of health care organizations. Quantum leaders must possess not only intellect, analytical ability, technical skills, and appropriate experience, but also the ability to understand and manage relationships, including their emotional dimension. To be fully effective, they must, first, master the required technical work skills; second, understand and intentionally choose those work processes most likely to achieve the desired outcomes; and, third, be able to form and sustain relationships—and they must do all this in an organization in which the interdependence of individuals and work processes is recognized (Figure 6–1).

Traditional leadership job descriptions generally do a good job of defining the necessary product- or service-specific knowledge, skills, and abilities. As for the second requirement, choosing the appropriate work processes, leaders often find it difficult to determine which interventions or processes will achieve the organization's goals efficiently. The object is to define and commit to value-based interventions. Too often organizations employ long-established processes that are outdated and do not contribute to reaching the desired outcomes in any way.

Consider the myriad times health care providers monitor and record vital signs and no intervention follows. Why perform these activities with such frequency? Perhaps just because "we've always done it this way." The reality is that taking vital signs, although it re-

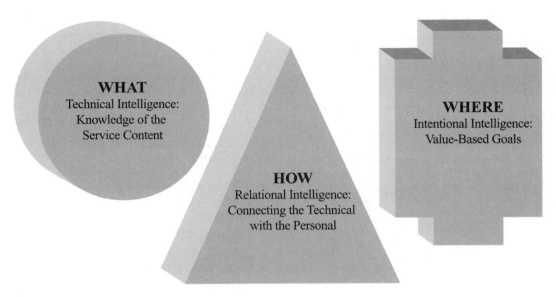

Figure 6–1 The Components of Leadership Effectiveness

quires skilled providers, seldom contributes to the outcome. Indeed, the need to show that taking vital signs frequently has real benefits for the patients deserves consideration. Providers are reluctant to give up long-held practices for fear of losing critical data and out of concern for the legal ramifications, but given the serious shortage of health care workers, any and all practices that do not obviously contribute to better patient outcomes should be evaluated for elimination. Leaders, especially in this new age, must ensure that resources are appropriately allocated, and that the work of each individual is aligned with the goals of the customers and the organization. In fact, all members of the organization must become skilled in selecting interventions that will further the organization's mission.

Purposeful (intentional) use of time, labor, and equipment is closely related to the third requisite, developing and sustaining relationships to support work processes. Proficiency at building rapport among members of the organization is increasingly seen as an essential leadership skill; effective relationships, it is now recognized, can substantially improve performance. It is also recognized that effective relationships require the participants to have some understanding of naturally occurring human emotions. The kind of emotional competence required by leaders (and others) is discussed in the following section.

THE NATURE OF EMOTIONAL COMPETENCE

Traditional leaders tend to look on the meaning or feeling side of leadership as its *soft side,* the work that is often subjective and difficult to teach or measure.

Emotional competence is more than a list of attributes. It is a collection of perceptions, behaviors, knowledge, and values that, for instance, enable a leader to manage meaning between individuals and groups within an organization. For health care leaders, emotional

> **Key Point**
>
> *Principles of emotional competence:*
>
> - *The individual members of an organization are interconnected and interrelated.*
> - *The individual members perceive their work as natural and a source of fulfillment and growth.*
> - *Creativity is inherent in the individual and in the collective wisdom of each team.*
> - *The individual members are motivated to contribute to meaningful goals and focus on self-esteem and self-actualization.*
> - *Leadership emerges from the combined active engagement of all members of the organization, not from the activities of a single individual.*

competence involves the interpretation and translation of personal feelings into the processes of the workplace. The key concepts of cognition, competence, emotion, intelligence, and volition are defined in Exhibit 6–1 to assist in understanding the essence of emotional competence. The characteristics and behaviors that make up emotional competence include

- self-awareness
- mindfulness
- openness
- impulse control
- personal humility
- appreciation of ambiguity and paradox
- appreciation of knowledge
- willpower
- compassion
- passionate optimism
- resilience

As an additional note, although it is often difficult to describe or measure the soft stuff in the business world, its absence is often very obvious. When negative outcomes result from the lack of the soft side of leadership, for instance, these can be described very clearly by nearly every leader. They include the negative consequences of not showing a regard for others as unique individuals, discounting the feelings of others, and being abrasive to or ignoring others, all of which tend to cause alienation and loss of support. A leader may

---

Exhibit 6–1 Key Concepts

- **Cognition:** Pertains to mental processes of perception, memory, judgment, and reasoning.
- **Competence:** The state of having suitable or sufficient skill, knowledge, and experience for some purpose.
- **Emotion:** The affective side of consciousness in which joy, sorrow, and fear, etc., are experienced. Emotions are distinguished from cognitive and volitional states of consciousness.
- **Intelligence:** The capacity for learning, reasoning, and understanding; aptitude in grasping truths, relationships, facts, or meanings; mental alertness and quickness of understanding.
- **Volition:** The act of willing, choosing, or resolving; the exercise of the will.

accomplish the technical side of a task quickly and in an exemplary manner, but a failure to consider the feelings of those involved usually will prevent the outcome from being sustainable and will diminish the commitment and motivation of the team in the future.

Self-Knowledge

Knowing what works for oneself enhances one's ability to understand what works for others in similar situations. In fact, self-knowledge is an important pillar of emotional competence. To achieve self-knowledge, leaders need to understand the quality of consciousness that they bring to the workplace and to recognize that, although they cannot always control events, they can control their thoughts.

They also need to realize that individuals each have unique patterns and perceptual filters that affect their interactions with others. This is not to suggest that every individual requires a psychoanalytical evaluation. The point is merely that leaders need to appreciate that they each have a preferred style of interacting, have their own sources of motivation and energy, and have unique ways of perceiving information and determining which types of information to consider. Leaders (and others) also have different communication styles (e.g., open, confrontational, assertive, and withholding) and different decision-making styles (e.g., autocratic, collaborative, participative, and consensus building). Numerous assessment tools are available to help leaders determine their degree of assertiveness, their type of creativity, and their styles of collaborating and communicating. (Table 6–1 presents examples of behavioral assessment categories.)

Self-knowledge is also about developing an understanding of and appreciation for ambiguity and paradox. Although uncertainty or ambiguity can have a positive value, as discussed in Chapter 4, not everyone is comfortable with the lack of clear and certain pathways. Learning to live with paradox or seemingly contradictory ideas becomes a significant challenge for the leader trained and experienced in the command-and-control leadership model. Yet leaders today must recognize that paradoxical situations are a normal part of the organizational landscape and do not necessarily have to be resolved through compromise. For example, contradictions and uncertainty create opportunities for leaders to explore perspectives that differ from theirs and to be confronted with new ideas and feelings. In short, far from being calamitous, paradox, much like conflict (see Chapter 3), offers formerly hidden benefits to the organization that is open to profit from it.

Table 6–1 Behavioral Assessment Categories

Source	*Categories*			
Astrology	Water	Fire	Air	Earth
Hippocrates	Melancholy	Sanguine	Phlegmatic	Choleric
Jung	Feeler	Intuitor	Thinker	Sensor
Merrill, Wilson, and Allessandra	Amiable	Expressive	Analytical	Driver
Performax	Steadiness	Influence	Compliance	Dominance
Cathcart and Allessandra	Relater	Socializer	Thinker	Director

The leadership role as it relates to relationships itself has a paradoxical aspect. Although people generally have a need to belong to a group for support and for reference, research indicates that effective leaders, despite spending most of the work time in contact with others, tend to have an inconsiderable need to belong to a specific group. Leaders instead tend to be self-reliant and to be comfortable acting as a dissenting voice or challenging the status quo. This is not to say that leaders do not create and sustain meaningful relationships. Rather, recognizing that integrating subjective meanings into the leadership data set is essential for achieving optimal outcomes, emotionally competent leaders use both personal relationship data and organizational data to inform their decisions. Note, however, that this is very different from aligning with a specific partisan perspectives or choosing sides in decision making.

Recently, Collins (2001) found that powerful leaders often possess a paradoxical mixture of personal humility and professional will. The combination of humble unpretentiousness and fierce, even stoic resolve is at odds with the traditional image of leaders as larger than life. Yet this union of modesty and willfulness has some obvious merits as a leadership style, especially for leaders in the coming age. Among other things, leaders who are both modest and willful tend to act with a clearly expressed openness to others, place people and their feelings first, recognize the positive and negative aspects of the current reality, sustain their faith in the organization's potential for success, channel their energy into the organization, and are disposed to develop successors rather than leave the issue of succession unresolved. They appreciate the traps inherent in short-term success and false optimism, and they are inclined to foster organizational learning because of their healthy skepticism of their own accomplishments. Besides documenting this unusual combination of leadership values and priorities, recent research has shown the overwhelming improvements in organizational performance that can result.

Openness to New Ideas

Leaders who understand their own decision-making and communication styles find it easier to appreciate other perspectives. They thus can take better advantage of the fact that every health care organization, because of its range of individuals, teams, and disciplines, is a repository of multiple viewpoints on everything needed to create cost-effective services, from the content of the services to the processes for designing and delivering them.

In addition, these leaders, by considering other viewpoints, are able to achieve a high level of emotional competence, which includes the ability to listen to what others have to say and integrate what is important into the organization's collective wisdom. Sometimes, because of the fast-paced, results-oriented environment in which they function, leaders are forced to learn how to maintain *suffering silence,* which is a form of listening in which the emotions that obstruct listening and the objective evaluation of ideas are suppressed.

Valuing of Knowledge

For leaders of quantum organizations, self-knowledge and openness to the opinions of others are closely related to the perception that new information is essential for growth.

Necessarily, besides developing a thirst for new knowledge, leaders also must acquire the ability to filter out insignificant information. In the current data-rich age, far too much information is available on the Internet, and more yet passes through every leader's hands. Filtering and managing new information nonetheless reinforce the undeniable passion of leaders to make a difference.

The greater a leader's self-knowledge and openness to new ideas, the greater the leader's confidence in making decisions. Emotionally competent leaders make decisions readily and enthusiastically, not because they believe they are always correct but because they understand that there is always a risk of error and that progress cannot be made without taking action. In fact, they strongly believe that unsuccessful outcomes or errors are opportunities for improvement and not something to be avoided or eliminated.

Compassion

Compassion is another main pillar of emotional competence. In health care, the emotional intensity surrounding trauma, birth, suffering, and dying makes compassionate service the intended norm. Providers and patients have indeed come to recognize the importance of understanding and sharing one another's feelings, including joy, sorrow, and all the emotions in between. Further, compassion fosters the kind of personal involvement that is necessary for providers and patients to develop strong and effective relationships and for providers to apply their objective (technical) knowledge and skills.

Interestingly, the powerful urge of providers to alleviate patient distress cannot prevent them from objectifying patients when they discuss patient issues. The patient becomes "the gallbladder on Hall 1"—a medical condition instead of a person. In contrast, providers who are emotionally competent learn to integrate the objectivity of the gallbladder disease with the subjectivity of the patient and to perceive the patient's unique needs and feelings about the disease and its impact on the patient's functionality. The patient remains a person and is not referred to as a room number or a diagnosis.

> **Point To Ponder**
>
> *Without feelings of deep sympathy and sorrow for others struck by misfortune and a genuine desire to alleviate suffering on the part of caregivers, patient care service would be no more than a robotic endeavor.*

In many ways, compassionate patient care is similar to compassionate leadership. For instance, the leader attempts to integrate the subjective, which here encompasses the relationships between the members of the organization, and the objective, which encompasses the work to be accomplished. In addition, although the leader should sympathize with an employee who has suffered a misfortune, he or she should refrain from attempting to resolve the employee's issues. Offering guidance and reassurance is appropriate and consistent with the principle of personal accountability, but attempting to manage another's situation is paternalistic and disempowering. The emotionally competent leader develops the ability to express sincere sympathy when an employee experiences adversity but does not cross the line into paternalism. The challenge is to integrate the subjective and the objective—to remain personal in the relationship with the employee while also considering the organization's needs and the employee's accountability for doing his or her job. In meeting this challenge, the leader avoids objectifying the employee (e.g., treating the employee as an attendance problem).

Consider this common situation. An employee with repeated absences is disciplined by a leader on the basis of an established attendance policy. The leader's goal may be compassionate leadership, yet the objective policy is allowed to get in the way. To act with compassion, the leader needs to inject subjectivity into the equation, which can be done by exploring the surrounding events (the context of the absences) and the employee's feelings. Compassionate leadership emerges when the leader looks at both the personal information and the objective needs of the organization in order to find an equitable solution. This is not to say that it is okay to fail to hold the employee accountable for meeting the expectations of the organization in some way. In fact, compassionate leadership is a broad enough concept to include dismissing the employee if the employee fails to make a sincere effort to do his or her job.

As shown by this example, compassionate leadership is sometimes hard to achieve. It is especially hard to achieve in a traditional organization, where work force numbers and productivity targets are determined by the chief executive officer (CEO) and handed down to managers for implementation. In difficult times, the CEO will usually mandate a reduction in the work force using one of two approaches. In the first approach, the CEO keeps distant from the process, causing the employees to view him or her as callous. In reality, the CEO may be very compassionate, but by not becoming directly involved in the process, he or she inadvertently appears indifferent. In the second approach, the CEO, having identified the work force reductions to be implemented, remains involved and available during the communication and early implementation stages. As a result, the employees perceive the CEO as compassionate and caring.

Presence

For any leader, being present—especially being available following any decision that has positive or negative implications for others—shows that the leader is connected with

> **Group Discussion**
>
> Imagine that in the midst of a recent blizzard, a health care organization is experiencing a serious staffing shortage. As the storm is forecast to continue, the employees who are at work wonder whether they should call the leadership team to inform the members of the shortage. At what point, if at all, should they contact the senior leaders? When should the senior leaders be required to be present at the organization? How would the leaders' actions likely affect the willingness of others to attempt to come to work? What impact would the leaders' presence have on the employees' morale? How long will the employees remember the presence or absence of the leaders?

the employees and is willing to participate with them in a common journey. Leaders with a low degree of emotional competence tend to be visible in the workplace following announcements of pay raises or new benefit packages and noticeably out of town when decisions that negatively impact members of the organization are first publicized. Being involved in managing the impact of all decisions shows that the leader is committed to the employees, is willing to claim ownership of the decisions, and is sensitive to the varied meanings of the decisions for the employees. Being absent, by contrast, conveys that the leader is uninterested in the impact of difficult decisions on others and is afraid of claiming the decisions. Leaders must realize that it is not only their technical skills or verbal communication that makes a difference, it is also their ability to show that there is someone at the top who cares about what is happening.

Employees who are facing layoffs will search for the linkage between the (objective) financial goals of the organization and the (subjective) impact of the work force reduction on their lives. In such a situation, the leader's physical presence and availability for dialogue is interpreted by the employees as compassionate leadership. Note that this is not to negate the importance of the role of middle managers; it is merely to point out that employees facing adversity seek to connect their subjective reality (e.g., the reality of being out of work) with the personal (subjective) responses of the chief decision maker.

Mindfulness

The emotionally competent leader is mindful of recurring situations, the past reactions of members of the organization, and the implications of these reactions. As a result, the leader is able to identify certain patterns of behavior and develop skill in understanding and interpreting these situations as guidelines for future behavior. In essence, the leader interprets the emotional reactions of individuals in recurring situations and ensures that he or she is present when another such situation arises. For example, a disaster of any kind requires the physical presence of the leader to support the employees emotionally. Seldom is the presence of the leader needed for the technical work of a disaster—or even desired! Yet the leader should have no question as to the significance of his or her presence when employees are emotionally impacted.

Nonverbal Emotional Competence

A leader's physical stance and actions carry nonverbal messages and can arouse positive or negative emotions. Imagine a group of people standing together in such a way as to invite new participants. Now imagine a group standing close to each other in an enclosed circle and speaking in hushed tones. The message sent by this arrangement is that newcomers are not welcome. Again, an extended arm, a handshake, and the offering of physical space are friendly behaviors, whereas turning one's back to an approaching person, folding one's arms, and speaking in hushed tones are inhospitable. The former convey feelings of acceptance, whereas the latter are rejecting and exclusionary. Or consider the unexpected entry of a competitor into a group of highly antagonistic opponents. The conversation may stop altogether or verbal confrontation may ensue, depending on the emotional state of all the parties. Emotional reactions are pervasive in any situation in which people are present, and dealing with these reactions requires great compassion and self-awareness.

Passionate Optimism

In this time of chaos and unending challenges, health care leaders often find it difficult to remain enthusiastic about the work to be done, and they may find it easier to see the cup as half empty rather than as half full. They may therefore need the refreshment afforded by reminiscing about the beginning of their careers, when their deep concern for patient care was the driving force of all their actions. During this earlier period, besides acting out of altruism, they undoubtedly believed they could truly make a difference. In fact, as new professionals, they were focused on understanding the seriousness of each patient's condition and identifying the treatment most likely to result in a favorable outcome. In spite of the challenges, hopefulness was their modus operandi. Emotionally competent leaders retain the passion of their early health care experiences and work diligently to guide others in developing and cherishing the same spirit of passionate optimism. This is not to say that they are immune from discouragement or unrealistic about the future. All leaders experience disappointment and disillusionment, but emotionally competent leaders recognize that successes and failures are both normal and that times of disappointment will eventually give way to times of breakthrough and achievement.

Maintaining a positive mindset means holding positive images rather than negative images and viewing all situations as blessings and/or opportunities. When the results are not desired or anticipated, leaders should look for lessons to be learned and value the information gained. A positive mindset stands in sharp contrast to a pessimistic worldview, which fosters passivity and a general unwillingness to take appropriate action in the face of adversity. Pessimism depletes the life force of all involved. Even in the worst of circumstances, leaders are challenged to find positive meaning for themselves and the members of the organization. And when positive meaning cannot be found, the most logical source of encouragement becomes each individual's support system, including family and friends.

> ### Point To Ponder
>
> *Thoughts on resilience:*
>
> - *Resilience is the capacity to cope with unanticipated dangers after they have become manifest and learning to bounce back.*
> - *To be resilient means being able to come away from the event with an even greater capacity to prevent and contain future errors.*
> - *Resilience is the capacity for improvisation, which allows the organization to expand exponentially not only with the range of actions in its repertoire but also the range of potential threats it can foresee.*
> *—Karl Weick and Kathleen Sutcliffe (2000)*

Resilience

Few leaders have acquired the skill set needed to manage personal disappointments as well as coach others in the management of their disappointments. Traditionally, individuals who receive bad news are expected to deal with it outside of the workplace. Yet, when a team jointly addresses the disappointments of individual team members, productivity is likely to be enhanced and work disruption minimized. Further, allowing time for the team to process disappointments and create effective coping strategies strengthens the emotional competence of the team.

Passion through Balance

Creating or restoring passion for work typically has a subtle impact at the outset, but eventually the results become very obvious. Passion often emerges from situations that seem overwhelming. Given the current rate of change and innovation, few can keep pace to their satisfaction. There is far too much knowledge available and not enough time or skill to winnow out the unneeded information. Reestablishing a proper balance requires a new filter for consciousness, a filter that allows one to sift through information and select only what is pertinent to the issue at hand. Also, leaders can find new comfort in accepting their limitations and the impossibility of reviewing all there is to know. They can also find comfort in realizing that if out-of-the-ordinary information is needed, it probably is available through the Internet. Establishing a balance between information input and available time is one component of the total equation, and it helps in creating the space needed for passionate optimism. Establishing a balance between work and personal life is another prerequisite for passionate optimism.

Passion is more easily sustained when the conflict between personal life and work life is minimal. Emotionally competent leaders act to ensure that employees do not feel they have to hang their personal values at the door when they come to work. Although the purpose of their activities is to assist the organization in meeting its goals, only when these goals are congruent with the employees' personal values will their enthusiasm survive. If there is a conflict between goals and values, the best strategy is to bring the conflict and the employees' feelings into view and work to minimize the conflict. Failure to address such conflicts quickly depletes the energy of the organization.

Noted leadership expert and philosopher Peter Russell has postulated that in the past it was difficult for people to develop passion and happiness because they had scant material possessions and few career options. For example, in pre-industrial times, 97 percent of Americans worked on the land. Life was hard and food was scarce. There was no central heating, and the water was not always healthy to drink.

Today, in contrast, grocery stores offer a bounty of food, department stores are filled with clothing and other goods, and hot or cool air is available with the push of a button. If we are unhappy or lack passion, therefore, the probable reason, rather than the absence of something external, is that we are experiencing an inner lack of meaning or sense of personal purpose. Society unhelpfully tells us that to overcome our unhappiness we must do something to meet an external need—buy new clothes or a new car or eat a well-prepared meal—but the void remains. As a consequence, people are increasingly recognizing that what they are missing is meaning in their life. Meanwhile, the drive for more technology and more material goods continues to accelerate. The challenge is not to negate the value of material well-being but to make a place for passion—to use emotional competence to create a balance between the material side of life and the emotional side.

Impulse Control

Full emotional competence encompasses impulse control or self-regulation—the ability to temper negative emotions. Emotionally competent leaders know how to share feelings appropriately and maintain dignity. Managing emotions is not the same as lacking emotions. Even the most emotionally competent leader experiences feelings of anger and frustration, but he or she is able to mediate and reframe them to minimize the misuse of energy. The common expectation is that the fundamentals of impulse control were developed in childhood and that anger and frustration are thus managed in a healthy way. Unfortunately, not every individual grew up in a family in which healthy impulse control strategies were handed down. Many instead learned patterns of behavior that were obstacles to personal growth and accountability, such as conflict avoidance and assumption of a victim attitude. These individuals need new skills and behaviors to function in high-stress environments.

As the need for emotional competence becomes more apparent, organizations are developing personal growth and development programs not only for leaders but for all employees and even members of the community. Not surprisingly, attendees of such programs identify nonworkplace roles, such as that of parent, spouse, friend, and community member, to which the skills they learn can be profitably applied.

> **Point To Ponder**
>
> Emotionally incompetent anger management: *Whenever you select anger as a response to someone else's behavior, you are withholding from that person the right to be what he chooses. Inside your head is the neurotic sentence, "Why can't you be more like me?"* Emotionally competent anger management: *"I will not give other people's behavior and ideas the power to upset me."*
>
> —Wayne Dyer (1976)

Leaders are expected to achieve personal impulse control and also to acquire the skills to coach others to develop and maintain impulse control. By generally remaining composed and positive in attitude, leaders are better able to support group processes and contribute to the accomplishment of the organizational work. They can still express strong and passionate feelings, but they keep themselves from losing control. Maintaining their cool also allows them to better manage other individuals who become emotionally upset or agitated. If someone does begin to get overly excited, an emotionally competent leader can respond in such a way as to de-escalate the loss of control and minimize the chance of emotional fireworks.

Interestingly, self-control is manifested largely in the absence of obvious outbursts. Being unfazed under stress or handling a hostile person without lashing out in return are indications of self-regulation and the ability to manage negative emotions. Controlled emotional behavior avoids misinterpretation of events through the lens of anger and minimizes the chance that a benign comment will lead to skewed perceptions through hostility.

Related Concepts

Several concepts related to emotional competence—emotional intelligence, character, and integrity—are helpful in understanding its underpinnings and significance. Although none is equivalent to or subsumed under the concept of emotional intelligence, they apply to the same set of phenomena. For example, although the concept of character is much broader than the concept of emotional competence, a person's character—the traits that form that person's nature—directly affects the person's ability to become emotionally competent. In general, an emotionally competent leader possesses a high level of emotional intelligence, a strong character, uncompromising integrity, a strong moral conscience, and an optimistic outlook on life.

Emotional Intelligence

Goleman (1998) has done groundbreaking research on the nature of emotional intelligence and its importance as a factor in achieving personal excellence. Emotional intelligence, according to Goleman, determines our potential for learning the practical skills of emotional competence. The five elements that make up emotional intelligence are as follows:

1. *Self-awareness* is the ability to recognize and understand one's moods, emotions, and drives as well as their effect on others.
2. *Self-regulation* is the ability to handle emotions so that they facilitate rather than interfere with the work to be done. People with this ability are conscientious, able to delay gratification to pursue goals, able to control or redirect disruptive impulses and moods, and prone to suspend judgment and think before acting.
3. *Motivation* is a passion to engage in work for reasons that go beyond money or status. It leads to a propensity to pursue goals with energy and to persevere in the face of setbacks and frustrations.
4. *Empathy* is the ability to understand the emotional makeup of other people. It allows a person to develop a rapport with a broad diversity of people and treat them according to their own emotional reactions.
5. *Social skill* is a proficiency in managing relationships and building networks. People with this skill are able to accurately read social situations and find common ground and build rapport.

Emotional competence, like other kinds of competence, is the possession of certain skills, learned or unlearned. As indicated above, emotional intelligence, like other kinds of intelligence, is the potential to learn new skills. Thus, a person who has emotional intelligence has the potential to learn how to be emotionally competent, whereas a person who has emotional competence already possesses a fair number of the appropriate skills.

Character

The term *character* is ambiguous. First, it can refer to the aggregate of features and traits that form the individual nature of a given person. The term has that meaning in such sentences as "What is her character?" and "He has a bad character." The term can also be used as a synonym for moral fortitude, as when we tell someone, "Show some character." To say that a person has character in this latter sense is to say that the person has the moral fortitude and discipline to exemplify the highest virtues of his or her time.

Integrity

Integrity is the quality of being morally upright and always acting openly and honestly. Individuals who have integrity consistently act on their own values in all situations and do not hide critical information, break promises, or fail to fulfill commitments.

THE EMOTIONAL RISKS OF LEADERSHIP

All leadership decisions are inherently uncertain and have the potential for error, as discussed in Chapter 5. But even if a leader fully understands that mistakes are unavoidable and accepts that he or she will make some wrong decisions, the emotional impact of making an error can be devastating. Historically, leadership education programs have offered the participants little preparation for managing miscalculations and missteps. The emphasis has been on success, not failure.

The emotional effects of failure faced by leaders on a daily basis cannot be eliminated. They can only be managed. In essence, the reputation of the leader is continually at stake. To manage emotional risk, leaders need a high level of emotional competence, including self-awareness, compassion, passionate optimism, and resilience. They typically must use their emotional competence to deal with things such as lack of feedback, inconsistency in the reactions of stakeholders, and employment insecurity, all of which have the power to cause confusion and emotional turmoil.

Lack of Feedback

Honest feedback given to a leader and recognition for work accomplished fuel the leader's passion for doing his or her job. Both are highly valued and sought after by most leaders (and also by most employees). On the reverse side, a lack of performance feedback causes stress and undermines the leader's confidence. So does a lack of acknowledgment from a supervisor, whether positive or negative. Not knowing where he or she stands with the supervisor is emotionally draining.

In addition, the more uncertain the leader becomes about his or her performance (because of the lack of feedback), the more likely the leader is to lose confidence in his or her decision-making ability and the more likely the supervisor is to continue to withhold feedback, leading to a cycle of uncertainty and negative emotional feelings. Failure to create the ideal team, achieve clinical goals, or meet financial targets all result in damage to a leader's ego. In such cases, timely feedback is critical to reversing negative outcomes, learning from the undesired outcomes, and relieving the leader's emotional stress.

Inconsistent Feedback

Imagine that the patient care standards committee develops a plan for patient restraint management with the intent of ensuring patient safety and meeting regulatory requirements. When the plan is presented to the medical staff committees, the medical committee quickly reviews and approves the plan, but the surgical committee recommends numerous revisions and withholds its endorsement. The leader of the patient care standards committee, faced with such different stakeholder responses, is likely to feel confused as well as less confident in his or her abilities. Yet the leader should keep in mind that, all too often, actions that are successful in one situation are disastrous in others, with no apparent explanation. In other words, the wide-ranging responses that different individuals or groups can have to the same action might appear as an impenetrable mystery that challenges a leader's ability to lead, but in such situations it is healthy to avoid being overly self-critical and to minimize the emotional insult. The best strategy is to focus on the context of the actions and reactions and to recognize that the values and goals of the stakeholders can vary widely, resulting in widely differing responses. In the case at hand, the leader's task includes not just creating an appropriate plan but understanding and managing the context in which the plan is proposed.

Employment Insecurity

In the typical organization, leaders serve at the will of the organization and can be removed without much notice or explanation. An employment contract will help in managing the processes of separation, but it cannot prevent the emotional damage resulting from the removal. Regardless of the health of the individual's ego, the experience is devastating. Expecting the individual to see the discharge as a business decision and not as a personal judgment is insulting and dishonest. Whenever someone's professional relationships are severed, membership in an organizational team is cancelled, or income is eliminated, it is, in fact, very personal.

Being discharged from a job or position often results in serious emotional trauma. In fact, heightened sensitivity to the experience can be seen as the downside of emotional competence. If the leader avoided all feelings and emotions, he or she actually could view the discharge simply as a business issue. The reality is that situations negatively affecting any part of an individual's life are personal and often painful. Compounding the problem for health care leaders is that people in health care are expected to provide care rather than receive care. Thus it is very difficult for them to handle being in need of support, sympathy, and compassion.

Although the emotional effects of uncertainty and employment insecurity are not unique to health care, the values of providers, especially the importance they place on caregiving, cause them to have heightened emotional sensitivity and often heightened vulnerability to emotional upset. Among the consequences are that providers, especially those who are emotionally incompetent, are predisposed to experience great stress, suffer a loss of confidence and passion, and feel incredible turmoil and disappointment. The solution to being exposed to emotional risk is to develop significant emotional competence. In addition, a leader undergoing an employment crisis can mitigate the resulting depression and sense of devastation by keeping in mind his or her skills and abilities and past performance and achievements.

THE BENEFITS OF EMOTIONAL COMPETENCE IN HEALTH CARE

The soft stuff—meaning and feelings—does make a difference in health care. That is not a controversial claim, but leaders are often unsure how the value of the soft stuff can be substantiated and translated into organizational effectiveness and a bigger bottom line.

Traditionally, leaders have examined care delivery from a purely technical perspective. However, the processes involved in providing care encompass both technical (quantitative) and human-related (qualitative) attributes, and thus a holistic perspective, one that includes quantitative and qualitative measures, is needed for evaluating care delivery.

Leaders know that technical skills are necessary for producing products and services and are essential for success. Leaders also know that defined, goal-directed (intentional) behaviors are essential. More recently, they have begun to realize that the relationships between members of the organization have an impact on effectiveness. Yet, all too often, they fail to see the interconnections between the technical aspect of work, the intentional aspect, and the relationships between the workers. It is only when leaders integrate the workers' essential technical skills, their goal-directed activities, and their ability to form meaningful relationships that optimal organizational effectiveness results (see Figure 6–1). In addition, treating the work to be accomplished as a nonreducible unit of service shifts the evaluation focus from the parts to the whole, where it properly belongs.

Group Discussion

The three components of integrated leadership—the technical, relational, and intentional—offer a framework for optimizing the use of resources. In a recent committee meeting, a new benefit for child care was introduced and added to the benefits package at the request of an influential board member. The benefit offers a fixed per diem reimbursement amount to pay for child care provided to the children of employees. It is uncertain if employees are interested in or will use this benefit. It is also uncertain how the value of this benefit will be assessed. Analyze the addition of this benefit from the perspective of the three components of integrated leadership. That is, identify the technical, relational, and intentional considerations that pertain to it. Based on the discussion of these considerations, recommend whether to add the benefit or reject its inclusion into the benefits package.

The value of emotional competence is evident in nearly every interaction in an organization. For instance, effective leaders possess a high degree of self-awareness, compassion for others, self-control, resilience, and passionate optimism, and this powerful combination enables them to achieve the most challenging goals and enlist others in completing the organization's work. Yet, it is difficult not only for the leaders themselves to measure the value of passion and emotional competence but also for board members, who tend to neglect these in the selection of CEOs, especially where the financial stakes are substantial.

Focused Hiring

Increasing evidence exists that choosing a leader should involve more than finding the candidate with the best history of financial performance, stock pricing, expense management, merger experience, and work force reductions. Many boards, however, still believe that if a candidate's achievements are notable, especially in the financial area, they cannot go wrong in hiring that candidate. The problem with this strategy is that many hard-nosed number crunchers are emotionally inept, and because they are—because they fail to listen to others, develop meaningful relationships, share honest feelings, and empathize with others—their leadership can harm organizational performance rather than improve it. In particular, their way of handling subordinates might easily cause an increase in turnover and a decrease in market share and net income. Cases in which this has occurred confirm that there is indeed a relationship between the emotional competence of an organization's leader (soft stuff) and organization's financial measures (hard stuff).

The cost of turnover has skyrocketed. In many job categories, the cost of turnover and replacement for one position exceeds $50,000. With health care annual turnover rates averaging 15 to 20 percent, the annualized costs are phenomenal. In addition, although many organizations assume the greatest turnover is at the staff level, in fact the greatest turnover is at the middle management level.

Researchers have found that the staged encounters of the formal interview process seldom reveal the real nature of any job applicant. Finding the applicant with the right fit requires spending extensive time evaluating the most promising candidates prior to hiring. Then, once the candidate with the greatest potential for success is selected, extensive time is required to integrate him or her into the organization. Recent evidence indicates that the more time spent with the candidates prior to hiring, the more likely the candidate with the best fit will be hired, the less likely that person is to leave the organization, and, as the new hire becomes more acculturated over the first year, the greater the job satisfaction he or she will experience. New interviewing processes and different types of questions are needed to identify the chemistry between an applicant and the members of the organization (Exhibit 6–2).

Improved Succession Planning

Another opportunity for leaders to utilize emotional competence is in succession planning. Currently, there seems to be a lack of qualified or committed candidates for health care leadership positions, and consequently organizations are wise to increase their efforts to ensure that the integrated skill sets of all management hires, not just the top leaders, are consistent with their needs. Because lower level managers will become candidates for leadership positions in the future, the skill sets and characteristics desired for these positions should be clearly defined and shared within the organization.

Successful leaders have a tendency to encourage their heirs apparent to model their behaviors, failing to recognize these behaviors will have become outdated by the time they resign. The challenges of each upcoming generation will be different, and so the best strategy is to create new pathways bridging the generations rather than expect later generations to conform to the values of earlier ones. Attempts to clone current leaders can only hold back organizations from moving into the future. As an example, retirement-age leaders who are currently instilling the principles of the command-and-control model into their likely successors may prevent them from traveling the same pathway as their peers (i.e., keep them from using more participative models, focusing on short-term goals, and eliminating middle-management positions through technological innovations).

Exhibit 6–2 Interviewing for Emotional Competence

These questions are asked of both the candidate and representatives in the current work environment. Interviewing team members compare responses for consistency and fit with the organization.

Directions: Select the most appropriate response.

	Never	Seldom	Sometimes	Always
1. Does the candidate have the ability to manage disappointment?	☐	☐	☐	☐
2. Does the candidate listen to others' ideas?	☐	☐	☐	☐
3. Does the candidate value the contributions of team members?	☐	☐	☐	☐
4. Does the candidate hold others accountable for their performance and promises?	☐	☐	☐	☐
5. Is the candidate comfortable delegating important tasks to others?	☐	☐	☐	☐
6. Does the candidate energize others?	☐	☐	☐	☐
7. Does the candidate spend time communicating the organization's vision and purpose?	☐	☐	☐	☐
8. Do members of the organization trust the promises of the candidate?	☐	☐	☐	☐
9. Is the candidate interested in the concerns of employees?	☐	☐	☐	☐
10. Does the candidate share information willingly and in a timely manner?	☐	☐	☐	☐

The incongruence of traditional health care leadership values with the values of the emerging generation of leaders may explain the common concern that talented leaders are being especially attracted to industries other than health care. Generational management is about understanding the meaning of the work for individuals of different generations. It is a form of diversity management—integrating the different beliefs and values of different age groups and not negating the beliefs and values of the emerging generation or attempting to make them conform to those of past generations. Emotionally competent succession planning allows current and aspiring leaders to make the skill sets of emotional competence, specifically self-awareness and passionate optimism, a permanent part of the organization and ensure that the feelings of individuals in the organization and the community are not suppressed out of concern for marketplace values.

Higher Productivity

Significant opportunities for increased productivity exist when emotional competence becomes an attribute not just of individual members but of the entire team. Given that the real work of an organization occurs within a team framework, the greater the ability of team members to truly work together, the greater the positive impact on organizational performance. Note that working together involves more than cooperation, participation, and commitment to goals. The team members must exhibit self-awareness, compassion, passionate optimism, and impulse regulation if they are to achieve their desired outcomes. According to Druskat and Wolff (2001), team success lies in the fundamental conditions that allow effective task processes to emerge and cause members to engage in these processes wholeheartedly. Three conditions—trust among members, a sense of group identity, and a sense of group efficacy—are essential to effectiveness. Without these, teams simply go through the motions of cooperating and participating, and members hold back rather than fully engage, reducing the level of effectiveness.

> **Point To Ponder**
>
> *When leadership is understood as a community development process, it will serve the many rather than the few.*
> —*Richard A. Barker (1998)*

Health care teams that recognize the interconnectedness of members and acknowledge the unique contributions of each to the delivery of services are able to make substantial contributions to the achievement of organizational goals. Specifically, they are able to help improve patient care outcomes, implement strategies in a shorter time, apply new knowledge as it becomes available, use organizational resources more productively, problem solve more creatively, and manage work processes more effectively. According to Orsburn and colleagues (1990), most organizations experience a 20 to 40 percent increase in productivity when employees are deeply involved in their work.

Selecting and mentoring individuals for team membership using the principles of emotional competence reinforces the benefits of effective teams. The object is to select members who are not just team players but also bring to the team varied interests and skills. To do this, it is helpful to look at the results of self-assessment exercises used to assist members in learning about themselves and other team members. These exercises can provide information about behavior patterns and the filters people use in their interactions with others. Understanding the unique characteristics of different team members facilitates the team's work and makes it more timely. Information on the following usually can be easily obtained:

- *Decision-making style.* Some individuals consider information and ideas objectively and logically, whereas others tend to be more subjective and value oriented.
- *Motivation.* Some individuals are energized by dealing with the outside world and thrive on personal interactions, whereas others are more comfortable thinking and reflecting and are disinclined to share an idea until comfortable with it.
- *Values.* Some individuals require facts and step-by-step processes and focus on the present, whereas others are more comfortable with insights and intuitions and focus on the future.
- *Orientation to outside information.* Many individuals strive for control and want as much information as they can get, whereas others tend to be comfortable with little information and letting things happen.

If all the team members are aware of each other's behavior patterns, interests, and background, the team will not only work together more effectively but be able to plan for future membership. For instance, if a behavior pattern is missing from the team (e.g., the reflective pattern mentioned under "motivation" in the above list), the team can try to identify candidates who possess it. The team can also target candidates likely to offer a range of ideas or have the skills to facilitate the team's work.

In addition to providing guidance in the selection of members, emotional competence increases the probability that team members will be able to hear each other's concerns and understand each other's feelings. By taking time to consider matters from each member's perspective prior to making a decision, the team, besides being able to incorporate the different perspectives into the final decision, recognizes each member's importance, thereby

Group Discussion

Giving feedback upward is the same as giving feedback downward or sideways (to peers), provided you establish an explicit contract with your boss to do so. The CEO of your organization has scheduled a leadership retreat at a time when the staffing is seriously low. The topic of staffing does not appear to be of interest to the senior leaders, or at least of less concern to them than other topics. Together with your team, create a plan to discuss this situation with the CEO. The goal is to give feedback to the CEO, a person with more power, authority, and/or experience than you. In the best case scenario, the feedback will enhance the effectiveness of the retreat and ultimately improve the organization's performance. The risk is that the feedback may be rejected by the CEO and may negatively impact your relationship with the CEO. The following list of steps can be used to guide your preparation for the "coaching upward" meeting.

1. Describe the situation (topic).
2. Agree on the specific objective of the session.
3. Share your assessment of the situation. Why is a change needed? How will the CEO benefit from the change? How will the organization benefit from the change?
4. Validate your assumptions with the CEO. Ask for comments.
5. Invite suggestions from the CEO.
6. Suggest possible solutions. Cover the full range of options.
7. Select a course of action.
8. Agree on the course of action. Identify the time frame for the expected change.
9. Identify specific steps to achieve the change.
10. Commit to action. Thank the CEO for his or her willingness to examine the issues and work to make the organization more effective.

improving the members' morale and willingness to cooperate. This process is very different than calling for a majority vote in the interest of expedience. Teams with high levels of emotional competence understand that consideration of the views of each member is a requisite of sustainable decisions. They try to obtain a consensus rather than majority agreement to ensure that all team members are behind the decision. The intent is never to remove the emotion from the process but rather to give every member a hearing to create trust and ultimately foster greater participation among members.

Coaching Upward

Coaching is a valued method of developing skills, but it traditionally has been used almost exclusively by superiors to assist those below them. The most challenging type of coaching—and the one ordinarily overlooked—involves providing feedback to individuals with greater authority. As the members of an organization become more emotionally competent, coaching upward becomes less challenging and is embraced more readily. Once the halo of the infallibility is removed from the most powerful positions in the organization, those in other positions can use the skills of coaching upward to give appropriate feedback, often averting serious negative outcomes as a result.

People generally appreciate constructive, timely, and sensitively delivered feedback that can be put to practical use. Despite this, people who give feedback frequently are tentative and unsure that what they are doing is appropriate. Giving feedback completes the circle of communication in an organization dedicated to managing the marketplace and the meanings attached to the individuals in the organization.

DEVELOPING EMOTIONAL COMPETENCE

Effective and accomplished leaders are often referred to as *born leaders* based on the belief that leadership skills are inherent or learned at an early age. Although some leaders may indeed have natural leadership ability, those who are not born leaders can acquire the necessary skills, including those that make up emotional competence. These latter skills, however, cannot be obtained by attending a one-day workshop. Rather, their development requires focused coaching, time, and experience.

Below, a five-stage model of development based on the Dreyfus and Dreyfus (1996) skill acquisition model is presented as a framework for understanding how emotional competence is obtained incrementally (Exhibit 6–3). Each of the five skill levels is described to assist readers in assessing their own level of emotional competence and continuing to mature toward the highest skill level. The following section describes emotionally incompetent behaviors that individuals sometimes exhibit and should seek to eliminate.

Novice Stage

In the first stage, the individual, despite having formal education in leadership, has no experience in the application of leadership knowledge and skills. The novice is a detached observer of the processes of leadership and, in regard to emotional competence, has at most a personal awareness of interaction styles and behavior patterns.

Exhibit 6–3 Individual Emotional Competence Skill Levels and Behaviors

- Novice (detached observer)
  - Formally educated in the principles of emotional competence
  - Aware of personal interaction styles and behavior patterns
  - Has not held a formal leadership position
- Advanced beginner (active participant)
  - Has increasing self-awareness but limited openness to the ideas of others
  - Tends to be judgmental
  - Has increasing confidence in ability to participate and make decisions
  - Begins to think and feel simultaneously; not always certain of the meaning of events or if there is a connection between an event and another's emotional reaction
  - Is easily discouraged and not always optimistic about the future
- Competent (integrated with the process)
  - Has emerging compassion for others
  - Exhibits authentic presence in teamwork; listens actively and critically to others
  - Is able to think and feel simultaneously and acknowledge the feelings of others
  - Gives both positive and negative feedback (a requirement of effective communication)
  - Is increasingly open to others' ideas
  - Gains comfort in challenging the status quo
  - Begins to develop the ability to control impulses
- Proficient (therapeutic engagement)
  - Has emerging sense of optimism and ability to manage negative emotions
  - Is able to read or experience chemistry between people (e.g., recognizes allies, identifies whom to trust, and recognizes nonsupport or hostility)
  - Understands the meaning of relationships
  - Has positive but realistic attitude; believes in the team's ability to accomplish the work to be done
  - Believes integrity is an essential characteristic
  - Has emerging passion for the process and the relationships among team members
  - Inspires others with passionate spirit and commitment
  - Begins to develop resilience to negative events
  - Exhibits increasing impulse control
- Expert (dialogic engagement)
  - Demonstrates self-awareness and utilizes self-assessment information to improve personal performance and to support and understand team members
  - Possesses strong resilience to the negative realities of the workplace and coaches others in developing similar skills; able to manage difficult information
  - Is able to think and feel simultaneously
  - Is open to others' ideas and viewpoints
  - Actively seeks opinions from team members on their task processes, progress, and performance
  - Actively coaches and mentors new members as well as current members
  - Exhibits well-developed impulse control

Advanced Beginner Stage

The advanced beginner is finally engaged in a leadership role, testing the knowledge and skills gained during formal education. The focus is on developing competence in coaching and mentoring and in relationship building. Although the advanced beginner's level of self-awareness is increasing, his or her main goal is to demonstrate personal competence and ensure satisfactory work. The advanced beginner is starting to think about group processes and how to integrate the emotions of others but is not always certain of the connections between an event and another's emotional reaction.

The advanced beginner spends little attention or time on understanding the reactions of others in the setting. Also, he or she is not always open to the ideas of others and tends to be judgmental. The advanced beginner is starting to become more confident as a decision maker but is discouraged easily and not always optimistic about the future.

Competent Stage

In the third stage, the individual is more experienced as a leader and is beginning to develop compassion for others. The individual is able to think about issues and simultaneously have feelings and acknowledge the feelings of others. He or she also now develops the ability to be present physically and mentally, attend to conversations with authenticity, and listen to and ask questions of team members with sensitivity to their emotions.

The individual is increasingly compassionate and open to the ideas of others and is less judgmental than previously. He or she also exhibits a greater ability to control impulses and begins to feel comfortable challenging the status quo.

Proficient Stage

Team leaders often hit an invisible wall at the competent stage and do not make it to the proficient stage. If this happens, the teamwork becomes rote and frequently is ineffective. Longstanding teams that meet without adding value to health care outcomes fit this category.

A team leader who reaches the proficient stage is noticeably more comfortable in the role and has a better grasp of the influence of relationships on team activities. The proficient leader is able to think and feel simultaneously and to read the chemistry between people, recognize allies, identify whom to trust, and sense where nonsupport or hostility is present. This leader is beginning to develop the ability to manage negative feelings and is generally optimistic, including about the team's ability to accomplish its work. Only rarely is the individual discouraged or negative about the future. Passionate optimism—the integration of a positive outlook and wholehearted commitment—becomes the norm. Finally, the proficient leader has increasing control over impulses and is developing resilience in the face of difficulties or crises.

Expert Stage

The leader at the expert stage uses self-assessment information to improve personal performance and support the other members of the team. Thinking and feeling simultaneously is the only way the expert leader knows how to act. As an accomplished team member, the expert leader not only is open to new ideas but seeks input from others. The expert leader actively coaches and mentors new members as well as current members in developing expert emotional competence skills. As a passionate optimist, the expert leader is highly resilient and at the same time possesses sophisticated impulse control.

Emotionally Incompetent Behaviors

In journeying toward full emotional competence, people will exhibit behaviors indicative of emotional incompetence. Given that incompetence is often easier to describe than competence, the following examples of emotional incompetence are presented as a means of indicating what emotional competence is.

Acting as Devil's Advocate

All too often people consider an issue or situation from the self-appointed position of devil's advocate. In most such cases, people assume this perspective for lack of self-awareness and understanding of their own point of view. They hide behind the role for any number of reasons—usually only known to them. Common reasons include lack of information, inability to support an idea while unsure how to express nonsupport, and desire to block the decision-making process.

Displaying a Bad Attitude

People who have a difficult time participating in work processes often display negative behaviors ranging from grumbling to shirking. They usually do not understand that such behaviors impede progress and decrease the overall morale of the group, or, if they do, they might refuse to acknowledge the effects of their actions on others or dismiss their behavior by claiming, "That's just the way I am."

Displaying a Superior Attitude

An individual with a superior attitude responds to comments with indignation and criticism. The individual also usually does not recognize the adversarial nature of his or her responses and their impact on others but views them as a necessary means for getting the entire group to understand its inadequacies.

Tolerating Errors

Tolerating errors or undesirable behaviors implies these are accepted. In many cases, the tolerance results from the inability of those in charge to react and correct the errors or behaviors and/or the organizational culture's lack of support for managing problematic behaviors. When an individual has failed to meet the relevant behavioral standards, managers and others in the organization must use the situation as an opportunity to reinforce the organizational culture and build better relationships.

Failing To Balance Work and Relaxation

Often leaders find themselves spending more time at work and less time at home, believing that the operation of the organization is more important than other priorities. Further, they commonly believe their presence is required for productivity to occur. They thus wind up spending excessive hours at work and neglect the other parts of their life, including recreating with family and friends. The focus on work tasks is characteristic of the advanced beginner level of emotional competence, whereas achieving a balance between work and family and community is characteristic of the expert level.

TEAM EMOTIONAL COMPETENCE

In creating team-level emotional competence, a team builds on the skills of the individual members and extends the focus to itself as a collective. The assumption is that the members have at least a basic understanding of team processes such as goal setting, agenda management, and communication. It is through these processes that the team members begin to feel confidence in each other and in the team as a whole, reinforcing successful team behaviors. Team emotional competence, like the individual variety, usually is developed incrementally in a five-stage process (Exhibit 6–4).

Novice Stage

A novice team consists of individuals coming together for the first time for a newly defined purpose. The members know very little, if anything, about each other and typically do not share common feelings or values—or if they do, they are not aware of their commonalities at this point. A novice team's focus is on understanding the purpose of the team and setting the ground rules.

Advanced Beginner Stage

In this stage, the team becomes more cohesive through establishing how to carry out meeting tasks such as setting agendas, recording the minutes, and ensuring that the ground rules are defined and followed. Jockeying for power often occurs at this level, but it tends to end once the team develops feedback skills and gets into the habit of recognizing the contributions of each member. The team makes a conscious and deliberate effort to (1) shift from valuing power as traditionally used to foster empowerment and (2) develop an awareness of the behavior patterns of each member. However, the members evidence little openness toward substantive ideas and dialogue. Their focus is on task completion and agenda management. They also are discouraged easily and are uncertain as to their ability to create meaningful change.

Competent Stage

A competent team is a compassionate team, and its compassion is reflected in its willingness to discuss every member's issues of concern. The team members have moved from trying to acquire individual power to acting as an authentic collective. They not only show themselves capable of thinking and feeling simultaneously but acknowledge each other's feelings and integrate them into the team's overall work. In addition, they set and follow ground rules that are realistic and support the team's work. The coaching and mentoring they do with each other are intended to foster behaviors that aid the team rather than to develop skills that are useful only outside of the team. Finally, the team's level of trust in itself grows, and the members begin to challenge the status quo and consider alternatives to the way things are currently done.

Exhibit 6–4 Team Emotional Competence Skill Levels and Behaviors

- Novice (detached observer)
  - Team is newly formed and consists of independent participants.
  - Members have no prior relationships with or knowledge of behavior patterns and emotions of other members.
- Advanced beginner (active participant)
  - Group guidelines are developed and understood by members (this transition stage reflects the shift from the use of individual power to integrated goals and unified or share support for goals).
  - Group cohesion is beginning to develop.
  - Team is mainly focused on meeting processes.
  - Team behavior patterns are beginning to emerge.
  - At times the team is overwhelmed and easily discouraged.
- Competent (integrated with the process)
  - Members are increasingly self-aware and sensitive to communication dynamics between members.
  - Team establishes realistic ground rules.
  - Members understand each other's skills and emotions.
  - Team routinely requests feedback from every member at the beginning and the end of the meetings.

  - Outcomes of the team's work are evident.
- Proficient (therapeutic engagement)
  - Team members understand the goals of the team and the relationship of their work to that of other teams in the organization.
  - Team members seek feedback from others in the organization following team meetings and bring feedback to the next meeting.
  - Team is passionate about its work and optimistic that it can make a difference.
  - Team shows tolerance for character failings.
- Expert (dialogic engagement)
  - Team members understand the team's goals and how they relate to the organization and community at large.
  - Team consists of experienced and mature members.
  - Team is able to integrate local and national regulations into its work.
  - Team often makes recommendations and moves beyond its specific assigned tasks to create better options for the organization.
  - Team terminates itself when it is unable to add further value to the organization.

As with individual emotional competence, there is often an invisible wall between the competent and proficient stages. Teams at the competent stage can meet the requirements for standard success but find it impossible to become passionately optimistic while recreating the future or to maintain resilience in the face of negative events. They accomplish the assigned work but seldom move beyond the assigned boundaries.

Proficient Stage

As the emotional skills of the team mature, it develops a sense of passionate optimism about the future. A proficient team differs from a competent team in considering the needs and priorities of the whole organization as integral to its work. All the members are aware of and understand each other's behavior patterns and use these patterns in developing a consensus on issues, encouraging each other to discuss difficult issues, and addressing the emotions that these issues tend to give rise to. At this stage, the team members are able to recognize each other's character failings as inevitable and to work to restore the integrity of relationships.

Expert Stage

For a team to arrive at the expert level of emotional competence is a highly desirable but rare event. An expert team is purposefully coached and mentored and requires ongoing support and validation if it is to be sustained. At this level of performance, the team not only embodies all of the characteristics of the proficient team but also considers the needs and priorities of the organization and the health care community and ensures that proposed team actions are congruent with the organization's culture and politics.

The members are aware of individual, team, and organizational emotions as an interactive whole. As a team, they have established norms that strengthen their ability to respond effectively to the kind of emotional challenges a group confronts on a regular basis. These norms are directed toward three goals: creating resources for working with emotions, fostering an affirmative environment, and encouraging proactive problem solving. In addition, the expert team embodies resilience to the realities of the environment. Finally, the team members, besides being individually aware of their inward- and outward-directed emotions and able to regulate them, jointly develop a level of group mindfulness.

Causes of Team Dysfunction

Teams that have existed for a long time commonly acquire behavior patterns that render them inefficient or nonproductive. For instance, they often leave assignments incomplete, allow malcontents to continue griping, pay scant notice to habitual tardiness and absenteeism, and go off on tangents that have little to do with their intended work. Each team has a natural lifespan, and when its work is completed, it should be disbanded or assigned another project.

It is also important to realize that a team may move along the developmental trajectory at an irregular rate and may even regress, such as when its membership and goals change. Further, it is common for a team's development to inexplicably halt before the proficiency stage, in which case the team never gets to the point of integrating its work with that of the organization, much less with the environment or the community at large.

To see how team development can be arrested, consider the breach between senior health care leaders and point-of-service providers that occurred following the implementation of managed care. As the reimbursement systems changed and the actual dollars paid to organizations decreased dramatically, significant expense reductions were needed. Nonetheless, in many cases the actual work increased. The point-of-service workers ranted and raved about the impact on quality and staff morale, yet the leaders demanded more and more expense reductions as external reimbursement continued to decline. The rift between staff and management widened, with little hope of relief.

Before the reimbursement levels were reduced, health care teams, although not yet at the proficiency level, were aware of the needs and feelings of all individuals, and their emotional performance could be rated as competent. Their work had two focuses: providing high-quality patient care and maximizing reimbursement. When reimbursement decreased, the teams fell even further short of taking into account the goals of all members (or the goals of the organization as a whole) and thus never reached the proficiency level.

In many ways, the course of events described resembles Levy's (2001) Nut Island effect. The Nut Island story is about a team of competent, highly committed employees who performed a vital, behind-the-scenes task. The team was adept at organizing and managing itself. Its self-sufficiency was taken for granted by senior management, and when it asked for help or tried to warn of impending trouble, it was ignored or put off because senior management, looking at its history of success, would assume it could handle the current situation. Consequently, an adversarial relationship began to develop between senior management and the team. Unfortunately, the team reacted in a way that worsened the problem. The team made it a priority to stay out of management's line of sight, which led it to deny or minimize problems and avoid asking for help. Eventually, the team began to make up its own rules to enable it to fulfill its own mission—apart from the mission of the organization as a whole.

Group Discussion

The Nut Island story (described in the text) encompasses a number of issues, including lack of teamwork, insensitivity to a team's context, and disharmony between the feelings of individuals in the local setting (the team members) and individuals at the system level (the senior managers). Can you use this story to elucidate adversarial relationships that exist between leaders and departments in your organization? If so, identify at least three strategies to mitigate the friction or hostility between the parties, using emotional competence as the framework. What outcomes would you select as measures of the effectiveness of these strategies?

At this point, both senior management and the team had distorted views that were very difficult to correct. The team members believed that they were the only ones who really understood their work and were unwilling to listen to outsiders attempting to help solve their problems. Management remained disconnected, believing that no news was good news. Only a significant external event could change the course of events. Neither the senior managers nor the team members considered the meaning of their work within the context of the entire organization or the marketplace. As a result, the team's level of emotional competence decreased dramatically.

MEASURING EMOTIONAL COMPETENCE

Most health care organizations know how to measure and document clinical outcomes, financial results, and market share. Most, however, are very uncomfortable assessing factors such as behavior patterns, compassion, passionate optimism, and impulse control. The reality is that individuals tend to measure what they are comfortable with and ignore those areas they are not comfortable measuring. Given that at least four characteristics have been identified that reflect emotional competence, individuals and groups have the opportunity to measure their level of competence in handling their own and others' feelings.

First, individual leaders should consider developing a reputation assessment and management survey (Exhibit 6–5) to help them formally manage their reputations. Reputation management has been done informally by many forward-thinking leaders on the assumption that how others perceive them influences their ability to impact organizational operations. By creating a personal sensitivity process for gathering accurate feedback, a leader can learn about his or her effect on others and gain useful information for developing a reputation management plan. Both self-perceptions and the perceptions of others provide a helpful perspective on one's effectiveness.

Self-knowledge allows leaders to begin the journey toward the highest level of emotional competence. In many organizations, leaders use a 360-degree evaluation to gain additional information about their leadership abilities. Although feedback from superiors, peers, and subordinates is important, the source of the feedback must be identified to reinforce the importance of trust and honest communication. Further, such assessments need to contain items for measuring behaviors and characteristics that reflect emotional competence, including self-awareness, compassion, passionate optimism, self-regulation, and resilience.

> **Point To Ponder**
>
> *The way to gain a good reputation is to endeavor to be what you desire to appear.*
> —*Socrates*

To help measure the emotional competence of teams, specific items related to self-awareness, compassion, passionate optimism, self-regulation, and resilience should be included in employee satisfaction and patient satisfaction surveys. The integration of individual and team information provides an overview of the emotional competence of the organization.

Exhibit 6–5 Reputation Assessment and Management Survey

1. Am I trustworthy?
2. To what extent do I trust others?
3. Do I practice what I preach?
4. Do I tell people who need to know what I am thinking and why I am acting in a particular way?
5. Am I dependable?
6. Do I listen nondefensively?
7. Am I able to find the grain of truth embedded in a criticism?
8. Am I visible and available when things are not going well?
9. Am I perceived as a hard worker?
10. Do I value the contributions of team members?

CONCLUSION

We live in complex times. To be successful, we need to think and feel simultaneously and to acknowledge our feelings and those of others. The goal of the quantum leader is to learn as much as possible from the past and gracefully and soundly move to more appropriate methods of managing the work of organizations. These methods include acting in ways that are sensitive to people's emotions to increase their active engagement with their work.

The ability to manage feelings is a skill no leader can be without. The first step toward gaining this skill is to understand what is important not only to oneself but also to others in the organization. Ignoring the feelings and behaviors of others is a sure way to impede progress. Although progress is usually incremental at best, quantum leaders always have an eye on the future while holding onto their passionate optimism as a sacred gift.

REFERENCES

Allen, K.E. 2000. Leadership as an emergent property of individual and group interaction. *The Inner Edge* 3, no. 6: 20–21.

Barker, R.A. 1998. The future of leadership research. *Futures Research Quarterly* 14, no. 1: 5–16.

Collins, J. 2001. Level 5 leadership: The triumph of humility and fierce resolve. *Harvard Business Review* 79, no. 1: 67–76.

Dreyfus, H.L., and S.E. Dreyfus. 1996. The relationship of theory and practice in the acquisition of skill. In *Expertise in nursing practice: Caring, clinical judgment, and ethics,* ed. P. Benner et al., 29–47. New York: Springer.

Druskat, V.U., and S.B. Wolff. 2001. Building the emotional intelligence of groups. *Harvard Business Review* 79, no. 3: 81–90.

Dyer, W. 1976. *Your erroneous zones.* New York: HarperCollins.

Goleman, D. 1998. *Working with emotional intelligence.* New York: Bantam.

Levy, P.F. 2001. The Nut Island effect: When good teams go wrong. *Harvard Business Review* 79, no. 3: 51–59.

Orsburn, J.D., J. Moran, E. Musselwhite, and J.H. Zenter. 1990. *Self-directed work teams.* Homewood, IL: Business One Irwin.

Weick, K., and K. Sutcliffe. 2000. High reliability: The power of mindfulness. *Leader to Leader* 21 (summer): 33–38.

SUGGESTED READINGS

Bennis, W., and J. O'Toole. 2000. Don't hire the wrong CEO. *Harvard Business Review* 78, no. 5: 171–176.

Forsyth, S., and M. Parish. 1999. The practical side of emotional intelligence. *The Inner Edge* 1, no. 5: 9–11.

Hansen, M.T., and B. von Oetinger. 2001. Introducing T-shaped managers: Knowledge management's next generation. *Harvard Business Review* 79, no. 3: 107–116.

Mecklenburg, G.A. 2001. Career performance: How are we doing? *Journal of Healthcare Management* 46, no. 1: 8–13.

Porter-O'Grady, T., and C.K. Wilson. 1998. *The health care team book.* St. Louis: Mosby.

Sandberg, J. 2001. Understanding competence at work. *Harvard Business Review* 79, no. 3: 24–28.

Quiz Questions

Select the best answer for each of the following questions.

1. Emotional competence is based on specific principles. Which one of the following is not consistent with these principles?

a. holism
b. Newtonian principles
c. Theory Y behaviors
d. emergent leadership

2. Leaders have resisted the notion that emotional competence is an essential leadership characteristic. The most likely reason for this resistance is:

a. the difficulty of measuring and evaluating the impact of emotional competence
b. the lack of theoretical support for the concept of emotional competence
c. the cost of integrating emotionally competent behaviors into an organization
d. the lack of employee support for the idea that emotional competence is important

3. The four attributes specific to emotional competence are:

a. self-awareness, integrity, passionate optimism, and compassion
b. self-awareness, passionate optimism, character, and impulse control
c. self-awareness, compassion, passionate optimism, and emotional intelligence
d. self-awareness, compassion, passionate optimism, and impulse control

4. Integrated leadership is a synergistic combination of technical, relational, and intentional skills. This combination leads to:

a. emotionally competent individuals and leaders
b. optimal resource use and positive patient outcomes
c. additional costs to the organization
d. improved employee satisfaction

5. Self-awareness—the understanding of one's personal behavior patterns and preferences—is a fundamental characteristic of emotional competence. Among other benefits, it leads to:

a. passionate optimism and compassion
b. impulse control
c. openness to others and an appreciation of paradox
d. character and integrity

6. The emotional risks of leadership are ever present and cannot be ignored. Sources of emotional risks faced by leaders include:

a. the lack of timely feedback
b. the lack of an employment contract
c. unacceptable levels of employee dissatisfaction
d. sharing decision making with team members

7. Emergent leadership is one of the underpinnings of emotional competence. Emergent leadership differs from the dyadic model of leadership in this regard:

a. The organizational chart for emergent leadership is a matrix.
b. Emergent leadership eliminates the need for a CEO.
c. Emergent leadership is based on the principle that high levels of organizational performance depend on the presence of a strong leader who defines the work of the organization.
d. Emergent leadership is based on the principle that high levels of organizational performance depend on the engagement of the members in the work of the organization.

8. Impulse control is one of the hallmarks of the emotionally competent individual. To develop this skill, the individual:

a. reframes negative feelings when necessary to maximize the use of his or her energy
b. learns how to apologize sincerely
c. recognizes conflict as normative
d. works to eliminate emotions in the workplace

9. Focused hiring is a way of selecting new employees that:

a. eliminates the need for external search firms
b. decreases leadership turnover
c. focuses on the fit between the candidates and the organization
d. identifies the candidate with the greatest potential for integrating into the organization successfully

10. Individual emotional competence develops gradually through the novice, advanced beginner, competence, and proficiency stages to finally arrive at the level of expertise. Individuals who have reached the competence stage are able to:

a. think and feel simultaneously while considering the opinions of others
b. project passionate optimism for the work of their profession
c. control their impulses effectively
d. coach others in the development of emotional competence

11. Team emotional competence develops through the same five stages as individual emotional competence. A team that has reached emotional proficiency is able to:

a. understand the skills and emotions of all team members

b. orient its work toward meeting the needs of the community

c. orient its work toward meeting the goals and needs of the organization

d. integrate local and national regulations into its work

CHAPTER 7

Toxic Organizations and People: The Leader as Transformer

The workplace can be a positive crucible, not a mind-bending and spirit-shattering one.

—*William Lundin and Kathleen Lundin* (1993)

Chapter Objectives

At the completion of this chapter, the reader will be able to

- Identify the common sources of toxicity and dysfunction in health care organizations.
- Analyze longstanding leadership behaviors that negatively impact organizations.
- Describe the negative impact of system toxic practice on employee performance.
- Describe the negative impact of career entrenchment and career entrapment on organizational effectiveness.
- Critique the 10 principles for minimizing organizational toxicity.

Because of the trend in health care toward restructuring, downsizing, and merging, organizational leaders are finding themselves increasingly challenged by dysfunctional and toxic situations. Health care organizations, as any other, are microcosms of society. The potential for the expression of positive and helpful behaviors or negative and interfering ones always exists. The reality is that there is no screen for dysfunctional behaviors when hiring, except for the most obvious. Dysfunctional behaviors come in various degrees and affect organizational effectiveness in a range of ways.

This chapter discusses dysfunctional behaviors that typically impair health care organizations, including antisocial behaviors, toxic mentoring, and neurotic and self-defeating behaviors. It also discusses organizational practices that are prone to dysfunction and organizational characteristics that reinforce dysfunction. To mitigate the negative impact of dysfunctional behaviors, it presents 10 principles designed to minimize organizational toxicity. These principles focus on reversing the dysfunctional behaviors of leaders and guiding them toward more appropriate practices that can transform dysfunction into health. Specifically, leaders need to become more self-aware, become more consistent in word and behavior, listen better, empower employees, and create new models for reward and recognition.

Health professionals are increasingly asking themselves the following questions: If healing is my profession and contribution to society, why do I feel so bad? Why are so many of my colleagues more discouraged with their work than ever before? Shortages of available workers, declining enrollments in colleges and universities, and the unstable financing system all continue to fuel the disfranchisement of health professionals. Employees are reluctant to trust one another and must be coaxed to interact. They are increasingly engaging in labor union activity as a means of mediating their pain. Care providers frequently are conflicted over whether to give care or withhold it. The care that is given is believed by many to be substandard, incomplete, and sometimes even harmful. The environment that is created by these problems tends to kill cooperation and creativity.

The complaints of colleagues, along with the newspaper headlines, might suggest that health care organizations are more toxic and in greater distress than many of the patients receiving health care services. Far too many health professionals, particularly leaders and point-of-service workers, are missing the energy and collaborative spirit that mirror health. Their psyches have been assaulted too severely and for too long by neurotic leadership styles, dysfunctional group processes, inappropriate superior-subordinate bonding, and abandonment. These unfortunate toxicogenic practices need to be swiftly reversed, for they are destroying the vitality of health care organizations.

Some may be tempted to attribute the distress of health care workers solely to changes in reimbursement policy and to look for the solution in a more palatable financing structure. The reality, however, is that the toxicity of health care organizations is not just a matter of reimbursement. Indeed, the silver lining of the prospective payment and managed care models may be that they can help expose the subtle yet pervasive toxins currently harming the health care system.

Health care organizations, for example, have been plagued by a delivery model in which (mostly male) physicians have almost total control, not to mention disempowering practices, a mentality of personal entitlement, and resistance to change. These factors, along with the increasing challenge of financing care and a philosophy of things first and peo-

---

Group Discussion

At the next team meeting, ask employees to identify at least two toxic behaviors in the organization that they believe should be changed. Consider the following questions: Can you clearly and objectively define the problem? If you were in charge, how would you change behaviors to make them less toxic? What indicators would you use to measure the change in behaviors?

ple second, cause organizational toxicity and nullify the essential values of healing and restoration of health. The job of organizational leaders is to identify the toxic behaviors and develop strategies to minimize their effects. Rather than attempt to determine who the guilty parties are—individuals or organizations (or both)—the challenge is to move forward and create the kind of culture that will lead to organizational health.

Some of the main differences between toxic and healthy organizations concern the issues of control, conflict, and adaptability. For example, an organization in which the level of toxicity is high can be characterized in this way:

- The employees are widely subject to forces outside their control.
- Because of their lack of control, the employees are more susceptible to illness.
- The leaders and employees try to decrease conflict rather than accept it as normal and as useful.
- The employees tend to become stuck and lose their ability to change.

The following is true of a healthy organization:

- The organization depends on group process and shared decision making to accomplish its work.
- The employees are basically relaxed rather than stressed.
- The leaders and employees recognize conflict as normal and treat instances of conflict as opportunities for gaining information and planning and implementing improvements.
- Individuals and groups become facile at adapting to changing circumstances.

HEALING IS OUR BUSINESS?

Paradoxically, the working conditions in health care organizations are generally not healthy. Many leaders are aware that changes need to be made, but not all of them understand that the cures for the toxicity in the health care system should come from within the system, in particular, from the health professionals who create and manage the system. If a better system is to be built, it must rest on the fundamental values of healers—restoring wholeness and a state of harmonious energy.

The principles that apply to the health of individuals also apply to the health of organizations. In the case of individuals, health is "harmony between the most basic cell and its environment in which there is abundant energy and the basic unit is effectively performing the function appropriate to its location in time and space" (King 1989, 30). In order to function properly, each individual cell requires a sufficient supply of nutrients and an efficient system of cleansing or waste removal (Figure 7–1).

An organization likewise requires nutrients (inputs) in order to provide health care: dollars, medical supplies, and human resources, for example. A healthy organization, like a healthy individual, can be described as an entity harmoniously connected with its environment and thus able to take advantage of the environment's available energy. All life requires a continual replenishment of inputs. A shortage or oversupply of inputs can result in negative outcomes. Too much food results in obesity (Figure 7–2), and too little results in the loss of mass and energy; the result in both cases is an impairment of the entity's ability to

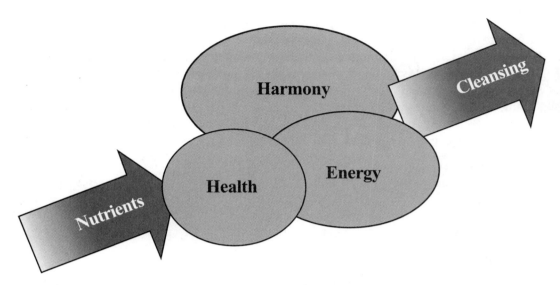

Figure 7–1 Adequate Nutrients and Adequate Cleansing Result in a Balance of Health, Harmony, and Energy

function (Figure 7–3). Similarly, a surfeit of employees or unrestrained financial resources lead to a lack of accountability and cause dysfunction. When there are no parameters on resource availability or use, there is no accountability—until the resources run out!

All organizations also require the removal of waste products in an effective and timely manner. When an organization is unable to remove waste, the buildup of toxins begins to

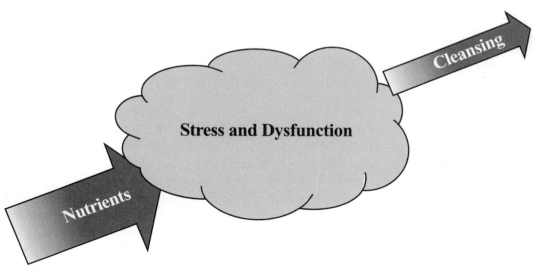

Figure 7–2 Excess Nutrients Lead to Obesity and to Stress and Dysfunction

Group Discussion

In both organisms and organizations, there is a healthy middle ground between an overabundance and a deficiency of inputs. From this perspective, consider whether there is a shortage of health care workers in your organization. Ask team members the following questions: Is there an excess of employees that are less-than-average performers? Is there a shortage of employees with appropriate skills to meet the contemporary needs of the organization? What are the missing skill sets? Develop a plan that focuses on improving the skills and increasing the number of employees. What indicators of organizational performance will be used to measure progress?

impede functioning. At some point, enough "cells" are affected to cause a symptom and bring the problem to conscious attention. For instance, the organization, by retaining policies and practices that no longer serve a purpose or add value, will become toxic from the buildup of these. The goal may be to preserve tradition, but the result is inappropriate resource use leading to dysfunction.

Whether the problem is under- or oversupply of nutrients or disturbance of the cleansing processes, an entity (an organism or organization) will experience decreased effectiveness and possibly distress. When an organization is unable to remove waste, the toxins begin to build up and impede functioning. Indeed, if an organization retains less than adequate employees or ineffective equipment, the processes needed for transformation will be ineffective and non–value-added work will continue to drain resources and act as a serious obstacle to doing the work that needs to be done. If the flow of nutrients to an organism is constrained or the organism's cleansing processes are inhibited, the organism will experi-

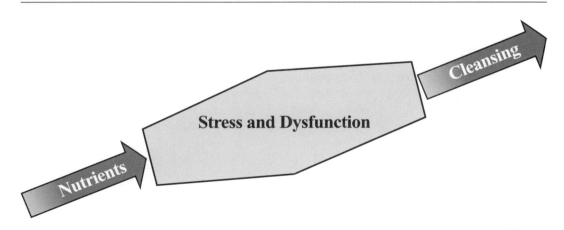

Figure 7–3 Inadequate Nutrients Lead to Loss of Mass and Energy and to Stress and Dysfunction

ence tension. In an organization, constriction in the flow of inputs (money, materials, or health professionals) will impede the work processes and cause dysfunction and damage.

The stress that results from balancing nutrients and cleansing occurs as a natural effect of resistance to change. Resistance, like stress, is not bad in itself. It enables us to sense our environment and to grow by working through challenges and accomplishing goals that stretch our talents and capacities for learning. But for these benefits to accrue, a dynamic balance between resistance and nonresistance must be maintained. Distress comes from rigid resistance, the kind that continues beyond the point of effectiveness and into the range where function breaks down. When practices that produce no obvious value are sustained because they have become ritual, not only does performance suffer but toxicity accelerates among the employees, often leading to the demise of the organization.

Toxicity in an organization can impact employees both physically and emotionally. Indeed, the field of psychoneuroimmunology has documented that there are links between feeling states and physiological responses. The emotions associated with caring—namely, hope, love, and joy—have been identified as ingredients in the remission of disease, whereas loss of hope or love and the failure to adequately cope with stress have been identified as factors in both the onset and exacerbation of the symptoms of major illness. In other words, the lack of caring or nurturing may be a primary causative factor in disease. Surely, there is a relationship between the lack of organizational caring and nurturing and the level of organizational toxicity.

Organizational toxicity is often unnoticed at the onset but slowly emerges as cynicism, declining morale, loss of creativity, and lower productivity. If its emotional component is not addressed, it can leave a toxic residue, preventing a complete return of function. The broken spirit never heals. That is, the unresolved or buried anger and resentment remain and thwart organizational efforts.

> **Key Point**
>
> *If you are not the master of your spirit and permit yourself to be demeaned, you are going to get sick unless something changes.*
> *—William Lundin and Kathleen Lundin (1993)*

Often the organizational response to toxicity mirrors the primitive response of granuloma formation. In a case of granuloma formation, the body does not deal with the underlying injury but instead walls it off with a fibrous deposit of cells. The injury merely appears to be mended, and no additional healing occurs. So too can an organization seal off a dysfunctional component while believing that it is taking proper corrective action. Unfortunately, this response prevents the organization from developing strategies for avoiding similar types of dysfunction in the future and also impedes work processes that should involve the dysfunctional component. The unresolved organizational conflict, like a granuloma, persists and affects every related decision in the future.

TOXIC BEHAVIORS

When an organization provides services in ways that subtly work against its stated goals, it violates its fundamental covenant with its employees and the community. At the same time, the organization's leaders and other members reinforce negative beliefs about the organization and further entrench the dysfunctional behaviors. The resulting toxic interactions become destructive to effective relationships.

Toxic or hostile work environments are recognizable not just by the presence of screaming, flaring tempers, and abusive language, but also by the less noticeable but often more damaging quiet demoralization that occurs. Unilateral decision making, the ignoring of requests, and the avoidance of unpleasant issues cause substantial toxicity, specifically, employee discontent. Furthermore, although chronically angry individuals and controlling supervisors regularly reinforce the toxicity, careless insensitivity to the impact of one's actions on others is one of the main causes. Leaders do not always stop and think!

The organizational culture, which of course has an enormous impact on decision making, leadership style, strategy formation, and organizational change, can be influenced in subtle and complex ways by invisible, longstanding psychological forces hidden from the individuals who experience them. These covert forces all too often produce organizational outcomes that appear to be extremely irrational and dysfunctional.

Health care leaders are seldom satisfied with the structures, processes, and outcomes of their organization. It is the complex, longstanding interdependencies between stakeholders that create both healthy behaviors and toxic behaviors difficult to untangle and remedy. Toxic behaviors within an organization seldom are the result of one individual process gone awry but rather are the culmination of many dysfunctions that form a syndrome of organizational pathology. Similar patterns of strategic and structural defects can be as dramatic and bold as they are toxic. If one top executive uses a neurotic leadership style, others will adopt similar behaviors. The result will be a poorly functioning, self-defeating organization.

This is not to deny that some mildly dysfunctional traits and behaviors can occur in moderation without causing significant difficulties. Most individuals exhibit low levels of shyness and depression and have a few irrational fears and suspicions. Major problems occur when these dysfunctional traits and behaviors dominate relationships between individuals.

Below, 10 sources of organizational toxicity are presented to help the readers gain an understanding of its dynamics and formulate strategies to decrease it (Exhibit 7–1). Note that the distinction between the toxic behaviors of individuals and organizational toxicity is artificial, because the work of individuals acting as a team is in fact the work of the organization.

Vertical Authority Structure

The structure of an organization, including its authority and decision-making parameters, can be a source of organizational toxicity. A vertical organizational structure, for example, frequently reinforces negative behaviors and serves as a defense against personal involvement. Leaders of vertically structured organizations tend to believe there is "an enemy out there" that must be managed, and they become driven by anger, fear, and suspicion. A vertical structure, besides encompassing a rigid hierarchy of authority, restricts communication, for directives must be handed down from the chief executive level to the staff through multiple layers of middle managers. Employees are discouraged from engaging in accountable behaviors, healthy dialogue, and creative thinking.

Exhibit 7–1 Ten Sources of Organizational Toxicity

1. Vertical authority structure	6. Tolerance of antisocial behavior
2. Inequitable reward and recognition practices	7. Toxic mentoring
	8. Inconsistency and dishonesty
3. Abuse of power	9. Imbalance between work and personal life
4. Lack of respect for the work force	
5. Failure to manage unmotivated employees	10. Advocacy gone awry

In addition, traditional vertical organizations require clear localization of decision making at the higher levels. Leaders often become obsessively vigilant because of their belief that subordinates and competitors cannot be trusted. Their paranoia also leads to the centralization of power and to excessive control over individuals and decision making. These organizations suffer from too much leadership, too many rigid procedures, too much documentation, and too much attention paid to keeping on schedule. Leaders in a vertical organization typically fear change and steadfastly defend ritualistic behaviors out of a desire for security.

The corporate culture in a traditional vertical organization typically suppresses individual creativity. Managed like a monarchy, this type of organization infantilizes its employees by expecting near-blind obedience. The rare exceptions tend to be organizations that have adopted a shared leadership model as a needed replacement for the traditional command-and-control model.

Vertical organizations recognize that creative people are expressive people but do not allow employees to be expressive at work. They think that emotional outbursts should be saved for the home. Later, when their emotions recede, the employees are supposed to produce new ideas. This expectation leads to a waste of talent—talent for the original thinking that organizations so desperately need for survival and success. Furthermore, as a result of the suppression of emotions at work, employees develop a desire to be managed, nourished, and protected by a leader, and their misplaced awe for the leader can lead to depression and guilt.

In a vertical organization, the different types of vice-president—senior vice-president, executive vice-president, assistant vice-president—connote varying degrees of authority and reflect an imbalance of power within the executive team. The practice of having several levels of vice-presidentship may be intended to allow for progression through the executive ranks, but in reality it minimizes the opportunity to create a mutually valuing and cooperative setting.

The separation of individuals into departments and divisions rather than functional units further reinforces power differentials. In this model, the core processes are specific to each department and are focused more on meeting departmental needs than on creating and delivering products and services to meet customer needs.

Reorganization within a vertical organization often results in mazelike reporting networks in which managers manage other managers and set precise communication expectations. If reorganization is a recurring phenomenon, the frequent changes in team size and membership will hinder the development of expert team behaviors. Also, the threat of losing organizational positions because of anticipated mergers and acquisitions has in some cases caused senior leaders to move in opposite directions, harbor personal agendas, and be minimally compatible with each other. As for the employees of a vertical organization, when greater productivity is expected at the same time that resources are decreased, they unsurprisingly become angry and disillusioned. The survivors of layoffs are frequently less productive, develop poor job attitudes, and often voluntarily follow their discharged coworkers into unemployment or to other organizations. Yet the essential vertical structure is retained regardless of the frequency of the shuffling or the complexity of the rearrangements. Power is retained at the top and distributed through departmental leaders.

Inequitable Reward and Recognition Practices

Another toxin found in most organizations is inequitable pay. It is important to note that few people are ever satisfied with their level of compensation. Nonetheless, although always desirous of more money, most individuals recognize that resources are limited and are only seeking equitable compensation. Compensation practices become toxic when rewards and recognition are inequitable or inconsistent.

Severely compressed pay ranges, particularly in nursing, limit financial growth while making other disciplines, such as law, engineering, and technological fields, more attractive. Also, limitations on annual compensation packages result in equal but minimal increases for all employees. Employees who do the requisite work without extending themselves, attend only mandatory continuing education programs, and miss work occasionally

Group Discussion

Compressed pay ranges and limited dollars for reward and recognition continue to challenge leaders in their efforts to motivate staff. In collaboration with members of your team, revise the current reward and recognition system or create an entirely new one. Make sure the system you design

- separates the compensation process from the performance evaluation process
- awards nothing to employees who have a mediocre performance rating
- includes nonmonetary rewards, such as preferred scheduling, weekend or holiday preferences, and inclusion in decision making
- uses objective measures of performance to determine the effect of nonmonetary programs on employee satisfaction and turnover and on patient outcomes

(although staying within the normal range) are awarded the same 3 percent increase as employees who receive numerous thank-you letters from patients, attend external continuing education programs, have perfect attendance, and participate on committees.

The challenge of using limited available dollars to pay employees appropriately for their different levels of effort is rarely taken up by leaders. Rather than awarding 0 percent to mediocre employees and 10 percent to exemplary employees, leaders use the across-the-board approach so that everyone gets something. Seldom are other rewards, such as preferred scheduling, used as alternatives for rewarding excellent performers.

Compensation continues to be highly subjective, particularly at the senior level. Compensation for leaders is often based more on market standards than on their performance as team members. Consequently, compensation practices can cause severe division, infighting, jealousy, and mistrust, particularly when the senior executive's compensation is 20 times greater than that of the entry-level employee.

Abuse of Power

The third toxin is abuse of power. Because the highest turnover occurs, not at the staff level, but at the middle management level, leaders scramble to fill positions at this level, often selecting expert nurses with little or no management experience. In such cases, reports of the new "manager from hell" may soon begin to circulate. In short, the wrong person has been promoted to a leadership position and then, with title and power in hand, runs into trouble. The problem of quickly finding candidates with adequate experience to fill leadership positions and guiding them to become effective managers is faced by nearly every organization. Indeed, the toxicity mainly results, not from the appointment of inexperienced managers, but from the failure to intervene early in the process of assisting appointees to develop the skills needed for their positions.

When a new manager belittles staff members in front of patients or other staff members, communicates by memo rather than face to face, changes policies without input from others, and is rude and thoughtless, the staff soon run out of patience. Some staff members may attempt to communicate the issues to the manager and the manager's supervisor, but any dialogue between the staff, the new manager, and the supervisor will typically result in ascriptions of blame—of the new manager by the staff and of the staff by the new manager. Eventually, the staff members resign or transfer to other areas without making clear that their reason for changing employment was the lack of collegiality and of a respectful and caring work environment. The senior managers generally assume the staff members were seeking better salaries, better schedules, or shorter commutes to work—easily recognizable concrete reasons—and fail to recognize the true reason, allowing the toxicity to continue and intensify.

Mandatory Overtime

Another example of abuse of power is mandatory overtime. Although health care by its very nature involves the delivery of vital services that cannot be turned off and on in line with the availability of staff, mandatory overtime in a predominantly female profession raises significant issues, such as the difficulty of meeting both professional and family responsibilities. Nurses often feel exhausted and discouraged when they leave work, power-less to effect changes to ensure safe patient care and overburdened by the overtime they are expected to put in. Like the shoemaker's children who had no shoes, health care work-ers have no health—or are being slowly stripped of the healthy balance between work and personal life they once had.

Intolerance toward Diversity

Because communication technology and supersonic travel have made the world smaller, the diverse peoples of the world are able to share ideas and learn new approaches to a mul-tiplicity of tasks. Yet health care organizations have commonly failed to integrate the mul-tiple cultures of their staff members and patients (e.g., by not giving due consideration to their dietary habits and religious beliefs). Many have also been reluctant to actively seek diverse perspectives by including representatives from all gender and age groups in essen-tial work teams. Instead, stereotypical executives—male and middle aged—continue to develop strategic, human resource, and budgetary plans. Thus, in spite of educational pro-grams designed to minimize discriminatory practices, more proactive efforts to increase the diversity of the work force are needed. This is especially important given that the com-munities served by the predominantly white health care work force are on average more than 30 percent nonwhite.

Lack of Respect for the Work Force

Leaders of health care organizations have been known to view staff members as expend-able nuisances—as the cost of doing business. They have been known to objectify their employees and give them little or no consideration. Leaders may fall into such attitudes out of fear of dependency and an associated sense of vulnerability. For instance, when they see dependency in their subordinates, they may experience anxiety, causing them to reject their subordinates.

Employees often feel like foster children, powerless and completely dependent. They never know what they are going to get until they are hired. If an employee does not like the organization, he or she, like an unhappy child, can daydream and pretend not even to be there. Or the employee can run away and live on the street (resign and remain unem-ployed). Or the employee can hope that a nice gentleman with a big heart will appear with the offer of a better job!

Lack of respect takes many forms, from obvious rudeness to subtle discourtesy. It can include being nonresponsive to employee requests, dismissing new ideas with a smile, refusing to discuss issues that are important to employees, and exhibiting a general lack of manners, such as failing to say, "Thank you."

Failure To Manage Unmotivated Employees

The fifth toxin is one that haunts even the best leaders. Finding the time and energy to work with unmotivated career employees can be overwhelming. The difficulty is not in rec-ognizing less-than-optimal performance but in continuing to work with these employees despite minimal success at guiding them to do better. The lifetime career syndrome—lack-luster performance by career employees unexcited or burnt out by their jobs—is one of the impediments to efficiency that leaders are required to deal with regularly.

New expectations regarding employment have emerged during the last 20 years. Organizations are not prepared to enter into lifelong partnerships with individuals. No longer can an individual expect a durable commitment as a condition of employment. The trend is for the terms of employment to be congruent with the needs and financial resources of the hiring organization. When these needs or resources change, the employee's services are likely to be terminated.

Of course, terminating the services of long-term employees has never been an easy task. Many employees stay with an organization out of desperation but do not remain committed to it in the way management would like. Rather than firing these employees, managers often continue to invest in them in the hope that the support given to them will reverse their attitudes.

Many organizations are in fact burdened with workers who want to leave but who, for a variety of reasons, stay nonetheless. Department managers and directors often whisper among themselves, cursing the organization's flaws, but stay on because they are afraid to leave or because the pay, if little else, is excellent. Furthermore, if they left, they would have to sacrifice imminent salary increases, paid holidays and vacations, and retirement benefits. Yet they do not identify with or feel emotionally attached to their current position and do nothing about changing the situation.

Research by Carson and Carson (1997) has confirmed that career entrenchment and career entrapment are actual phenomena of organizational life. Career entrenchment is the tendency to stay in a vocation because of the investment already made, psychological preservation, and a perception that there are few career opportunities. Entrenched or entrapped employees have an established way of life, usually have good salaries, and know the challenges of the workplace. Leaving their jobs would create uncertainty as well as loss of identity and loss of income. Career entrenchment perpetuates itself, for when an employee becomes reconciled to staying in a career despite unhappiness with it, the employee is likely to invest further in the career, becoming more entrenched.

Individuals who are dissatisfied with their career usually engage in one of four coping strategies to manage the associated stress: They will either leave the career, openly discuss entrenchment with their employer, remain loyal to the organization while hoping for improvement in the future, or retire on the job (Exhibit 7–2).

People choose to enter a career based on their interests, preferences, and evaluation of opportunities. Once a person has selected a career, he or she then invests money and effort to achieve success. Typically, the person will periodically look at whether the career chosen truly offers adequate opportunities for meeting the person's needs and achieving his or her goals. If it appears to do that, the person will continue to invest in the career. On the other hand, if it does not, the person may change careers, especially if the level of investment to date has been low (a high level of investment might incline the person to remain in the career to justify the investment).

A career change also can be involuntary, as when an employee's job becomes obsolete or the employee is underutilized. Career changes sometimes cause only minimal disrup-

Exhibit 7–2   Career Entrapment Strategies

- *Exit:* An active strategy in which an individual leaves a career to change fields, retire, or withdraw from the labor force.
- *Voice:* An active strategy in which an individual constructively tries to improve conditions through verbalization of concerns.

- *Loyalty:* A passive strategy in which an individual passively but optimistically waits for conditions to improve.
- *Neglect:* A passive strategy in which an individual allows conditions to deteriorate through reduced interest and effort, tardiness or absenteeism, increased errors, and ineffective use of working time.

Source: The Academy of Management Executives, by Kerry D. Carson and Paula Carson, Vol. 11, No. 2, pp. 62–76. Copyright 1997 by the Academy of Management. Reproduced with permission of the Academy of Management in the format textbook via Copyright Clearance Center.

tion in lifestyle and sometimes major upheavals. For a person to see a potential new career as viable, he or she must perceive the career as desirable, be willing to invest in the career, and have a reasonable opportunity to enter it.

Most individuals attempt to select careers that match their personal interests. When a good match does not occur, the individual, besides having little passion for the work and being unsatisfied, is likely to be ineffective on the job. Unfortunately, whether a career is really congruent with an individual's personal interests is not always immediately evident, and thus mismatches and their negative consequences cannot always be avoided.

In the steady-state career prototype, an individual selects a career in late adolescence or early adulthood using a minimal amount of information, is trained in the career, and maintains the necessary performance skills for remaining in the career. Interestingly, some careers in which a high proportion of the professionals fit the steady-state model, including nursing, teaching, social work, and law enforcement, often result in burnout.

Group Discussion

Which came first, the lack of interest in nursing or the toxic conditions in the workplace? Together, the serious nursing shortage, the reluctance of nurses to recruit others into nursing, unmanageable workloads, the lack of valid and reliable workload systems to measure patient care needs, compressed pay scales, and the increased attractiveness of other professions have broadened the challenge of maintaining a viable health care work force. Create a flow chart of the nursing supply that reflects these conditions and any other that you believe affects the shortage. Where are the leverage points for increasing the supply? Where would you begin? What resources are needed? What outcomes are to be expected from the interventions you recommend?

Daily confrontation with human suffering and death, in conjunction with lack of autonomy, heavy caseloads, court-ordered mandates, inadequate salaries, and frequent interpersonal conflicts, understandably causes many individuals in these careers to want to escape.

Career entrapment occurs when a person is deeply entrenched in a career because of prior investment in career development, psychological attachments, and a sense of obligation. Among other things, the emotional bonds forged in coworker relationships and the intimacy of a mentor-protégé relationship may be difficult to give up. As the career tenure lengthens, the person spends greater energy rationalizing the decision to stay and convincing himself or herself that success is within reach. The person also may experience social pressure to continue in the current field or have a low propensity for risk taking (a career change obviously carries risks, including the risk that the new career may be no more fulfilling than the last).

Paradoxically, whereas dismal labor and market conditions and high unemployment negatively impact turnover, they can positively impact the process of changing careers. The pressures of depressed economic conditions often provide the impetus for entrapped or entrenched employees to seek other employment opportunities. Further, an economic crisis can cause an organization to retrain employees, thus providing them a chance to escape unfulfilling positions.

Individuals who experience career dissatisfaction and distress are susceptible to anxiety, anger, and depression. The anguish of boredom and tedium associated with work tasks often leads to rumination, resentment, melancholy, and an accompanying sense of hopelessness, with negative consequences for the organization.

Tolerance of Antisocial Behavior

Much has been written about deviant or antisocial behaviors in the workplace. Sexual harassment, dishonesty, rumor mongering, withholding effort, and stealing are of obvious concern, as they reduce group effectiveness, among other consequences. In addition, the failure of leaders to recognize antisocial behaviors as inappropriate and try to minimize these behaviors has a negative impact on the social climate and the general moral conduct of employees.

According to Robinson and O'Leary-Kelly (1998), the social context largely determines how employees think and feel about aspects of their work environment and how they behave. In particular, a positive relationship exists between a given individual's level of antisocial behavior and the level of antisocial behavior of his or her coworkers. This should come as no surprise, because individual group members working in a shared social environment will receive similar social cues (cues perhaps indicating that certain types and levels of antisocial behavior are acceptable). In addition, when a new employee enters an established group, the extent of the group's antisocial behavior will affect how likely the newcomer is to develop similar behaviors. Typically, the newcomer will adjust his or her personal behavior to fit the work environment or eventually leave the organization. Indeed, the longer an employee remains in a group, the greater the chance he or she will behave in accordance with the group's standards of behavior.

Another factor that impacts the level of a group's antisocial behavior is the degree of task interdependence (i.e., the extent to which the group members must coordinate their individual efforts). Enhanced interaction allows the members to more easily acquire the social information that will determine their subsequent behavior. In other words, the higher the level of interaction, the greater the likelihood that group members will take each other as role models.

Of course, in any work group, it is always possible that some members will perceive themselves to be significantly different in some important way from the majority, feel dissatisfied with their poor fit, and want to withdraw from the group. In the case of antisocial behaviors, since these, by definition, violate social mores, it is even likely that some group members will feel alienated by antisocial behaviors prevalent in the work group as a whole.

Toxic Mentoring

Mentoring has long been extolled as a means of guiding the development of inexperienced employees, but not all mentoring results in the growth of the mentee. Some leaders in fact believe that mentoring is an ill-conceived method of continuing past practices—ill-conceived because it obstructs necessary adaptations to changes in the work environment, the marketplace, and society at large. In their view, rather than seeking out a wise elder as a guide to corporate life, an aspiring leader should read a lot, listen a lot, work a lot, and observe a lot. That way, according to Geneen (1997), the young leader will learn a lot on his or her own and not be spoon-fed antiquated wisdom gained from someone else's past. It is worth noting here that the workplaces of America are filled with industrious and upright citizens on a treadmill to nowhere because they are so intent on playing it safe.

Toxic mentoring can also result when an aspiring leader seeks to please an experienced leader that he or she has idealized. If the mentor (the experienced leader) does not assist the mentee in developing his or her own identity and leadership style, the mentee could be misled into following the established path of the mentor. The main danger here is that, once the mentor is no longer on hand as a guide, the mentee might become empty and powerless and unable to progress.

Another hazard of mentoring occurs when an experienced leader idealizes an aspiring leader and places unrealistic hopes on him or her. The mentor will then give the mentee overly ambitious assignments that frequently remain uncompleted. Finally, some mentors attempt to transfer their defense mechanisms to their mentees or at least convince them of the need to approach situations from a defensive and hostile posture rather than a posture of openness and inquiry. In such cases, the mentoring process is more a cloning process than a means of growth and development.

The point that aspiring leaders must keep in mind is that they need to take the initiative rather than travel the same old route, be decisive rather than defer to a higher authority, expose themselves to failure rather than make peace with mediocrity, and seize opportunities rather than retreat from them.

From a somewhat different perspective, toxic mentoring exemplifies the negative side of transferring one's experiences. It is impossible to approach new people or situations with a blank sheet, so we use our past experiences, positive or negative, and the stereotypes we have inherited to fill the pages (Exhibit 7–3). A good mentor tries to keep the slate as clean as possible. The mentee needs to make personal assessments and form personal opinions using his or her own emerging leadership lens.

Toxic mentors typically base perceptions not only on current practices but also on early childhood experiences. They make judgments about individuals and situations before examining the circumstances and the available data. They often put forth negative profiles of individuals that include derogatory references to the individuals' gender, age, culture, mental capacity, physical stature, or religion.

Effective mentoring is truly circular in nature. Sharing experiences from the past with aspiring leaders is as important as sharing experiences with colleagues and superiors. Mentoring upward, sideways, and downward reinforces the importance of lifelong learning and makes the point that wisdom and insight are not limited to those with tenure. The healthy mentor encourages self-assessment, open and nonjudgmental examination of issues, and reevaluation of decisions as new information becomes available.

Rather than selecting and promoting others of their own image, experienced leaders need to ensure that aspiring leaders gain an appreciation of the substantial personality differences that leaders can exhibit and the importance of diversity in personality and methodology for creating optimal solutions.

Inconsistency and Dishonesty

Leaders frequently add to the toxicity in an organization by being inconsistent in word and action and by telling white lies. In general, employees respect and are willing to follow leaders who act in accordance with their values, principles, and beliefs. When a company identifies balancing work and leisure as a goal, it will usually focus on the employees' time at work and develop initiatives giving employees work-hour flexibility. But if the company at the same time is not filling vacancies and is asking employees to do more with less, the added flexibility is counteracted by the extra 5 or 10 hours of work that each

---

Exhibit 7–3 Toxic Stereotypes

1. Female leaders cannot understand financial situations and cannot sustain company solvency.
2. Older leaders cannot be effective because they do not have technical competence.
3. Younger leaders cannot hold senior leadership positions because they do not have enough experience.
4. Members of our church will make better leaders because we know we can count on them.
5. Avoid members of certain ethnic groups when selecting new leaders, as some are too expressive.
6. Overweight leaders will never concentrate on the business of the day.
7. Avoid selecting leaders for your committee who require too much time to make decisions, as they think too slowly.

employee must put in weekly. The company's message becomes ambiguous, and, worse, when the employees complain, management will see them as ungrateful, making the employees feel that the executives just don't get it.

Ambiguous or contradictory messages are quite common and usually sow confusion. The recipients of these messages begin to feel angry, insecure, and entrapped. For instance, if one employee has a clearly superior performance review but is given the same compensation as mediocre performers, the contradictory message—performance both counts (because it is measured) and does not count (because superior performance is not compensated)—will likely demoralize the employee with the outstanding record.

Although people are ordinarily uncomfortable with conflict, their discomfort reduces their opportunities to learn more about the differing positions and viewpoints of colleagues. This in and of itself is enough to support the notion that conflict should be considered normal, but there is another very important reason. People's lack of comfort with conflict and confronting the truth has resulted in the "white lies of leadership" syndrome. White lies, in fact, have become all too common in performance reviews, the selection of candidates for positions, and explanations for downsizing given to employees (Malloch 2001).

The performance review process continues to be a struggle for most leaders, especially identifying strengths and areas for improvement in an honest and meaningful way. Reviewers find it difficult to discuss inadequate performance openly and kindly, particularly if the deficiencies have been persistent and have never been addressed. Leaders generally wish for performance problems to disappear from lack of attention so that they do not have to deal with the issue or engage in uncomfortable dialogue. To avoid confrontation, leaders will sometimes rate mediocre behavior as above standard—or to equalize the distribution of a limited compensation package, they will routinely rate the performance of all employees as above standard. Regardless of their intent, these types of misevaluation are forms of dishonesty.

Truth telling is also difficult when a job candidate is not picked for the position. Unselected candidates are often told the chosen candidate had better credentials, more experience, or more education. Although this may be true, there is usually more to the decision. Factors such as personal appearance, aggressiveness in the interview, or non-support from a colleague often play a role in the selection process, but information about such issues is rarely shared, preventing the candidate from learning how to better prepare for the next interview. Holding back critical comments, even if done out of kindness, takes control away from employees and can be seen as a form of autocratic leadership behavior.

Finally, leaders often tell white lies when explaining decisions to downsize or eliminate positions. Most often they claim the decisions are not personal or about the employees' competence but rather based on financial considerations. The truth is that downsizing is often used to weed out mediocre or dissident employees. It is also used as a way to cover the effects of poor management, such as when leaders fail to adapt to incremental changes in the marketplace or neglect to retrain employees to meet emerging needs. Nothing is more destructive to the morale of an organization than the chronic recycling of human beings, especially in an industry that espouses health as its service.

Imbalance between Work and Personal Life

For many people, the boundary between work life and personal life has all but collapsed with the advent of the Internet. Technology has opened up new doors to new experiences, and the condition of being without something to do is almost inconceivable. Idle hands or stilled minds are believed to be inappropriate—the devil's workshop. Individuals nowadays spend much of their time learning new ideas or deciding what to do next. Being in demand is a sign of importance and value, and new communication technologies allow people to seek out and contact each other in new ways. Palmtops, pagers, and home shopping networks increase the role of scheduling in our lives and divide our days into ever smaller segments. Yet, there is evidence that technological advances are not really increasing efficiency. It is important to realize that technology is not always adept at solving nontechnical problems—a better timepiece does not eliminate chronic lateness.

> ### Point To Ponder
>
> *Extremes of up and down are interrelated. Excessiveness ushers in disorder and disaster, which lead to burnout and fatigue as we walk the way of personal destruction. In leading others, there is nothing better than moderation. Leisure is good, yet too much can lead to restlessness and boredom. Work is important and beneficial, yet in abundance it can cause havoc in other aspects of life. Avoid the temptations of overdoing and overextending, no matter how enticing and attractive the pulls and lures might be.*
> —*Chungliang Al Huang and Jerry Lynch (1995)*

Perhaps high-speed living is toxic to human beings. So much time can be put into arrivals and departures that not enough is left over for the experiences themselves. Raising children, developing relationships, and creating art are not tasks that lend themselves to being done speedily and efficiently. The high-speed world of technology has separated individuals from contemplation and slow-knowing—the process of reflecting creatively rather than relying on the mere analytical horsepower of technology. The amazing data-analyzing capabilities of computers have turned contemplation into a seemingly old-fashioned pastime. The focus is on problem solving. Dwelling on issues to see if they might lead to deeper issues is seen as inefficient and self-indulgent.

What we know is that neither technology nor efficiency can acquire more time for anyone; time is not something one had or lost, it is what one lives in. The reality is that, for most of us, there will never be enough time. The real challenge is to develop a balance between work and personal life and to work to maintain the desired balance.

The challenge of finding enough time to function effectively in work and at home is even greater for female leaders. Because organizations desire the senior management profile to reflect the composition of the marketplace, they are on the lookout for competent women to hire. The problem experienced by female leaders is that women remain the primary family managers and spend nearly twice as many hours on household and childcare responsibilities as men. The conflicts of interest created by playing a leadership role and acting as a mother make it nearly impossible for women to remain as executives without failing to meet their full responsibilities in one or both areas and suffering a noticeable lack of balance between work and personal life. More flexibility in the workplace and an increase in the participation of males in child rearing will be needed to end the male orientation of the workplace and bring about a true partnership.

Interestingly, some people think the main challenge is not too much work but overstimulation. According to this view, there are too many demands and not enough sensible priority setting. If people had a healthy selfishness, they could step back from the minutiae of their work lives and find a good balance between responsibilities—one that allows them to be true to their personal values.

Reactive Advocacy Gone Awry

Health professionals find solace in serving patients and acting as advocates for them, but advocacy, when it is reactive, can sometimes be a source of toxicity. Consider the following scenario. The family of a patient in a critical care unit recognized that all interventions were futile and informed the nurses and attending physician that they wished to cease treatment. Keeping the patient comfortable was their only goal at this time. On the next shift, the consulting physician examined the patient and determined that he needed respiratory support. The physician then proceeded to intubate the patient. Given the power and reputation of the physician, no staff member challenged his actions, even though they were contrary to the family's wishes.

On the next shift, the returning nurse realized that the wishes of the family had been violated and called the attending physician, who in turn removed the respiratory support. The nurse expressed a feeling of accomplishment, although she was concerned about receiving a tongue-lashing from the consulting physician because she had gone over his head.

Advocacy leadership in health care is a proactive process. Its purpose is to create the conditions for patients to receive the care they desire. It involves much more than removing the barriers as they are identified; in fact, the goal of advocacy leadership is to avoid having barriers in the first place. Unfortunately, *reactive* advocacy is the kind of advocacy that has become commonplace in our world of ambiguous values. When traditional leaders take action to alleviate unhealthy situations, they feel accomplished and complete, despite often failing to identify or address the basic problems.

Consider the following. To thrive in the global economy, the United States requires a democratized work force. Despite coming far in a journey that began with slavery and the cruel exploitation of child and immigrant labor, the country still has numerous organizations in which most of the workers are alienated and apathetic. Further, our social institutions, including our schools and churches, have notably failed to fill the values void that pervades all sectors of society. The workplace, according to Lundin and Lundin (1993), may be the logical place to fill this void. It may be, but health care organizations often operate on the assumption that health care is a commodity rather than a service, presenting their leaders with the challenge of designing and implementing strategies to cure them of their toxicity.

Widely touted theories of transformational leadership are based on the belief that leaders have the power needed to transform a low-performing organization into a high-performing organization. This belief is itself based on the classical model of system control, which is inconsistent with the concept of organizational transformation. If one knocks down an anthill and rebuilds it, that is restructuring, not transformation. If the ants sprout wings and move to the trees, that is transformation. Thus, a quantum leader who is truly a transformer needs to approach the organization from a very different perspective—in other words, to avoid change strategies that amount to merely rearranging current structures, policies, procedures, and reward systems. Rather, a transforming leader creates a new and improved system that allows individuals to contribute to their fullest potential in order to deliver the most effective health care possible. And there can be no idea of asserting control in the traditional sense.

Some individuals are closer to being naturally gifted healing leaders than others, but almost everyone can be helped to reach their full potential for care and compassion. People can and do change. They find capacities they did not know they had. The fact is that healing traits are dormant within everyone. These traits are expressed in times of great joy, happiness, love, or compassion, when the spirit of caring and optimism overpowers any negative feelings.

The final challenge for quantum leaders is to avoid the obvious trap of believing that organizations are inherently toxic and that their job is to eradicate toxic behaviors wherever they are found. Their main focus should instead be on recognizing new beliefs and behaviors, understanding their implications, and integrating those that appear to be beneficial into current practice.

The solution to the problems that plague health care today lies in building bridges between the disciplines and recognizing the imperative to practice in such a way that environment-health connections receive primary consideration. Physical healing takes place through a multifaceted process in which the fabric of the body repairs and regenerates itself. So too can organizations heal.

TEN PRINCIPLES FOR MINIMIZING TOXIC BEHAVIOR IN ORGANIZATIONS

The first step in minimizing the negative effects of dysfunctional behaviors is to recognize that these behaviors exist and that their elimination requires a commitment to discarding the toxic past and redefining what should be. One of the reasons that effective organizational change is often so difficult is that it involves taking authority, status, prestige, and security away from those in power, threatening their self-image, and provoking resistance. But there is no other choice, because many of the toxins originate in misplaced authority and power.

For the work of transformation to begin, the organizational culture must support, as its main value, the common good rather than self-interest. Organizations steeped in bureaucracy and paternalism will experience a difficult transformation requiring persistent effort. For others, the journey may be somewhat less complex and traumatic. The model of seven evolving levels of organizational culture described by Barrett (1995) can serve as a guideline for organizations in monitoring their progress on the journey toward supporting the common good (Exhibit 7–4). Although these levels are progressive, an organization might regress at different times in the journey.

Exhibit 7–5 contains a list of 10 rules useful for combating toxicity in an organization. By following these rules, which are discussed below, leaders will be able to reduce the potency of the sources of toxicity described above or eliminate them entirely.

> **Key Point**
>
> ***Healing manager:*** *A person who helps others grow emotionally and intellectually—the emotional pathway from chaotic relationships to total quality relationships.*
>
> *—William Lundin and Kathleen Lundin (1993)*

Principle 1: Know Thyself

For the leader of an organization, the most important rule for minimizing dysfunction is to know what he or she stands for and what behaviors he or she finds unacceptable. Barrett (1995) makes the point that whatever a person identifies with, that person cares for. When people identify with family members, they give them support. When they identify with their environment, they protect and nurture it. When they identify with their organization, they give it their very best. Further, when they enlarge their sense of self by identifying

---

Exhibit 7–4 Seven Levels of Corporate Culture

---

1. *Survival consciousness:* The organization is focused on profits and typically uses an autocratic, uncaring, and fear-driven culture.
2. *Relationship consciousness:* Benevolent, paternalistic culture with a focus on internal communications. Fears at this level can lead to internal competition, blame, and manipulative culture.
3. *Self-esteem consciousness:* A desire to be the biggest or the best. Hierarchal power structure with goals of order, efficiency, productivity, and quality. Strong results orientation.
4. *Transformation:* Self-discovery, vision, mission, and awareness of values. Beginning of focus on equality and diversity.
5. *Organization consciousness:* The focus is on integrity, trust, creativity, intuition, innovation, freedom, and generosity. Efforts abound to create conditions for cohesion, community spirit, and mutual accountability.
6. *Community consciousness:* Voluntary environmental and social audits and support for local community and businesses. The search is for long-term sustainability.
7. *Global/unity consciousness:* The organization contributes to resolving social, human rights, and environmental issues beyond the local community. The focus is on ethics and a search for truth and wisdom.

Source: Reprinted with permission from R. Barrett, *Liberating the Corporate Soul,* © 1998, Richard Barrett. Published by Butterworth-Heinemann.

Exhibit 7–5 Ten Principles for Minimizing Dysfunctional Behaviors

1. Know thyself.	6. Build relationships on respect.
2. Walk the talk.	7. Act as an agent of transformation.
3. Be willing to listen.	8. Screen job candidates for dysfunction.
4. Value the truth of the whole.	9. Expect accountability.
5. Empower employees.	10. Reward value-adding behaviors.

with their organization, they develop a greater sense of responsibility toward it and link its welfare with theirs.

Knowing yourself is more than identifying your patterns of decision making. It includes identifying your values, your outlook on life, and the importance you place on integrity and the work ethic. The leader who believes that employees are basically honest, hard working, and optimistic about the future is quite different from the leader who believes that employees will do only what they absolutely must, tend to be less than truthful, and are typically negative about the future.

Leaders need to listen to what others have to say about them and to look carefully at their style of communication and the way they treat point-of-service workers. The words that others say about them are not always easy to swallow but cannot be ignored. As leaders, they are honor-bound to respond and make the changes necessary to improve their reputation. Interestingly, most leaders will listen to negative feedback up to a point and will permit some change. The goal, however, is to pass through a make-or-break threshold of anxiety about having to change, trust others, and renounce autocratic behavior. Getting through this threshold helps everyone in the organization, whereas backing away from making the necessary changes allows the damage to continue.

Leaders should look at themselves, confront their emotions, and acknowledge the pain and resentment of employees. How much of the pain are they accountable for? When an intimidating senior manager says to an employee, "I want to know how you see me," the employee might still be reluctant to answer honestly out of fear of retaliation. If a leader discovers that others are afraid of being open, he or she must make the effort to eliminate the toxic behaviors that cause their fear, such as yelling, criticism, and negative feedback.

Personal assessment often allows leaders to gain an appreciation of unexplained discrepancies between how they are viewed by colleagues and by family and friends. At work, even though people look the same, what they become in the eyes of others is seldom the same as how they are perceived in their personal life. It is possible, for example, for an individual to be considered competent outside of the workplace but incompetent at work—or vice versa. Although self-assessment and dialogue with others can clarify paradoxical perceptions, they cannot eliminate the disparities.

As leaders journey through the self-assessment process, they may find that meditation is useful for relaxing and regaining a healthy balance. Relaxation is not just the relief of tension but the foundation of self-healing abilities. By learning to relax, people build confidence in their ability to control their body, feelings, and thoughts. They become aware of having more choices in how to react and how to feel. They also become more aware of what kinds of things, people, and thoughts tend to produce tension—an important first step in learning to deal with these sources of tension constructively. In addition, relaxation interrupts habitual negative thought patterns and clears the mind.

Principle 2: Walk the Talk

The second rule for reducing toxicity is to walk the talk—or act in accordance with expressed values. If leaders did in fact walk their talk and consequently did listen to employees, would it be necessary to have suggestion boxes? If they really had an open-door policy, would they have to sell it so emphatically? Building trust between two individuals requires the words and actions of each to be congruent. The trust that leaders are able to acquire by walking their talk will encourage innovative behaviors by employees, minimize the potential for discrepancies between expectations and reality, reinforce their perceived integrity, strengthen the confidence that employees have in the appropriateness of future interactions, and reinforce the bond between the leaders and employees.

In times of chaos, the importance of constancy of values increases. Although the health care environment and marketplace present regular challenges for health professionals, the mission and values of health care remain unchanged. The values of respect, compassion, confidentiality, patient advocacy, accountability, competence, continuing knowledge development, supportive work environments, and collaboration remain constant beacons of light for those who work in the field.

Creating a team (or committee) to act as conscience of the organization could serve to assist all employees in evaluating their success at walking the talk. The committee, an extension of the traditional ethics committee, would provide an ongoing critique of leadership decision making to ensure that the decisions arrived at were consistent with the values and norms of the organization. In addition, it could give careful consideration to potential conflicts between formally stated organizational values and unavoidable financial or business pressures as well as issues related to all types of harassment, coercion, and discrimination.

> **Point To Ponder**
>
> *Passion is manifested in a commitment of energy and a personal investment in an effort so strongly felt that adversity cannot diminish the effort. Passion sees the leader through those inevitable times of toughness, darkness, and slow change.*
> *—Tim Porter-O'Grady (2000)*

As an example, recent downsizing efforts, despite the organizations' professed respect for the dignity of all individuals, resulted in a significant loss of dignity by the employees who were laid off. If instead these organizations had used their power appropriately, acted to protect human rights and dignity, and taken organizational and societal issues into consideration at the outset of their decision making, they could have responded to the financial pressures in a way that minimized the negative impact on employees and thus minimized the resulting organizational toxicity.

Given that the traditional compact between employers and employees—in which long-term job security is traded for loyalty—is becoming extinct, a new compact needs to be fashioned to ensure that employees are not victimized or wind up working in a trustless environment. In other words, the employer-employee relationship needs to be reconceived. Although it is true that promises of long-term employment and associated benefits are inappropriate in the current marketplace, employers and employees should openly and honestly discuss the nature of the work, expected changes that will impact the work, and ways in which employees can remain useful to the organization. If an employee leaves the organization, the termination of employment should be the result of a mutual decision rather than a unilateral act by either the employer or the employee.

Principle 3: Be Willing To Listen

Listening, active listening, is not just a matter of hearing, for instance, employees' feelings of loss, anger, or survivor guilt; it also encompasses taking these feelings to heart and not dismissing them as merely trivial. The leader who is an expert at listening believes that every employee is a source of unique information critical to the organization's success.

Shared leadership is one leadership model that is especially conducive to active listening—and to healthy dialogue. Also conducive to active listening is the horizontal organizational model, in which teams of individuals are involved in organizationwide, cross-functional core processes.

Listening is an essential part of effective problem solving and decision making. Leaders in quantum organizations use active and critical listening skills to gain a full understanding of problem situations. To acquire the depth of understanding they need, they must explore multiple issues and gather myriad data, both of which tasks begin with critical listening.

Group Discussion

If you could whisper one thing in the ear of your organization's leader, what would it be? Would it concern specific toxic behaviors? Look at what other people in your group would want to whisper. Would their questions and comments be like these?

- Why don't you react to that behavior?
- Give us a sign that you understand and truly care about employees in our organization.
- Why don't you fire that person?
- How will I ever know if you are satisfied with my performance?

Consider the differences and similarities in the questions and comments and identify at least two strategies to correct the problems you have identified.

Principle 4: Value the Truth of the Whole

The power to be gained from understanding both sides of an issue often goes unappreciated. Instead, an individual will strive to have others believe and support a particular point of view—his or her own. In the quantum organization, understanding multiple perspectives and balancing differing opinions is particularly helpful for arriving at optimal decisions. The challenge for the quantum leader is to cherish the fruitful opposition between order and creativity and to escape the grip of either/or thinking. Multiple perspectives are essential for understanding the whole. Often, the whole truth is a paradoxical joining of apparent opposites, and if the whole truth is desired, the opposites need to be embraced as a unit (Exhibit 7–6).

Perhaps one of the most challenging tasks involved in arriving at the truth is error management. Errors, although always part of the whole reality of a situation, have been historically cast aside, leaving only the successes to be remembered. Learning to integrate errors and absorb their lessons promises to be a long and arduous journey.

The emotional pain that is caused when an error is committed is often contagious and leads to self-defeating behaviors. Employees begin to have doubts about their own competence, and new mistakes appear to come out of nowhere. All too often these mistakes result from insidious lapses in judgment that occur when knowledge is steeped in the apathy and immobilization of emotional pain. Open and honest management of the whole of the situation—successes and errors—will serve to reinforce positive practices and minimize the potential for continuing errors and patient injury.

Finally, the leadership team should have room for a whole constellation of personality styles to ensure the effectiveness of its decision-making practices. Healthy organizations typically seek to include a broad variety of leadership personality styles so that multiple perspectives can be considered and no single one can dominate in the creation of strategies and structures, thereby minimizing the potential for group think.

Exhibit 7–6 The Community of Truth

- We invite diversity into our community not because it is politically correct but because diverse viewpoints are demanded by the manifold mysteries of great things.
- We embrace ambiguity not because we are confused or indecisive but because we understand the inadequacy of our concepts to embrace the vastness of great things.
- We welcome creative conflict not because we are angry or hostile but because conflict is required to correct our biases and prejudices about the nature of great things.
- We practice honesty not only because we owe it to one another but because to lie about what we have seen would be to betray the truth of great things.
- We experience humility not because we have fought and lost but because humility is the only lens through which great things can be seen—and once we have seen them, humility is the only posture possible.

Source: The Courage To Teach: Exploring the Inner Landscape of a Teacher's Life, P.J. Palmer, Copyright 1998, Jossey-Bass Inc. Reprinted by permission of Jossey-Bass Inc., a subsidiary of John Wiley & Sons, Inc.

Principle 5: Empower Employees

Leaders of quantum organizations work to empower employees and ensure that they have the freedom to make suggestions, grow and mature, and become sensitized to themselves and others. The corporate social democracy they practice is much different than the corporate elitism associated with centralized power. Instead of the chief executive and managers thinking for everyone, all individuals in the organization think. Instead of a mission statement being handed down, all employees should participate in the creation of the organization's vision, mission, and values, because they do the work and deserve the right to define these critical elements.

Leadership expertise is easily identified in action but difficult to describe in its richness. The wisdom of leaders is similar to the clinical wisdom of clinicians described by Benner, Hooper-Kyriakidis, and Stannard (1999). It includes the essential skills of grasp (comprehension), inquiry, and forethought. It is this wisdom that leaders who want to serve as transformers need to acquire.

Obtaining these skills requires significant leadership experience. Leaders who have this level of experience become expert at problem identification and solving and are able to act in situations that are ambiguous, underdetermined, unexpected, and/or markedly different from their preconceptions. Grasping involves making qualitative distinctions, doing detective work, recognizing changes, and developing relevant knowledge bases. Inquiry involves knowing what questions to ask. Expert leaders learn to use their knowledge, experience, and intuition to anticipate crises, risks, and vulnerabilities that may affect the organization or its employees.

For example, in implementing a program, the timing of events is often crucial to success. During a period when employees are demoralized from downsizing in other local organizations, a wise leader would not choose to reduce benefits and cause additional stress. Although it is possible to view this decision as motivated by expedience, political cowardice, or unrealistic optimism, it is more likely to be based on a grasp of the organization's entire context and a realization that traumatizing employees further will be counterproductive in the long run.

Forethought is another component of leadership wisdom that emerges after significant experience dealing with common situations as well as unanticipated events. It is basically the ability to anticipate likely eventualities and to take the appropriate actions—an ability seldom articulated despite the fact that it is pervasive in the everyday actions of expert leaders. These leaders subconsciously project possible situations that may result from particular conditions. Then, by being extra attentive and using their ability to recognize patterns and sense the relevance of events, they are able to prepare the organization for the most probable of these situations.

Empowering employees is a career-long journey of mentoring. The goal is to transfer leadership wisdom not only to aspiring leaders but to all employees. Along this journey, expert leaders provide tools for employees to do their jobs well and to help them feel successful. They try to create a culture of respect based on the belief that employees who feel successful and appreciated in the workplace will truly leave their work, both physically and mentally, at the end of the day and will thus be better able to manage their time and achieve and maintain a healthy balance between work and personal life.

Principle 6: Build Relationships on Respect

Each and every interaction between employees and between employees and patients should be directed toward achieving therapeutic outcomes. No relationships characterized by disrespectful behavior, insulting language, or emotional harm can be tolerated. Respect for employees is an expectation that is never open to discussion. No individual ever has the permission to be rude or abusive to any other individual. The fundamental right of every person to be treated in a manner that reflects the inherent value of human beings is the guiding principle of all human relationships.

Following are rules that leaders should keep in mind to help ensure that their relationships with employees and the relationships between employees are essentially therapeutic:

- Behave so as to preserve every person's dignity.
- Encourage employees to talk with each other to learn more about each other's opinions before reaching a conclusion.
- Encourage self-improvement.
- Give employees feedback on their performance.
- Be open to new ideas.
- Encourage employees to do their best.
- Compensate employees fairly for the work they do.

These next rules apply to the relationships between care providers and patients. Because their purpose is likewise to help ensure that these relationships are fundamentally therapeutic, they need to be followed by the care providers:

- Probe to uncover the rationale for any decision that a patient makes.
- Recognize that family members and friends can have a significant impact on a patient's ability to manage his or her own health.
- Consider a patient's cultural beliefs before providing care.
- Consider a patient's spiritual beliefs before providing care.
- Empower patients to avoid unnecessary dependency or overtreatment.
- Recognize that clinical and behavioral outcomes affect each other.
- Support a patient's choice to use culturally based healing practices.
- Be fully present and listen to each patient.
- Assist each patient to develop or sustain his or her ability to cope with life situations.
- Identify each patient's feelings about his or her illness and expectations for recovery.
- Encourage patients to participate in self-care programs.
- Recognize that a patient's choices should guide the plan of care.

Principle 7: Act as an Agent of Transformation

Quantum leaders encourage employees to be self-reliant and to take charge of their careers, not only their current jobs. They assist employees in overcoming the negative effects of career entrenchment or entrapment, such as dissatisfaction and ineffectiveness. Quantum leaders also:

- Encourage employees to voice concerns and work collaboratively to identify and address dissatisfaction.
- Do not threaten retaliation when employees express negative emotions or opinions.
- Recognize that there can be discrepancy between ideal career progression and reality.
- Seek to transform career pathways into a progressive career management program.
- Recognize that employee loyalty has advantages and disadvantages (e.g., loyalty can be merely passive and result in skill atrophy, boredom, and depression).

In addition, quantum leaders encourage employees to engage in extra-role activities that are not directly compensated but can decrease employee stress while simultaneously benefiting the organization. Acting as a mentor outside the organization is an example of extra-role citizenship work that can decrease the frustration of entrenched employees while reducing stress and meeting affiliation needs.

Quantum leaders understand that entrenched employees who attempt to cope with their career issues through loyalty or by acting as a constructive voice do contribute to work force stability and reduce turnover costs. These employees often can be jarred from their entrenchment by giving them the opportunity to be involved in special projects, by permitting job rotation, by facilitating downward or lateral moves, by training them in cross-functional roles, and by allowing temporary reassignments (Exhibit 7–7).

Career development programs can assist employees in using the "constructive voice" approach to dealing with career entrenchment. Retraining and redeployment programs further assist employees in managing their careers and thereby help the organization sustain its viability. Employees in organizations that avoid career management are less likely to discuss career issues affecting their performance.

Finally, when all else has failed, it may be necessary to remove an employee who has retired on the job. Employees who have lost the motivation to develop and grow become increasingly less productive and focus on noncareer activities at the expense of the organization. They therefore need to be counseled to seek employment opportunities outside of the organization.

Exhibit 7–7 Organizational Strategies To Minimize Career Entrenchment

- Offer generous severance pay packages to fund employees' explorations into new careers.
- Offer tuition reimbursements and time off for employees to attend classes while still employed.
- Give employees time to rotate to other positions in the organization so they might explore another career option within the relatively safe confines of the organization.
- Discourage linear career paths and emphasize psychological success.
- Ensure that employees do not feel as though they are violating the organization's trust as they investigate new career options.
- Allow employees who leave in good standing to return if their new career plans fail.

Principle 8: Screen Job Candidates for Dysfunction

New employees represent a significant investment for the organization, and job candidates require more scrutiny than they currently receive. To help in screening job candidates, leaders should identify specific dysfunctional behaviors that have a negative impact on organizational performance and, with the assistance of human resource experts, should develop new approaches to interviewing and selecting employees. The 10 principles for minimizing toxic behaviors under discussion in this section are likely to be useful in these endeavors, as are the six questions presented in Exhibit 7–8. In addition, these questions are appropriate for ongoing use to prevent or decrease dysfunction among current employees. Getting regular feedback from employees about their assignment preferences and current frustrations assists leaders in developing a good working relationship with them.

Principle 9: Expect Accountability

Accountability is more than the background against which everyday decisions are made. In fact, the way in which accountability is created, negotiated, communicated, and evaluated lies at the heart of an organization's operations. Unfortunately, years of entitlement philosophies have created workers who park their brains at the door and are comfortable with being rewarded for simply showing up. According to Connors, Smith, and Hickman (1994), the concept of accountability has been poorly defined in the popular press and in the literature on business. Consequently, most people think of accountability as something that happens to them or is inflicted upon them. They perceive it as a heavy burden, although they also view it as something that is applied only when something goes wrong or when someone else is trying to pinpoint the blame for a problem. Connors, Smith, and Hickman suggest that instead accountability should be defined as

> an attitude of continually asking "what else can I do to rise above my circumstances and achieve the results I desire?" It is the process of seeing it, owning it, solving it, and doing it. It requires a level of ownership that includes making, keeping and proactively answering for personal commitments. It is a perspective

---

Exhibit 7–8 Interviewing To Minimize Toxicity

1. Tell me about your preferences for assignments, delegating, and managing authority.
2. How frequently do you believe feedback and updating of work are needed?
3. What is your major frustration in your current job? What are the major frustrations in the jobs performed by those you have supervised?
4. What would make you comfortable in overriding my authority and decisions?
5. What type of people and financial support do you require to ensure that your job is done well?
6. What are the perceived strengths and weeknesses of this organization?

that embraces both current and future efforts rather than reactive and historical explanations.

Accountability systems, to function properly, require the clear delineation of individual behaviors and supporting management practices. Both individual accountability and system accountability are necessary to support the values of integrity and transformation and to foster therapeutic relationships. Individuals in a quantum organization are not threatened by the expectation for accountability but rather need accountability to perform at a high level.

Principle 10: Reward Value-Adding Behaviors

The opportunity now exists for leaders to shift the focus from return on investment to cost-effectiveness and create new rules that lay the groundwork for value-based reward and recognition programs. First and foremost, health care leaders are called on by the economic community to use resources in a way that ensures health care value. No longer can care providers give the best of everything without any financial accounting.

Health care leaders and providers are now required to examine services within the value equation. If resources are limited, does every patient symptom require intervention, particularly if little or no improvement in the patient's clinical condition is likely to result? Just to ask this question is a challenge for providers and leaders schooled in an environment characterized by increasing growth of and access to the health care system. Provision of as many services as possible was the sign of the successful leader. Unfortunately, there was no accountability and no control in the fee-for-service payment system. The result is well known—the exhaustion of resources.

Health care services need to be appropriate to the conditions being treated, focused on outcomes, and consistent with the wishes of the patients and families being served. The buyers and users of health care want to know they are getting value for the resources expended. They want to know that something good or better will happen because of the purchase of health care services—that the users' health will be improved. They also are demanding that the choices made by care providers are rational and based on evidence.

Given the expectations of buyers and users, health care leaders need to create an organizational context that will support the desired services and direct the rewards and recognition of the organization toward efforts that will be able to meet these expectations. In addition, the success of care providers in improving the health of patients or community members and in managing their own health needs to be recognized and rewarded.

In a quantum health care organization, the care providers work to ensure that the patients

- experience an improvement in their clinical condition, possibly including increased physical functioning, greater tolerance of activity, improved ambulation, and/or reduced pain
- improve their ability to care for themselves, including performing wound care, taking medications on schedule, maintaining a nutritious diet, and eliminating properly
- learn more about their condition and its treatment, including their own treatment regime, appropriate procedures, potential complications, and emergency interventions

- are aware of the elements of a healthy lifestyle, including proper nutrition, weight management, activity, stress management, sleep, safety, infection control, and disease screening

The main tasks of the leaders of a quantum health care organization include

- hiring and developing a work force capable of achieving the patient outcomes listed above
- retaining and continuing to develop the care providers needed to meet the organization's future needs
- creating a system in which providers and leaders can influence the context of care provision based on their understanding of what is needed and what they are capable of doing (e.g., providers and leaders both need to be able to actively intervene to improve communication, understand potential situations likely to unfold, and alter the context as necessary)
- fostering therapeutic relationships between leaders, providers, and patients that focus on the values and beliefs of the patients, develop the inner capacities of the patients and providers, involve patients in decision making, and make room for self-responsibility

Organizations might find it helpful to use the topic of organizational toxins and ways of minimizing behavioral dysfunction as the theme of a leadership retreat. In such a retreat, the participants could be challenged to identify toxins in their department or the organization as a whole and then consider strategies to reduce the toxicity using the above described principles.

CONCLUSION

To counteract the toxicity that currently exists in health care organizations, leaders need to return humanity to the workplace. There is nothing easy, however, about creating the proper context for providing health care services. An organization is an open system consisting of inputs, throughputs, and outputs, all of which can be healthy or toxic. The work of delivering care is complex and emotional. Care providers deal with human beings at their most vulnerable, requiring of the providers a high level of personal involvement and commitment.

What is terrifying about dysfunctional organizations is that employee emotional pain is accepted as a natural phenomenon. Employees are expected to live with discomfort as a condition of employment. The real mystery is the continual denial by leaders of a connection between employee pain and service quality. It seems to escape many leaders that employee dissatisfaction leads inevitably to patient dissatisfaction and that, conversely, there is a correlation between contented employees and gratified patients. Even when they accept this correlation, leaders find it difficult to create the conditions and practices that increase both employee and patient satisfaction.

The aim of leadership is not to create a workers' paradise but rather to engender an organizational culture that allows for organizational transformation and for the employees' performance to live and grow. It is the obligation of the leader of a health care organization to push toward organizational health so that the will of the patient is respected. To do this, the leader needs to demonstrate a willingness and ability to cultivate self-transformations as well as transformations in others on a continuing basis.

The obligations of leaders and employees are interconnected. Neither group can be successful without both of them meeting their responsibilities. Leadership is never an either/or situation. Further, leadership is a rational service performed by rational people directed toward achieving sensible organizational objectives. However, the reality is that these rational people carry with them past experiences laden with neurotic styles, negative transference, superior-subordinate entanglements, and untenable strategies. Not surprisingly, unless the leaders recognize this and foster appropriate behaviors, the result is persistent dysfunction.

Finally, leaders need to forget about ever finding enough time. There will never be enough time for all of the things that individuals want to do. Rather, the challenge is to find a healthy balance between the things of importance: work, family, and hobbies.

REFERENCES

Barrett, R. 1995. *A guide to liberating your soul.* Alexandria, VA: Unfoldment Publications.

Benner, P., P. Hooper-Kyriakidis, and D. Stannard. 1999. *Clinical wisdom and interventions in critical care: A thinking-in-action approach.* Philadelphia: Saunders.

Carson, K.D., and P.P. Carson. 1997. Career entrenchment: A quiet march toward occupational death. *The Academy of Management Executives* 11, no. 2: 62–76.

Connors, R., T. Smith, and E. Hickman. 1994. *The Oz principle: Getting results through individual and organizational accountability.* Englewood Cliffs, NJ: Prentice Hall.

Geneen, H. 1997. *The synergy myth.* New York: St. Martin's Press.

Huang, C.A., and J. Lynch. 1995. *Mentoring: The Tao of giving and receiving wisdom.* San Francisco: Harper Collins.

King, S.K. 1989. Removing distress to reveal health. In *Healers on healing,* ed. R. Carlson and B. Shield. Los Angeles: Jeremy P. Tarcher.

Lundin, W., and K. Lundin. 1993. *The healing manager: How to build quality relationships and productive cultures at work.* San Francisco: Berrett-Koehler.

Malloch, K. 2001. The white lies of leadership. *Nursing Administration Quarterly* 25, no. 3: 61–68.

Porter-O'Grady, T. 2000. A call for leaders. *SSM* 6, no. 10: 10–12.

Robinson, S.L., and A.M. O'Leary-Kelly. 1998. Monkey see, monkey do: The influence of work groups on the antisocial behavior of employees. *Academy of Management Journal* 41: 658–672.

SUGGESTED READINGS

Carlson, R., and B. Shield, eds. 1989. *Healers on healing*. Los Angeles: Jeremy P. Tarcher.

Hardy, R.E., and R. Schwartz. 1996. *The self-defeating organization: How smart companies can stop out-smarting themselves*. Reading, MA: Addison-Wesley.

Kets de Vries, M.F.R., and D. Miller. 1984. *The neurotic organization*. San Francisco: Jossey-Bass.

Palmer, P.J. 1998. *The courage to teach: Exploring the inner landscape of a teacher's life*. San Francisco: Jossey-Bass.

Quiz Questions

Select the best answer for each of the following questions.

1. Toxic behaviors in health care organizations:
a. are behaviors and practices that work against the delivery of health care services
b. are engaged in specifically by individuals fearful of accountability
c. can be remedied easily once the toxins are identified
d. result from established rituals rather than faulty communication

2. Much like physical toxins that cause illness in individuals, toxic behaviors cause illness in organizations. The following is true of both human illness and organizational illness:
a. Illness results from an imbalance in the amount and type of nutrients and cleansing activities.
b. Additional nutrients will lead to the restoration of health.
c. Routine cleansing of waste is an effective means of restoring health.
d. Health is the absence of dysfunction.

3. Toxic behaviors in health care organizations are caused by:
a. decreased financial support due to the advent of managed care
b. the personal characteristics of the leaders and employees coupled with the realities of the marketplace
c. a lack of leadership development
d. poor parenting during the leaders' developmental years

4. Vertical organizations are often considered toxic because:
a. the departments do not communicate with each other
b. the customer (or patient) is not the first concern
c. the vigilance of the senior leaders is not appreciated by the employees and other leaders
d. authority and decision making are localized at the top

5. As a management practice used in health care organizations, mandatory overtime:

a. is an appropriate means of responding to staffing needs where life and death situations frequently occur

b. shows an unjustifiable lack of consideration for the need of employees to balance work and personal life

c. is a matter best handled through legislation at the state level

d. should be up to each organization to use as it sees fit

6. An employee who feels entrenched or entrapped may well experience hope when:

a. the organization brings in a new leadership team

b. the employee is released from the expectation that he or she will perform community service

c. the employee is rotated to a different position to explore another career option within the confines of the organization

d. a new employee benefits package is implemented

7. Tolerance of antisocial behaviors has a negative impact on the social climate and general moral conduct of employees. Antisocial behaviors can be minimized when:

a. group interaction is encouraged and work tasks are shared

b. individual members of the group confront the offending employees

c. these behaviors are discouraged by the organization's leader

d. employees with a history of antisocial behavior are not allowed to join groups in which antisocial behavior is absent

8. Individual accountability is best described as:

a. the ability to give the reasons for one's actions upon request

b. something that happens to or is inflicted upon an individual

c. ownership of one's behaviors

d. the process of seeing it, owning it, solving it, and doing it

9. If leaders are inconsistent in word and action, employees will:

a. wonder whether their decisions will be respected

b. view regular communication as unimportant

c. feel a lack of support from the leaders

d. feel entrapped, angry, and insecure

10. The importance of therapeutic relationships between employees and leaders is not always recognized. The expected outcome of such relationships is:

a. improved communication and more productive interaction

b. more accurate medical documentation

c. preservation of confidentiality

d. improved job satisfaction

11. Advocacy is often misunderstood by leaders, especially when efforts are expended to repair a broken system. It is best to view patient advocacy as:

a. the process of creating the necessary conditions for patients to receive the care they desire
b. the proper responsibility of an ombudsman within the health care facility
c. a means of quickly addressing the situations in which patient requests were not honored
d. a desirable but often unattained phenomenon

12. Self-assessment is an essential task for a leader who wants to transform his or her organization. For this type of leader, the goal of self-assessment is to:

a. create a sense of identity with the organization and motivate the leader to do his or her very best
b. discover both positive and negative behaviors that impact performance
c. share personal flaws with other employees
d. identify continuing education needs

CHAPTER 8

Transformational Coaching: Leading the Membership Community

Ours is a brand-new world. Time has ceased, space has vanished.
We now must lead a global village.

—Marshal McLuhan

Chapter Objectives

At the completion of this chapter, the reader will be able to

- Recognize the key elements of coaching within a fast-paced organization in highly charged and changing times.
- Translate the characteristics of transformational coaching into the planning and implementation of new skill formation.
- Describe the needs of teams in a system and explain the importance of team leadership.
- Identify the fundamentals of the learning organization and the dynamics of learning leadership.
- Name the steps of revolutionary and innovation coaching and how it applies to the role of the leader.

Great changes are occurring in the format and the work of leadership. Much of the work of leaders is directed toward helping others confront the vagaries of major changes occurring in the work and structure of the workplace. Leaders must exhibit a new set of skills to create the conditions for new accountabilities while ensuring positive outcomes. The mental models and performance expectations of staff will require heavy retooling to ensure that they are able to thrive in the new work environment. Leaders will learn some of the elements of leading in this new environment and the steps necessary to get staff engaged and motivated to change and grow in a context demanding a different way of delivering health care.

Leadership is not so much who you are as what you do with who you are. Leadership is not a state of being. It is instead a set of internal tools possessed by a person with the energy and skill to use them well. Much of the work of leadership in this new century will consist of transferring new skills to the people who live and work in organizations.

Because this is a time of great change, increasing complexity, and fast-moving advances in technology, people are finding it increasingly difficult to meet the new demands that are arising. Social and technological forces are conspiring to create the conditions that affect how people work, relate, and plan for their own future. The role of the leaders in this process is to live the positive experience of change and master the ability to engage the questions and challenges that accompany change. The staff are watching closely to see how the leaders embrace and engage the challenges of change, for it is by observing how leaders do this that the staff create a vision for their own adjustment to change. The leaders' role-modeling of adjustment to change encourages them to adapt to change and gives them the necessary techniques.

> **Key Point**
>
> *Leadership requires a level of self-knowledge and vulnerability that makes the growth experience visible to others.*

FROM RESPONSIBILITY TO ACCOUNTABILITY

In the coming age, responsibility will no longer be the key element of work performance. Historically, a worker's performance was judged to be acceptable if the worker simply did what he or she was supposed to do. For the performance to be evaluated as excellent, the worker had to do this work and do it exceptionally well. In the 20th-century workplace, the focus on responsibility was prevalent in every aspect of the definition of work and the measurement of performance. There were several ways that this focus was structured in the workplace.

First, job descriptions were often laundry lists of functions and activities. In other words, they zeroed in on the activities of work rather than their product.

Second, performance evaluations reviewed the work someone did—the functions of work and the ability of the person to do the work. The person's behavior and the ability to get along with others were included in the list of "competencies." How well the person did the work, not whether the work was worthwhile, determined whether the person was to be specially rewarded for doing it.

Third, the evaluation of work tended to concentrate on the quality of the work processes—how the work was done and how many errors were committed. It also looked at efficiency, or the amount of time the worker expended in delivering a service or product as compared with the average.

Slavish attachment to process has been an earmark of the 20th-century workplace. Process improvement, process evaluation, process measurement—these all concern what workers do rather than what they achieve. One reason for this may be that, in health care, the relationship between outcome and process has never been well understood.

In the new century, work is starting to be looked at from the perspective of its outcomes. Research has shown that focusing on outcomes alters work processes and the elements of the work. Indeed, it is now clear that all processes gain their meaning from their results or products. In other words, a process is considered valuable to the extent it relates "tightly" to the desired outcome. Much effort is now being expended on investigating the "goodness of fit" between work processes and their intended outcomes and improving the fit where possible.

In short, it is the Age of Accountability, and the major role of leaders is to move people and organizations from responsibility to accountability—from a narrow focus on processes to a perspective that encompasses processes and results (Exhibit 8–1). In the Age of Accountability, leaders are expected to ensure that all of the components of the "fit" between processes and results come together into a complete vision of the work and its products. Among other tasks, they need to define expected outcomes for all actions and activities and to establish aggregate performance measures for evaluating the work performed by teams.

This movement toward the appreciation of outcomes requires a tremendous reorientation of the work and the workers. For the whole of the 20th century, the emphasis was on functions and work processes, whereas now it is on creating sustainability in a time of rapid technological change. Focusing on work processes is no longer a viable strategy, because each has such a short life span. The appropriate goal is to define the critical integration between means and ends, products and processes. This must be done with an understanding that sustainability is not resident in the work or even the incremental product of a given process or time. It instead results from a continuum of efforts that, when connected together, indicate the journey to be taken to improve the conditions or quality of life.

Accountability is always internally generated. It rests first and foremost within. Specifically, accountability is the result of a person's commitment to advancing, improving, growing, adapting, and enhancing his or her own life experience. For that person, accountability is generated out of the energy that the person brings to the exercise of living, whether at work or other realms of life. In addition, accountability depends on individuals' having complete ownership of what they are and what they do and on their making a com-

---

Exhibit 8–1 Responsibility versus Accountability

Responsibility (20th Century)	**Accountability (21st Century)**
• Process	• Product
• Action	• Result
• Work	• Outcome
• Do	• Accomplish
• Task	• Difference
• Function	• Fit
• Job	• Role
• Incremental	• Sustainable
• Externally generated	• Internally generated

mitment to take their talents, energies, and skills and apply them in ways that make the circumstances of life better for themselves and for others.

In an organization, in particular, accountability depends on the members' joining in a concerted collective effort to achieve the organization's ends. If each person brings his or her energy, gifts, skills, and knowledge to bear fully on the work to be done, the outcomes of that work are assured. Everyone in the workplace has a right to expect all the other employees to be committed to applying themselves and using their skills and talents to the fullest. Furthermore, everyone has a right to expect that each team member (or employee in a group work context) will have a positive relationship with the other members and exhibit the same level of energy and commitment to the work and the products.

> ## Point To Ponder
>
> *Accountability requires that people have ownership over their work. Consequently, the organization must recognize that it does not control the work that people do but simply provides the context within which they do it.*

Leaders have the obligation to make certain that the processes and structures needed to support ownership of the work are fully present. Each of the three main components—structure, relationship, and process—should be directed toward facilitating ownership so that the organization's work can be sustained and advanced. If the energy and desire of the worker cannot be maintained, it is impossible to sustain and advance the work of the organization.

> ## Key Point
>
> *In an organization, the leader has the responsibility of creating a sustainable structure for work and ensuring a good fit between the organization's goals and processes. Congruence here guarantees that the system functions as it should.*

The principles of human action and interaction must be clearly understood and applied. Human beings are dynamic and complex beings. When the commitment and motivation of employees are at high levels, conflicts and other challenges arise. The work processes in place must be designed with the understanding that such challenges are normal and to be expected. They should also be designed to anticipate these challenges and address them in a way that increases the probability of good outcomes and sustains the work and the relationship between the employees.

The recognition that the vagaries of human behavior and relationship are normal is critical to the role of leadership in an accountability-based organization. The leaders of such an organization must be aware of the whole spectrum of human dynamics and be capable of managing the vagaries of these dynamics. They must have tools and techniques to maintain the energy and focus of the workplace and its members in a way that advances the work and the achievement of desirable outcomes.

One of these techniques is to establish the expectation that principles will be consistently applied and that accountability will be maintained. If this expectation is made clear to all members of the organization, along with a commitment to not permit behavior inconsistent with this expectation, the members will try to live up to the expectation and act appropriately. In accountability-based work processes, the range of acceptable practices and behaviors is enumerated and articulated by the members, and processes for creating consistency are available to help members address those issues outside the agreed framework. Membership in a work group, like membership in any other collaborative enterprise, requires that the expressed expectations for the members be complied with; otherwise, the goals of the group will be threatened or be only partially achieved.

In regard to accountability, Conners, Smith, and Hickman (1994) discovered that, in any given workplace, there are behaviors that are below the line and behaviors that are above the line. Which ones fall below the line and which above depends on the particular culture and context of the workplace. The two sets of behaviors must be clearly outlined by the members to form a framework for the principles that determine the rules of engagement in the work relationship. The structure and process of leading and managing must be designed to ensure that the above-the-line behaviors are sustained. When the below-the-line behaviors emerge, the processes and methodologies in place must "click in" so that these behaviors can be addressed quickly and effectively. Quick response to behavioral variances is essential to prevent subsequent and sometimes irresolvable problems.

The dynamics of relationship and work are highly complex and variable. It might seem good if the framework for human behavior in the workplace were permanent and unchanging, but a permanent framework, besides being impractical, would also be boring. It is within the course of relationships and interpersonal demands that the vagaries of life always have an impact. Personal patterns of behavior and changing patterns of interaction challenge the best work environment.

> **Point To Ponder**
>
> *Typically, about 90 percent of the leadership role is devoted to managing relationships. If a leader determines that managing relationships takes up a much smaller percentage of work time than that, the leader may need to reassess her or his priorities.*

Leaders are always trying to read work situations. They assess the demands and the dynamics of intersecting and interacting variables and make judgments about how they

> **Group Discussion**
>
> *Responsibility* and *accountability* often are used interchangeably, but they actually have different meanings. Based on the analysis of accountability in this chapter, compare how to change behavior in an accountability-based organization and how to change it in a responsibility-based organization.

affect the work being done and the relationships between the workers. They know that these variables will create challenges for work relationships and functions—challenges that they will be required to address. Although research is being done in the area of accountable behavior and organizational considerations, it is a work in progress. Thus, leaders need to continually review this research to gain up-to-date information on how to ensure that work processes result in desired outcomes.

TRANSFORMING WORK AND THE TRANSFORMING WORKER

During the current era, the major leadership task is to change the mental model of and framework for work. In all segments of society, work and the workplace are changing too fast for most people to keep up. It is up to the leaders, therefore, not only to guide the transformation of work (see Chapter 1) but to help people make the adjustments that the transformation requires.

For transformation to occur, there must be a fundamental change in thinking. Workers must realize, for example, that they must completely reconceptualize their roles. Most people are satisfied with establishing an accustomed pattern of work and set of rituals. Eventually they become so used to the pattern and rituals that they see them as essential to the work. Indeed, they begin to see the work from within these and ultimately become suspicious of anything that threatens what has become normal for them. Despite the fact that their adherence to patterns and rituals may impede necessary changes, leaders who are agents of change should not criticize them. Leaders who are trying to bring about certain changes often become so unhappy with people's attachment to rituals that the rituals themselves become the visible representation of people's unwillingness to change.

After all, people's attachment to the routines of work does ensure that the work not only gets done but meets certain standards of performance. Their attachment may obstruct improvements in quality, but it does virtually guarantee the performance of the activities necessary for the work to be accomplished in some fashion. In fact, even in transformation, leaders are looking to establish new patterns of work, even if the patterns will soon need to be further revised because of further rapidly changing circumstances. Not only that, but leaders often want workers to establish the same kind of attachment to a new pattern even though they complained when the workers were attached to the old patterns.

There are also organizational dangers to transformative thinking. This type of thinking is characterized by a willingness to seriously question all current processes and can threaten organizational stability. During transformation, leaders engage the staff and other stakeholders in a dialogue and hear things that would not normally be expressed. In fact, to make the transformation succeed, the leaders must be open to new ideas and willing to listen to all kind of responses from the full range of stakeholders. Even the thinking that underpins the changes must be subject to question and exploration if their implementation is to be appropriately rigorous and thorough. The environment necessary to support this kind of thinking creates a level of challenge and instability that even the leaders may not be comfortable with (Figure 8–1 and Exhibit 8–2).

The process of transformation requires an environment in which creativity and change are embraced. In other words, discourse, deliberation, dialogue, consensus building, and

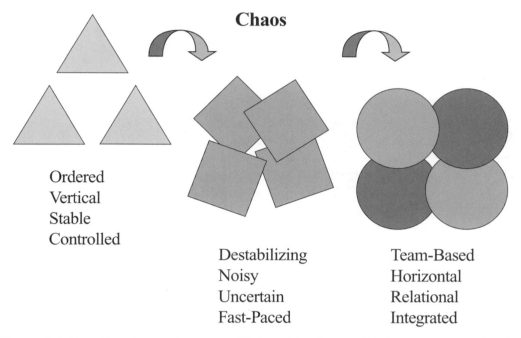

20th-Century Work   **21st-Century Work**

Chaos

Ordered
Vertical
Stable
Controlled

Destabilizing   Team-Based
Noisy   Horizontal
Uncertain   Relational
Fast-Paced   Integrated

Figure 8–1 Transition from 20th-Century Work to 21st-Century Work. The transition involves moving through the stages of change from predominantly vertical organizations to more horizontal systems.

experimentation must be viewed as safe and appropriate strategies. Leaders must create this environment before they can expect to see innovation and engagement with change become routine in their units or services. If the staff do not feel safe in the presence of change, they certainly will not feel comfortable making change.

Group Discussion

In the emerging world of health care, the major leadership task is to transform people's attitudes and insights regarding the changes that are required of them. On a flipchart, list changes that affect what health care providers do and also list attitudes toward the demand for change. Order the attitudes based on their potential influence and discuss how a health care leader could go about altering two of the most important in order to smooth the transition to new ways of working.

Exhibit 8–2 Causes of Transformation

• Destabilized environment	• New financial realities
• Noise	• Demand for new behaviors
• Culture of change	• Work process changes
• Loss	• Shifting technology
• Emerging reality	

Living in an environment of horizontal relationships and accountability-based controls rather than of management-driven decision making and vertical controls is a different experience for all parties. The former type of environment, however, is essential for transformative thinking and acting. There is no research that suggests that rigid vertical control structures lead naturally to change and innovation. On the other hand, there is a whole body of research that indicates that an open, inclusive, and accountable work structure creates numerous opportunities for creativity and innovation.

> **Key Point**
>
> *There is a whole body of research demonstrating that an open, inclusive, and accountable structure for work creates extra opportunities for creativity and innovation.*

Biology has lessons for organizational survival. Biological research shows that growth and adaptation are required for life to continue. If the environment changes noticeably because of some cataclysmic event or the accumulation of small alterations, plants and animals will either adapt or cease to exist. Indeed, past changes form the foundation for future changes, and adaptation to earlier changes determines the level of adjustment to future changes.

The same is true of organizations and other forms of social life. Even minor changes can upset the delicate balance that allows certain kinds of organizations to thrive and can turn the environment into a threatening place for them. In order for organizations to survive in this world, many of the processes and behaviors, rituals and routines, that have their foundation in the 20th century must be replaced by new processes and behaviors. The transition will require true leadership and a transformational format for radically altering everything that workers know and do.

EVOLUTION AND REVOLUTION

The only difference between evolution and revolution is the rate of the change process—the amount of time it takes for the changes to occur. Certainly, technology, because of its high rate of innovation, can be said to be undergoing a revolution, but the resulting changes in society are occurring at more of an evolutionary pace. It takes much longer to incorporate social and behavioral changes than to implement technological advances. Yet, both types of change must be accommodated, and people have to be able to adjust at both a fast rate and a more studied rate. The challenge is to know which is which and to attach the right rate of accommodation to the right process.

Leaders in an organization need to be able to recognize the demand for change in enough time to respond correctly—at the right time and in the right format. Of course, not all changes are known far enough in advance to allow an appropriate and timely response. Nonetheless, the chance of responding correctly will be increased if the leaders assess the probability of any reasonably likely change and consider its expected effects. By anticipating the kind of changes that will occur, developing an understanding of their conditions and circumstances, and passing this understanding on to the staff, the leaders will help ensure that the staff can react appropriately. In short, leaders must be signpost readers and be able to articulate trends clearly enough to create a picture of their impact.

Leaders must also be transformational agents. In coaching staff members to embrace necessary changes, leaders must show the same tone, enthusiasm, and skill in adaptation they expect from others. Seeing the signposts is simply the first step in transferring the information to the staff in a way that puts accountability for response into their hands. Leaders must be able to see systemness and complexity as normal conditions of change and adaptation (see Chapter 2). Through expressing their accountability for witnessing and previewing the potential for change, the leaders prepare the staff to deal with the right change at the right time and in the right circumstances.

Transformational coaching requires leaders to engage in an array of activities that move employees through the process of responding to essential changes in a way that embraces the changes and achieves desired outcomes. In fact, leaders are responsible for creating a system of response to essential changes and then creating a structure and process for these changes to occur as lived or operational experience. Transformational coaching is more of a system than a process, and it is in applying the components of this system that leaders can ensure a dynamic, ongoing framework for adaptation and engagement.

THE LEARNING ORGANIZATION

An organization's ability to adapt to change depends on how open and responsive the social and organizational context is to change and to the dynamic processes of learning. If the organization values change and learning, the vagaries of change will be less traumatic and incidentally dynamic. Research, however, has shown that there are rules of engagement even in creating a true learning context.

Chris Argyris (1999), in his review of the research, indicated that there are some basic criteria for success at any level of organizational learning and change. The focus must first be on behaviors and attitudes. Identifying the fundamentals of behavior and the factors that influence specific behaviors is critical for creating a context and process for change. Once these behaviors and attitudes are identified, the focus switches to the vagaries that affect particular behaviors or recurrent patterns of behavior and through them affect the way work is done or the way it is adapted to new realities.

The system developed for addressing behaviors must include a mechanism for reducing the number of continuing counterproductive activities and self-fulfilling patterns of behavior that keep the participants from fully engaging with the changes they must make. Behaviors that are inconsistent with both norms and expectations will find room to exist if not addressed quickly and efficiently. They even stand a chance of becoming the norm and will in any case compromise the environment and participants in a way that obstructs adaptation to the necessary changes. The noise that results will create a further impediment to the participants' ability to engage with the changes and thrive.

Focusing on the behavior of participants gives leaders an image of the mental and emotional "maps" that are in operation. These maps can then be used as a beginning point for the process of making meaningful and sustainable change. Leaders need to look critically at the participants' mental maps to determine from them the pattern of response they have helped to create. In fact, this pattern of response—the participants' theory-in-use—has a more dramatic impact on the participants' engagement with essential change than do the behaviors themselves.

When leaders approach participants to discuss their mental maps, they do need to be cautious. These maps form the contextual framework out of which behavior flows. The theory-in-use is simply the conceptual constant that the person draws on to explain, justify, and retain sufficient commitment or energy to a particular course of action. In this highly individual context, the person seeks to provide a solid values or belief foundation that can give meaning to a position or specific action. Often the theory-in-use is identified as the rationale or justification the person uses for his or her actions. This theory-in-use has only an inferential relationship to the truth. It relates more to the individual's sense of truth or interpretation or application of truth than to anything that may actually be true. Regardless, it is vitally important to the person. It is the theory-in-use out of which that person acts and it gives a reason for the action. In this issue, leaders find that much of a theory-in-use is undiscussable, for it concerns who the participants perceive themselves to be even to the point of being perceived as a part of their identity. A person's role and sense of self in the role and the person's relationships with others and the organization create a foundation for the person's pattern of behaviors. However, because every person's theory-in-use is expressed in his or her pattern of behaviors, the patterns of all participants must be directly addressed if the behaviors necessary to learning, adaptation, and meaningful change are ever to be evidenced in the organization. This awareness of person's theory-in-use helps the leader understand and address particular behaviors and gives a clearer context to an individual's personal struggle with change.

Almost every organization fails to maintain adaptability over time. The main reason is that organizations, although they might change what people do, usually fall short of changing how they think. Because the conditions of change are now so prevalent, not to change the thinking of people has ceased to be an option. Nurses, for example, must learn to practice in a world where long lengths of stay and long-term patient relationships no longer define nursing practice. Nurses who complain that they do not have time to do what they need to do for patients have failed to realize that their grievances reflect an outmoded mental model of nursing. Hospital lengths of stay will continue to shorten, the aged will be cared for in ways that do not require their institutionalization, new pharmaceuticals will radically alter how patients get treated, and so on. In this instance, the role of leaders is to assail the old mental model and create a fluid enough foundation for nurses' expectations that they give up their old expectations and acquire new ones.

Physicians also need to be aware that the circumstances that brought them into medicine no longer exist. The unilateral, responsible but nonaccountable practice modalities that once defined medicine are disappearing, to be replaced by accountability-based, outcome-oriented, rational, complex, and multifocal modalities. The health care system is rife with the dissatisfactions of physicians who say they can no longer practice the medicine they know. What they have

> **Point To Ponder**
>
> *Failure to thrive is not uncommon in times of great change. The main reason is that organizations, although they might change what people do, usually fall short of changing how they think.*

failed to recognize is that the 20th-century manual and mechanical model of medicine has died. The one that is emerging, driven by all the improvements and enhancements in therapy and treatment, has altered forever what medicine is and how it will be practiced. In order for physicians and others to enthusiastically and energetically engage with the changes affecting medical practices, their mental models must be confronted directly and in a manner that allows them to identify the discrepancies between what they think they know and the current reality.

In earlier books (Porter-O'Grady 1992, 1994; Porter-O'Grady and Finnigan 1984; Porter-O'Grady and Krueger Wilson 1995), we enumerated the structural components and context necessary to create the scaffolding for sustainable change and full participation. Now we are joining a host of contemporary leaders in declaring the importance of empowerment, shared decision making, self-direction, and shared governance and urging the replacement of traditional organizational and management constructs with currently relevant models of workplace organization.

To gain a fuller understanding of how to adapt to the changes that are occurring, leaders must create an environment that fosters learning. In doing this, they should keep the following in mind:

- Learning must be oriented to the actual experience of the learners in their own environment.
- The purpose of learning is to ensure growth, improvement, and adaptability.
- People need to be empowered to take charge of the design of their own learning and to alter their roles and behaviors in response to what they discover.
- The organization must be willing to allow experimentation and risk taking so that innovation becomes a constant.
- Learning requires time, and the organization must therefore allow staff the time they need to pursue new knowledge.
- People need to feel that they are growing and improving. Therefore, learning should always be directed toward giving people new skills that are relevant to their job activities.

Learning can be single-loop or double-loop. In single-loop learning, the learning process is implemented as designed and the outcome is achieved as anticipated. Single-loop learning deals with the apparent, the visible, and the symptomatic. In double-loop learning, the governing variables, the driving forces, the root causes, or the foundation for action are

> ### Key Point
>
> *Being open to the dynamic processes of learning and change is a requisite of adaptability. The leader is always testing the system to see how much the staff engage with the demands of change and how quickly their roles adjust to new performance expectations and to the chaos and vagaries of changing the way work is done.*

understood and applied to the process. In addition, the participants are familiar with the process of learning and incorporate it into their own learning activities as an ongoing part of delivering health services. Double-loop learning is essential to address sustainable solution-seeking and achieving enduring results.

For learning to occur, especially double-loop learning, participants must understand their own theory-in-use (or automatic reasoning processes). Most people bring their own reasoning processes and preexisting notions to any learning situation and will even look for things that validate their preexisting notions. The mother of one of the authors is a smoker of many years. When confronted with the fact that long-term smoking leads inevitably to illness and death, she will invariably identify those rare creatures that are long-lived lifelong smokers. When reminded that she can name these people because so few are still alive, the logic escapes her. Her theory-in-use forces her to identify the circumstances in which her premises and beliefs can be confirmed and reinforced, giving her, in her own mind, no reason to change her pattern of behavior.

All people have preexisting notions and a propensity to try to validate them. Leaders (or anyone else acting as a coach) must recognize the importance of identifying and describing these notions sufficiently clearly to be able to address them and even use them as vehicles for personal learning and change. The goal of coaching is to help people acquire new ideas that will validate the experience of change and more accurately reflect the prevailing reality, ensuring that they will have a place in it.

> ### Group Discussion
>
> How many of us really know why we believe what we do or act as we do? The members of the group should each identify a statement about their professional work that they believe and two reasons for believing it. What is the theory-in-use in the application of this belief? Do others understand the statement in the same way? Is it really rational to believe the statement? Helping others change means knowing your own rituals and routines and the rational basis for acting on them.

The final step in the learning process is to generalize what has been learned and reinforce it through applied action. Using new knowledge is the best way to incorporate it into the foundation upon which the processes of work are built. Furthermore, integrating the new knowledge into the foundation will lead to additional new learning and to another revision of the foundation, allowing the workers to achieve higher levels of performance and personal satisfaction.

Leaders need to understand that for double-loop learning to occur, they must create a culture that promotes the necessary processes and risk taking. This means that every role at every level of the organization—from the very highest levels of authority to the point of service—must be involved to some degree in the learning process and make use of available learning tools (Exhibit 8–3). In other

> **Point To Ponder**
>
> *Adults learn most easily when they can apply what they have learned. The best approach is to teach them on the job so that they can apply their new knowledge then and there. Likewise, they accept changes most easily when they can act on the changes immediately.*

words, the organization must live the learning process in everything it does. When an organization fails to embrace learning, the reason often is that a genuine culture of learning and adaptation was not designed and structured into the life of the organization. Dynamic adaptation and learning are simply unsustainable in any organization that does not have a vibrant learning culture.

All learning is essentially individual. It begins at the personal level before it can become organizationwide. Therefore, each member of an organization must be expected to engage in learning activities, and the structure of the organization should even make it impossible for members to survive without pursuing new knowledge. The need for all members to become more knowledgeable is especially great now because of the reconfiguration of systems and enterprises that is occurring. Leaders, through coaching, can help staff change the language in use and find the right questions to ask—those that reflect the current reality, for it is in this reality that the answers lie.

People are so strongly socialized by their past relationships and experiences that it is difficult to alter behaviors resulting from their socialization. When people come to work, their socialized behaviors come with them and are acted out. Leaders must recognize that socialization is a critical factor with regard to change and make sure it is incorporated into the structure and dynamic of learning. By engaging employees in a discussion of the effects of socialization on their behaviors and incorporating that discussion into the learning equation, leaders will be more likely to get the personal changes necessary to generate the shifts in work processes and outcomes.

Exhibit 8–3 Action Learning Tools

- Computerized scenarios
- Case studies
- Comparative modeling
- Video presentations
- PowerPoint presentations
- Storyboards
- Clinical exemplars
- Virtual classrooms
- Satellite interactive sessions
- Group practice sessions

ORGANIZING FOR TRANSFORMATION

Leaders know that behaviors do not change accidentally or upon request. The context or culture of the organization or unit plays a major role in determining what behaviors occur and how they become modified. The leader of a unit, for instance, must have in place a uniformly applied set of expectations to ensure that the patterns of behavior are consistent. Further, the expectations and associated patterns of behavior must be congruent with the environmental demands that drive the work of the unit to ensure that responses to the demands are quick and appropriate. Finally, the interplay between behavior and structure must be such that the prevailing operational processes reflect it and can use this intersection as a way of advancing organizational effectiveness.

Another essential leadership task is to establish, together with the unit's members, some basic foundations undergirding the unit's functions. To do this, the leader must continuously assess the patterns of relationship, interaction, and personal and professional behavior within the context of the expectations defined for them. In the culture of adaptation, there are clearly understood and consistently applied processes that assure each participant that the agreed parameters are up front and continuously applied.

The leader should be aware that the purpose of these processes and structures is not to keep people happy. In many organizations, the goal of keeping people happy actually has become an impediment to making them happy. In fact, the knowledge that the leader expects employees to be happy can create conditions that ensure that they are not.

Happiness is not something that can be achieved through organizational means; it is instead a personal matter. What is within the leader's purview are those things that keep the employees motivated, invested, involved, and satisfied with what they are doing. The leader's best chance of creating an environment in which employees are all of these things is to set expectations that are high but not so high as to prevent the employees from consistently meeting them and even surpassing them. These expectations and the structures and processes developed to ensure they can be met form the framework for advancing the organization's goals and those of the people who make it up.

The leader also has the responsibility to ensure that certain basic requirements for learning and adaptation are in place:

- The members of the unit must be informed of the prevailing rules for personal behavior, personal interaction, and problem identification.
- There must be a mechanism for calling the parties to the table when a problem occurs or an issue arises. This mechanism must become the unit's normal means for first responding to problems and issues.
- There must also be a routine mechanism for discussing and critically reviewing each issue that affects the staff. The purpose of this mechanism is to give the relevant parties an opportunity to play an active part in the deliberations and decision making intended to resolve the issue.
- Shared decision-making models should be used for empowering the staff and giving them a role in dealing with issues for which they are accountable.
- There must be a forum and method of resolution for conflicts between members, concepts, plans, or processes. These conflicts must not be allowed to continue unad-

dressed for long periods of time. In the case of conflicts between individuals, the goal is to return the parties to a productive and active relationship with each other. If a good working relationship cannot be established, there must be a mechanism for separating the parties.

- Staff should be involved in the strategic and tactical activities of leadership. In particular, they should participate in decisions that define their future, thereby gaining ownership of their work.

Besides building appropriate processes and structures, the leader has the responsibility of stimulating the members of the unit to achieve high levels of performance. This can be done through building a shared vision and helping the members see that their work is a significant part of a great enterprise. The leader must realize that everyone wants to be a part of something important and to make a meaningful and sustainable difference. The leader keeps the members as focused on the purpose of their work as on its processes. The members should not become so fixed on the work itself that they lose sight of why they are doing it.

> **Key Point**
>
> *When gathering people together, the first step is to clarify the rules of engagement. Although this can be tiresome, people must be reminded of the expectations regarding interaction and communication. Deliberations break down most often because the parameters for dialogue were not reinforced and adhered to.*

Structure is a critical element in the creation of a meaningful and motivating work environment, for it provides the context for behavior and sets the parameters determining how the processes of work unfold. A good structure enhances personal interaction, problem solving, learning, and adaptation and keeps alive the human dynamics that energize and give meaning to the work. In the absence of such a structure, none of this can be assured (Figure 8–2).

DEALING WITH THE LACK OF TIME

"Not enough time" is perhaps the most widely heard mantra in the workplace today. In the past few years, it seems as if work has expanded and time has been compressed. Although time has not literally shrunk, dramatic changes during this period have affected people's perception of both time and work.

First, work generally has become more complex. Although the purpose of a job may be the same, what it takes to do it has changed radically. There is simply more to the job than there used to be. In health care, for example, managing the continuum of care so that the proper services are provided in a timely fashion requires communication and interaction with a whole host of professionals and use of numerous resources that are new on the scene. The need to do work speedily and effectively has also increased the intensity of the work and made time even more of a concern.

Leaders and staff need to look at the issue of time differently. For many years, work was looked at as a process that had no beginning or end. As a result, it became an end in itself,

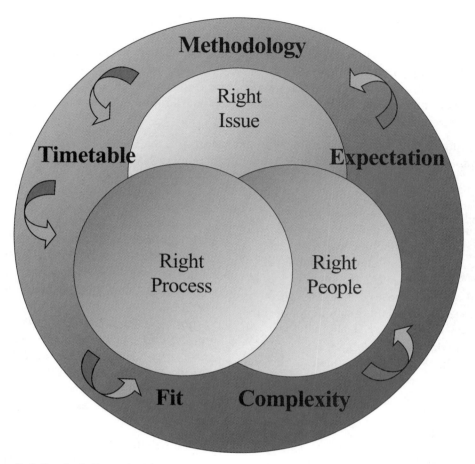

Figure 8–2 Leader's Focus in Times of Complexity. When moving through the change process, leaders must focus on core elements.

and the usual goal was simply to be efficient and do what had to be done on time. The issues are now more profound and require a different mental model for their resolution. Rather than looking for more resources or time, leaders are confronted with the questions about who should be used and how they should be used—questions about being different in a world that is changing before our very eyes. The fact is that resources, human and other, are not available in the same numbers and format they once were. The questions are no longer about more of anything. Looking for more resources, people, or time is not likely to help get more of any of these resources. The issue is no longer about doing more with less; there are instead questions about doing and being different in a world that is becoming different before our very eyes.

In other words, leaders need to challenge the prevailing framework. For instance, besides realizing themselves that resources are finite and not as readily available as formerly, leaders must repeatedly point out to the staff that the value of work is embedded in outcomes, not processes. They must also recognize that nurses and physicians are challenged with having to validate their treatment decisions by providing evidence that their choices were either less costly and less resource intensive than comparably effective treatments or had better results than other possible treatments. For most of their years in practice, health professionals never had to prove that there was a functional relationship between what they did and what occurred. Nowadays, there is no future for health care treatments for which such a relationship cannot be demonstrated.

Work in this new era requires more flexibility and fluidity than previously. The old notion that work should have fixed time and function parameters is no longer realistic. With wireless technology, a health care provider can be anywhere and still be reached for advice or follow up. When does a provider's job really begin, and when does it really end? It is now the responsibility of the individual to determine his or her workload and availability and the extent of the work period. In the past, people went to a workplace, did their jobs, and went home. Nowadays jobs go with the jobholders wherever they go, and there are no parameters defining the jobs more narrowly.

> ### Point To Ponder
>
> *Leaders can have a big impact on problem solving merely by eliminating the word* more *from the dialogue. As long as people think that* more *resources—more money, time, people, capital, equipment, and so on—will solve their problems, they will not put enough imagination and creativity into the mix to discover sustainable solutions.*

Leaders must now begin to apply tools to staffing that allow the planning and utilization of staff to be more flexible. They must also consider job candidates with an eye to their skill sets and personality characteristics to ensure that they increase the organization's adaptability. The notion of "goodness of fit" applies to people just as it does to roles. Scheduling around workload is now a critical method of staffing. So is contracting for workload—bringing staff on board based on an agreed workload and paying them for the workload rather than for time and function. These methods give staff more control over their work life and over their life outside work.

The revolution in communications gives staff members more documentation and information-gathering options, not to mention unprecedented access to each other. The hands-free earpiece or headset allows providers to connect with others at a wide variety of times rather than just during a few set periods (e.g., rounds). Finding someone, reading the chart, and documenting information have become easier with the new telephone and personal digital assistant devices now common in the workplace.

Because of the increase in specialization, health professionals have become more interdependent. No one can be an expert in everything, and the members of a health care team must identify and make use of each other's expertise, fashioning a strong clinical network in the process. The leader of the team helps the other members become both more self-reliant, where appropriate, and also more interdependent. Rather than being a manager in the traditional sense, the leader is instead a colleague who creates the possibilities and conditions for real advancement and learning.

Time and resources problems do not always have easy answers, and what might work in one part of an organization will fail outright in another. The organization's leader should realize that all problem solving is ultimately local and that those individuals who own a problem must be the ones to discover and implement its solution. Therefore, the leader needs to push the staff members to find their own solutions and to identify processes that work for them and can be sustained in their environment. The key here is ownership. Those at the top of the organization do not know how to resolve all of the difficulties that arise at the point of work. It is rather the staff members who know how to handle problems there, and the leader's job is to make them understand that they are expected to own the problems that arise, apply the appropriate methods and tools to solve them, and then utilize the necessary means to evaluate the outcomes and sustain whatever benefits they have achieved. The leader, of course, keeps his or her eye on the results, knowing that outcomes drive all processes and that all processes are disciplined by sustainable outcomes.

> **Key Point**
>
> *Staff members must be allowed to find the solutions to their own problems. The role of the leader is not to solve problems but to make certain that the staff have the insights and skills necessary to solve them. The one absolute unforgivable is to take care of other people's problems for them.*

Leaders are often required to play the role of coach, and they bring to this role not only insight and skill but passion as well. In fact, by exhibiting energy and drive, they encourage others to stay invested in their own activities and commitments. They act as living examples of the excitement that results from engagement with the challenges of the times.

Coaches, including leaders acting as guides or counselors to staff members, find their greatest reward in helping others develop and move in the direction they need to go. They become invested in the achievements of those they are helping to learn and experience the learners' gains as gains of their own. Following is a summary of issues that arise in coaching and that leaders acting as coaches in a team situation need to keep in mind.

- Having a genuine interest in people means having an interest in their becoming the best that they can be. Every team leader, therefore, needs to make sure that the other members know and feel the obligation to advance themselves and become full participants in the process of learning and adapting. The individual team members are accountable for thriving, and the leader must always keep this truth in front of the team members' eyes.
- Coaching team members is not the same as raising children. The team members are always fully accountable for their own development. The leader provides assistance in the form of tools and support but does not take on the burden of accountability for the other members' growth and advancement. The leader's role is to remind the team members of relevant expectations and parameters for action and to support them in meeting those expectations.

- When acting as coach to the other members of a team, the leader does not acquire possession of their work. Nor does the leader own the staff's relationships and interactions or the outcomes of their efforts. The leader is on the alert for staff attempts to transfer possession of these to ensure that the ownership remains where it belongs. The leader is like a circuit rider, moving continuously around the periphery of the team, observing, interacting, assessing, and identifying. When issues, deficits, or concerns arise, the leader is ready to transfer skills, insights, and tools to the team members in a way that makes it clear that they have what they need to deal with their problems and advance their own work.

- The team leader is not in control of the lives of the other team members or of the circumstances in which they do their work. The leader is their colleague rather than their manager, and the coaching role is one of partnership. The team leader's job is to keep the other members connected, invested, and aware and to help them develop to the point where they can operate with little outside intervention. In a transformational time, the leader is always pushing at the edges, helping the other members recognize the changes that are occurring, the issues that are arising, and the best methods for resolving them. The leader is in back, pushing the team into its reality, not in front, pulling it into his or her reality.

- The leader is the chief learner on the team. By modeling her or his commitment to the "way of learning" as a way of living, the leader helps create a learning culture and shows others how to embark on their own journey. The leader is always curious, searching, reading signposts, transferring information, raising issues, and pushing the parameters. The leader sees learning as a dynamic, as an essential constituent of living and relating, and becomes for the team a visual representation of learning in action.

Because the work of transforming organizations is so critical in these times, leaders in their role as coaches must exhibit the attitudes and behaviors of change and adaptation. In living the process of change, they perhaps do more to further the ability of others to handle change than they do by their explicit instruction. People need to see leaders dealing with change so that they have someone rather than something to identify with. They look to leaders to humanize the experience of change by growing and adapting themselves, for by seeing others who are successfully adjusting to change, they become more comfortable carrying out their own personal journey of transformation.

THE LEADER AS REVOLUTIONARY

As mentioned repeatedly, the health care system is at a critical moment. New thinking, different models and processes, and whole new technologies are pushing the system toward a huge transformation. Yet there is so much in the way—a long history of now outmoded patterns, rituals, routines, and infrastructure. To help carry out the transformation, each leader must become a revolutionary in residence.

The skills of revolution are different from those of evolution, because, in a revolutionary context, time is compressed, it is already too late, the options to thrive are significantly threatened, and leaders and personnel are almost paralyzed by their circumstances. The leader of an organization in this case has the job of initiating a number of processes so that the organization as a whole can engage with the radical changes occurring and implement adaptations in a timely fashion. Of course, the leader cannot do it alone. A coalition of like-minded revolutionaries is necessary for substantive change to occur. Indeed, the leader, acting as a transformational revolutionary, will seek to widen the circle of "conspirators" until the whole organization is conspiring to transform itself and its processes to meet current demands. Following is a description of several steps a revolutionary leader goes through to ensure that adaptation becomes the modus operandi of the system.

> **Point To Ponder**
>
> *The only real difference between evolution and revolution is the pace of change.*

Create an Argument for Revolution

The organizational leader must create a vision of the transformation, for what the transformation is and does is critical to getting people mobilized. The leader thus gathers together like-minded leaders within the organization to make a statement about the efforts entailed by the transformation—essentially a vision statement. The forces at play, the impact of events, the changing circumstances, the altered financial configurations—all these jointly determine how the current mental model should be revised and what needs to be done. The organizational leader then collects data to validate and refine the vision statement. The statement must show a clear connection between the conditions and the response and indicate why the conditions are so compelling as to make nonresponding a nonchoice. It must not only describe the conditions but also explain the response, citing the critical factors that will influence the organization's position in the future.

> **Group Discussion**
>
> As a group, identify one major change that needs to occur in the health care system. Make sure that the change is significant and radical. Using a flipchart and pasting the pages on the wall, create a plan for revolution around the identified change. Identify the various constituencies and conspiracies that will be necessary for building momentum. Evaluate whether the plan is revolutionary enough and how and where to start its implementation.

Develop a Charter for the Future

After clarifying the conditions demanding transformation, the leader and his or her co-conspirators must develop an agenda for the future. This can be likened to a map of the territory through which the system must now travel. The goal at this stage is not to devise a detailed program for change but to articulate the themes and signposts indicating the organization's proper direction. The "charter" should consist of a simple and clear point-by-point enumeration of the factors and themes of becoming. It should contain engaging terminology so that key words and phrases like "creating a sustainable partnership" or "building the health journey" can be pulled out and used to generate energy and enterprise throughout the organization. It should also indicate obstacles that are in the way of achieving the goals of the charter and that the conspirators will need all of their commitment to overcome.

Build the Conspiracy

The transformation process has no meaning and will die an ignoble death if the conspiracy does not continuously expand. The charter starts to gain life when the organization embraces it as its work. The role of the leader is to make sure that commitment to the transformation moves outward into the far reaches of the organization. All the key players, informal and formal, at all places in the organization must embrace the charter, take ownership of it, and move it to the next levels of application. No formal mechanism of generation is required. Those who "get it" are brought on board when they are ready, and then they do their part to find and lead others who can "get it" as well. As might be guessed, the various organizational committees, from medical staff committees to management councils, are great vehicles for publicizing the vision and expanding the conspiracy.

This kind of revolution cannot be secretive. Everyone eventually must be on board to help in the creation of a preferred future. The work of the conspiracy is merely to stimulate this journey for all members of the organization, from those at the point of service to those in the boardroom. Joining the conspiracy to operational processes already underway is a good mechanism for getting the charter on the table of those who most need to engage with it.

Be Strategic and Patient

There are no enemies in this revolution—only those not yet part of it. The conspirators must understand who the stakeholders are that they need to bring on board in order to give the charter both life and legs. They must also understand when to approach these individuals and groups or include the charter in their work.

Further, they should know the local politics of communication and action and identify what strategies are best for addressing specific challenges and circumstances. Getting specific individuals to perform certain required actions (because of their relationships, positions, or skills) is a part of the strategic process of managing the charter and guiding it through the political landscape. Indeed, one-on-one interactions with key players are as important as group meetings. In approaching key players, the conspirators will need to translate the charter into their language to obtain their acceptance and advocacy. Key players have to be able to see how the process benefits them and advances their own opportunities and circumstances—that is part of the political process.

Seek out Significant Champions

As the conspiracy grows, it must incorporate champions able to take the charter further on its journey. The transformation process is like a relay race: Different runners with different skills are required at different points in the process. The organizational leader must be able to anticipate the new focus, person, or skill necessary for getting to the next stage and must ensure that each is applied in the right format and at the right time to move the process along.

As in most conspiracies, movement toward the goal is not along a straight line. Backward or horizontal steps are occasionally required to refresh or expand the process. In addition, as progress occurs, the kind of champions needed will often be found at new locations. That is as it should be. The conspirators must celebrate any support that will move the transformation along to the next stage and increase its chance of success.

Make Sure That Small Successes Occur Early and Often

Successes must take place along the way to maintain momentum. Creating a plan for substantive change and getting the whole organization to embrace it is a long, gradual process, and people will remain unmotivated if they perceive their efforts as unlikely to make a difference. Even small accomplishments show that movement has occurred, and without some "deliverables" the organization is sure to lose interest before it gets very far. The accomplishments give the transformation process "legs" and ensure that the process's champions will be able to overcome objections and opposition in a manner that allows them to incorporate new ideas into the process and convert possible opponents into supporters.

Make the Transformation the Mainstream Activity

The goal is to enable the whole organization to thrive well into the future. The conspiracy is simply a means of ensuring the organization's survival at a time when the organization appears to be missing an opportunity to prosper. Thus, the conspirators must always keep in mind that the purpose of their efforts is to benefit the organization, not themselves. They also must avoid becoming so committed to the conspiracy that their attention is diverted from the real end and their energies wind up misdirected. Once the conspirators have attained their objective—to make the transformation the central activity of the organization—the nature of their endeavors shifts toward initiating work processes related to the new reality. The conspirators must now fully embrace the character, context, and content of the new reality, which means redefining the work, retooling the workplace, and focusing on the conditions that will allow the organization to thrive. In a sense, the conspiracy has now become the new reality.

Of course, the talk, in this section, of a conspiracy is merely a way of highlighting the focused commitment to fundamental change that leaders in an organization must have when options are limited or opportunities are being missed. It pinpoints the sense of urgency the leaders must impart to the entire organization to get everyone to make the kind of effort needed to ensure the organization's ability to thrive in a highly charged and changing set of circumstances. The leaders, acting as change agents, must stimulate the staff and other stakeholders to raise their own levels of energy and refocus their efforts. The "conspiracy" enlists them in an effort that is greater than they are as individuals, giving them a sense of meaning and purpose and generating the energy, emotion, insight, spirit, and commitment they will need to adapt and grow. Focused commitment and strong motivation, along with appropriate processes, methodologies, and techniques, round out the requisites of revolutionary transformation.

INNOVATION COACHING

A team leader has the responsibility to create the right conditions for the team and its members to learn and grow. In fact, the main purpose of team leadership is to ensure the team members can develop and become what they must in order to thrive in shifting circumstances. The achievement of this goal, of course, requires the team leader to overcome existing obstacles to effective coaching (Exhibit 8–4).

To become successful in the new age, leaders and staff members must be able to relate to the processes of transformation so that they see them as the essence of their work and not as mere responses to a demand to do things differently. Adaptability is as much an attitude as it is a way of doing business, and the goal of leaders should be to help everyone *be* different, not just perform new job activities. After all, in this era of revolution, it is not just the work that is changing, it is the very workplace itself—the conditions, elements, and technologies of work.

Because the working conditions are being substantially altered, leaders must ensure that the differences do not escape the attention of those who do the work. They need to help the workers revise their mental model of work and turn *every* one of them into a revolutionary. In other words, they need to publicize the fact that innovation is now a way of life and help the workers develop the skills and attributes they require to live that way of life and become part of the transformation of the workplace (Figure 8–3).

Exhibit 8–4 Impediments to Effective Coaching

Use of power
- Inadequate power
- Autocratic application of power
- Lack of empowerment
- Nonstrategic use of power

Self-image
- Poor self-esteem
- Unclear role
- Psychological flaws

Knowledge
- Undeveloped knowledge
- Learning needs
- Inexperience
- Lack of personal technique

Problem solving
- Inadequate worldview
- Intolerance of diversity
- No clear process
- Situational solutions

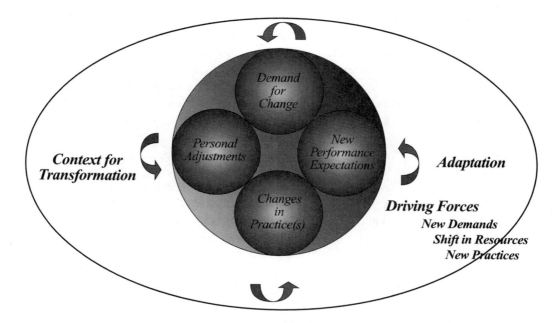

Figure 8–3 Innovation as a Way of Life. The leader focuses on the central components of personal transformation to ensure each person can embrace change.

To convert work into innovative effort, leaders need to follow several rules, discussed below. They should also keep in mind that the workers not only must figure out the emerging context for their work and relationships but must create the structures and content for the journey itself.

Set the Bar High

Leaders need to convince workers that expectations for their performance are high but not so high that they cannot be met. The challenge is to set expectations that prevent the workers from falling back on old behaviors and practices but that also do not discourage them. The expectations should stimulate the workers to engage in different thinking and to change the very nature of the work.

Another way of saying this is that the transformation of work requires the new models for thinking, a new context for work, and goals that demand new ways of working. The goals should not be so easily attainable that the workers can retain their old ways of doing things.

Be Clear about Who You Are

In the new world of work, people need to redefine who they are and what their definition of success is. For example, hospitals, which were originally defined as places where the sick were cared for, have been redefined as places where health care services are delivered. The range of services that fall under the rubric *health care* differ from the range that fall under the rubric *caring for the sick.*

Because of alterations in the health services landscape, health care leaders must highlight the changes in the context of work and the implications for its performance, including the new demands that have arisen. They must then revise the structures and processes of work to meet the new demands and assist staff in adjusting their insights, attitudes, and behaviors appropriately. Staff members must live the image of the organization in all they are and do. Making sure that staff members see the shift and can live the new perspective in their work and relationships is a critical element in the journey into the future.

Treat Transformation as a Mission, Not a Job

The staff of an organization must not simply change the way they do their work but also change the way they live their work. Therefore, the organizational leader, acting as a coach, must be able to explain how to live and work differently using the broadest and clearest language possible. Transcending simple notions of labor, the leader creates an image of health care delivery as having a purpose beyond its immediate effects. By showing how work efforts can influence the world of health care, the leader transforms the performance of work by an individual into the pursuit of a mission. People want to support good and noble causes that take them outside of themselves and also want to view their efforts as having a profound value. The leader can help them take this leap from the mundane to the honorable and incorporate a sense of mission into the very fabric of their work activities.

> ### Key Point
>
> *The leader must be so consumed by the organization's mission that transformation becomes second nature. In addition, by being committed to this mission, the leader presents a visible example of transformation in action that has the power to inspire others to transform themselves and their job activities.*

Expose Staff to Different Messages and Different Messengers

To motivate the staff, the leader must give them encouraging messages that differ from those they have heard all along. The leader must also communicate new expectations and provide opportunities for the staff to learn what they need to know to meet these expectations. The encouragement and the expectations communicated must be consistent with the transformation upon which the organization has embarked. The goal is to stimulate the staff to think about how to do their work more effectively.

New voices should also be allowed a hearing. Young workers, workers who are quiet and reserved, and workers from outside the particular work group should be included in the collective dialogue. The leader should do as much as possible to "push the walls" to move people out of their comfort zones and stretch into new ways of thinking and doing.

Create an Egalitarian Organizational Structure

Hierarchy should be minimized in times of great change. In fact, in the new age, hierarchy has little value. Horizontal relationships, defined not by position but by role, are the cornerstone of accountability. The leader of an organization must therefore facilitate relationships with those he or she depends on for planning and performing the organization's work.

In other words, the leader must value the work and the worker equally. Each worker has a contribution to make, and the leader's job is to get each to offer innovative ideas on how to improve methods and processes, for the workers are the ones who know best what produces results and what does not. The leader therefore needs to make it safe and easy for workers to become part of the collective dialogue and put forth suggestions. Barriers to interaction, sharing, and challenging simply cannot exist if the spontaneous communication of ideas is to become the organization's modus operandi. Ideas are an important form of capital for any enterprise and they can come from any place. In order for them to be released, the organization's culture must make it not only possible but routine.

Put Money Where the Ideas Are

In order for an idea to be implemented, some level of financing is required. Although not every idea is worth supporting, funding for good ideas must be available, for the staff need to know that their ideas have the potential to go somewhere and make a difference. If their ideas are ignored for lack of funding, they will eventually go back to old routines and refuse to contribute. If their ideas, on the other hand, are taken seriously and investigated, they will continue to make suggestions.

The funding or budgeting process must make it possible to explore ideas and innovations to an extent commensurate with their likely utility. Out of 1,000 ideas, perhaps only 10 will ever be used, but those 10 could not have emerged unaccompanied by the rest. In short, the exploration of all ideas is critical to the discovery and application of the few that do become part of the organization's practice.

Let the Talented Experiment

It is impossible to apply new thinking by rote or through using a "straight line" approach. Talented people must be gathered together and supported. This means, among other things, allowing them to take risks. The outcomes of ideas are often unpredictable, and thus a certain amount of trial and error will be necessary. Ideas must be tried and possibly modified before their worth can be known. If an idea, after a period of trial, is shown to be not beneficial, then it should be discarded.

Nothing should be set in cement. Strategies should be implemented and then modified as necessary. Structures and permanent processes should be avoided, since they create barriers to necessary revisions. In addi-

> **Point To Ponder**
>
> *Experimentation is critical to innovation and adaptability. An organization not willing to experiment is doomed to failure.*

tion, there must be enough creative people in the organization to ensure that innovative thinking occurs. Constant attention to bringing in and keeping such people is critical for sustaining the transformation. The leader must be comfortable with those who are bright and creative and come up with ideas that challenge the leader to think and act differently.

Allow People To Share in the Fruits of Their Creativity

This is perhaps the most challenging notion for health care leaders. For some unfathomable reason, the practice of rewarding people for their contribution has not become common practice within the health care arena. However, people own their creativity and ideas and lose interest and move on if their ownership is not honored. Keeping creative people means investing in them, and investing in them means rewarding them for their innovations.

Creative people often do not seek to be compensated financially. For them, seeing their originality have an impact can be reward enough. Nonetheless, the leader should acknowledge contributions in a meaningful way. Although a bonus is the most recognized and established kind of reward and should be seriously considered, there are a host of other kinds, including public acknowledgment (celebrations and events), publishing the work inside or outside the institution, gainsharing (sharing the rewards), and shared ownership. Whatever rewards are defined by the organization, the reward granted to an individual for a given contribution should fit the needs of the person and the kind of contribution. Remember, highly creative people are looking not for long-term permanent positions but for opportunities to express their gifts and talents. Keeping them on as employees will depend on whether the organization's culture provides them with an ability to create, grow, and advance.

The leader is always attentive to the need to keep the organization moving and able to respond to current demands (Figure 8–4). Creating the environment, structure, and processes necessary to ensure the organization's adaptability is the leader's single most important task. Because inventive people are essential to the organization's ability to respond to new demands, the leader is forever looking for, challenging, and rewarding such people in an effort to maintain a pool of creative talent (Figure 8–5).

MAKING INTEGRATION WORK

Because of the systems-oriented dynamics of health care, making things fit together is very important. The leader of a health care organization must be able to evaluate the fit between elements and improve their fit wherever possible (Exhibit 8–5). When a merger or alliance occurs, however, creating proper fit can be a great problem. People bring to the new entity their past ideas, commitments, cultures, and notions of how the work is to be done, and they resist or find it difficult to create the level of integration that is required. Much of the energy of the leader is devoted to making the new arrangements not just workable but productive.

Perhaps the greatest concern is the speed with which things seem to happen today. Although time itself has not accelerated, the extra complexity of work has made it difficult

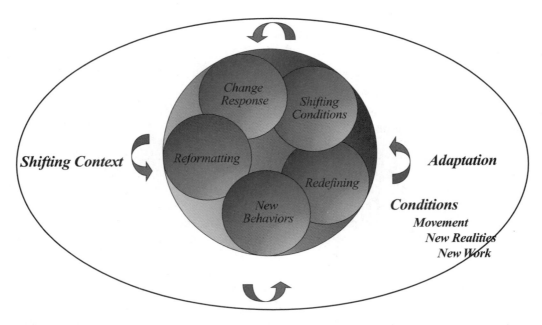

Figure 8–4 The Dynamics of Continuous Adaptation. The leader ensures that each element of adaptation is addressed by those whose work must be transformed by new realities.

to accomplish tasks at the pace once expected. Because staff are finding they no longer have enough time to do what they used to do, the leader must help them replace their focus on doing lots of things to doing the right things.

Group Discussion

A common topic of discussion today is the nature of true integration. As a group, brainstorm the basic elements of integration. Identify areas where group members disagree. Break into two debating teams of two or three members each and have each team take a position and argue for it. The remainder of the group will critique the debate and evaluate the arguments. After the debate, the group members should discuss how their view of integration has been altered or reinforced. Finally, identify three or four common elements of integration that can be used as criteria to determine whether integration has been achieved.

In the old days, health care providers did a lot of things for patients. In fact, this reality drove the definition of caring. Today, although caring is still central to health care, it is expressed differently. The independence and accountability of the users of health services

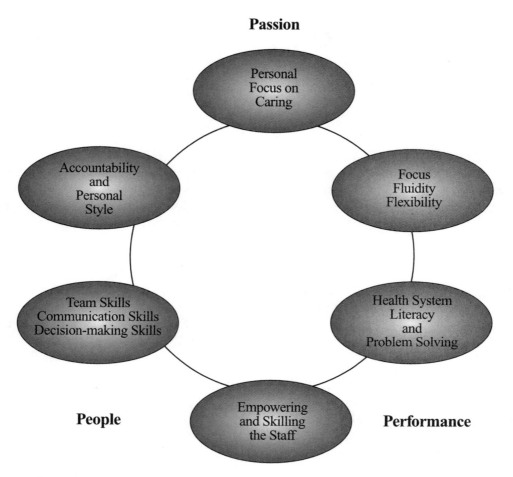

Figure 8–5 The Elements of Personal Transformation. Change is not complete until the cycle of transformation is complete. The leader brings personal passion to moving people to a new level of performance.

are now as important as the services delivered by care providers. People must acknowledge their responsibility for their own health and be empowered to act in the right way at the right time to ensure their well-being. Providers consequently are faced with a different mix of activities and priorities and must recognize that doing everything for patients is not the best way to render needed assistance.

To many health professionals, the idea that patients are responsible for their health borders on heresy. At the very least, it goes against a long tradition. Nonetheless, in this age of consumer control and accountability, the complexity of health care and the added demands on the providers' time require many of the tasks to be placed in the hands of the patients. This transfer of responsibility, of course, changes the character of the provider-patient relationship.

Exhibit 8–5 Elements of Integration

• Goodness of fit	• Focus on the whole
• Role congruence	• Interdependence
• Alignment	• Accountability
• Integrity	• Orientation toward outcomes

The leader must ensure not only that the transfer of responsibility is carried out but that providers and patients change their attitudes, beliefs, and practices accordingly. Replacing the expectation of "doing for" with the expectation of "doing with" is an arduous task, not just for staff but for patients as well. Patients, too, have grown up with a certain image of health care and certain expectations of what they should obtain from the health care system, and they can feel disappointed when these expectations are not fully met. They, too, operate with a dependency model according to which they surrender responsibility, accountability, and control to health care providers in return for being taken care of. In fact, their surrender of these things sometimes facilitates their descent into conditions and lifestyles that contribute to the illnesses for which they seek treatment.

> **Key Point**
>
> *The health care system is changing in fundamental ways, and so providers and patients need to act differently and "expect differently." The providers, in particular, need to change their own behaviors and expectations and educate the patients to change theirs.*

Today, part of the health care provider's role is to alter patient expectations of "being taken care of." Part of the health care leader's role is to work with providers in creating a new model of health care and revising the patient-provider relationship. The ultimate goal is to help providers use their time more effectively and appropriately in delivering care and providing services to those in need.

In particular, providers must focus on teaching and otherwise empowering patients to see more and do more in their own interest. They must also involve family members or significant others in the delivery of services and in counseling, supporting, and caring for loved ones in need of assistance.

In order for these changes to occur, health care leaders need to focus on four important responsibilities. These are described below.

Speeding up Processes

Time is of the essence. Providers have less and less time to talk with patients about their health care needs and provide appropriate services, and therefore providers and patients must make better use of their time together. For example, follow up now means making sure patients can gain access to the resources they need (i.e., connecting them to a network of resources, including sources of information, that can guide their actions when they are no longer within the health care system).

As noted, the locus of control is in the hands of the patients (where it really belongs), and the providers must make sure that it never shifts away from there and that the patients have what they need to do the right things for their health. Health care leaders have the task of helping staff become comfortable with this reality and guiding them into practices that will allow patients to make the best decisions and carry out those decisions. For the transition to the new provider-patient relationship to occur, both staff and patients must develop new skills or skill sets.

Orchestrating the Dynamics of Change

Making the shift to new ways and new roles is difficult for everyone. Complicating the situation is the fact that new rituals and routines must replace those that reinforce behaviors suitable for the older model of service. Staff members, having lived for so long with the more traditional dependent practices, now need approaches, tools, and skills to help them initiate and sustain new behaviors. Leaders must ensure that they develop and use these in ways that fit their culture and experience with change. By exchanging best practices with other settings, staff members can connect with others who are busy creating and constructing methods and models for improving services and changing their relationships with those they serve.

Building Relationships

Everything is built on good and sustainable relationships. The most important leadership task is to ensure that everyone is "singing off the same song sheet." Keeping an organization's staff on target and focused on its mission is difficult yet critical work. The leader continually tests, challenges, and extends personal and collective relationships with stakeholders throughout the process of changing behavior. When things get tough or stuck, the leader's only resource may be the personal relationships he or she has developed during this process. Identifying with the difficulties and vagaries that the staff are undergoing and supporting them through the changes they are having to deal with will be critical to sustaining their efforts. Testing, stretching, evaluating, renewing, supporting, and challenging are steps in the normal cycle of action, relationship, and response that every leader needs in his or her tool chest (Figure 8–6).

Putting Necessary Structure in Place

New behaviors are not sustainable without accompanying structural supports. We learned from the chemical dependency movement that addressing an addict's behavior is not enough—the environment also must be changed. Creating a context for behavior means building an environment that leads to desired behaviors. Having the workers themselves fully participate in the creation of their environment increases the chance that they will take ownership of the appropriate behaviors and achieve the desired outcomes.

Leaders often fail to pay close attention to the structural realities, allowing staff to fall back into old patterns of behavior. Creating structures that limit old patterns and foster preferred

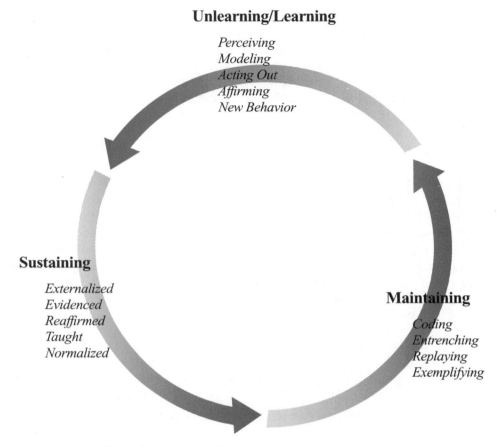

Unlearning/Learning

Perceiving
Modeling
Acting Out
Affirming
New Behavior

Sustaining

Externalized
Evidenced
Reaffirmed
Taught
Normalized

Maintaining

Coding
Entrenching
Replaying
Exemplifying

Figure 8–6 Cycle of Transformational Learning

patterns, along with rewarding the performance of desired behaviors, can make the difference between an effective workplace and one that is unproductive and problem filled. As an impetus for positive change, structure is at least the equal of behavior itself.

> **Point To Ponder**
>
> *Behavior changes cannot be sustained without structural supports in place, and leaders must pay as much attention to these as to the changes themselves.*

HITTING PROBLEMS HEAD ON

People who do not approach problems proactively acquire a "firefighting" mindset. Unfortunately, because of the large number of problems and issues that confront leaders daily, they often end up spending more time on daily skirmishes than on substantive issues. Their firefighting, by leaving their real responsibilities unattended, simply begets more fires to fight.

Some ways of dealing with problems allow leaders to do their transformational work. Indeed, problem solving can be a source of growth and can support a leader's transformational work. The trick is not to look at problems situationally and attempt to resolve them within the context of the situation but instead to investigate the circumstances in which they occur. Rather than filling holes in the staffing schedule on the spur of the moment, for example, a leader should identify and address the underlying causes, for otherwise the problem will occur again, often in a form more difficult to resolve.

A patchwork approach to problems creates more problems than it solves. It also creates problems in related but remote parts of the system. When a process is broken, other processes that interact with it pay the price. For instance, a delay in lab testing will result in a delay in treating patients. In a complex system, problems can cascade through the system, causing difficulties for everyone.

Leaders, in dealing with problems, should follow a few simple rules. Although simple, they are often forgotten, to the detriment of the problem-solving process.

Group Discussion

Tracy Polus, the head of the respiratory department, had a difficult time confronting behavior problems. Always using the third person when discussing such problems, she could often be heard saying, "When a person does . . ." or "If someone would . . ." or "If people could. . . ." The staff never really knew if she meant to refer to their behavior in particular or to the behavior of people in general. Eventually they began to discount her comments, and, because no one else was dealing with problematic behaviors, relationships in the department suffered. What recommendation would you give Tracy? How could she change her own behavior to make her a more effective manager? Is there a type of developmental program that she should undergo? Is it too late for her to establish new ground rules for her staff? What would some of the ground rules be?

Solve Problems Selectively

It is unbelievable how many leaders take on, all at once, the full range of problems affecting their organization. Not all problems can be or need to be solved immediately. Leaders must approach problem solving like any other deliberative process. In particular, they must develop strategies for prioritizing problems and bringing order and focus to the effort of addressing problems critically.

Because problems are omnipresent and impact everything that people do, leaders must look at the relationship between problems, explore the way in which they interact, and then decide the order in which the problems will be addressed. Not every problem has the same weight or the same ability to obstruct work and the achievement of desired outcomes.

Key Point

Not all problems can be solved quickly, so the leader of an organization must prioritize problems to make sure the critical ones are dealt with immediately. People problems always come first, relationship problems second, and external problems last. Structure and process problems are ongoing, as are the procedures for handling them.

Setting up a list of problems to be dealt with first is a necessary step in the problem-solving process.

Work on the Fundamental Problems First

Many leaders believe that they should work on the most urgent problems of the day. Yet problems that seem small and unessential can be the source of these seemingly more critical problems, and if the root problems are not taken care of, all of the others caused by them will not get resolved either. In addition, problems that appear to be critical to people in the midst of a crisis usually turn out to be mere symptoms of more fundamental problems. Thus, an important goal in problem solving is to determine which problem is a root cause and which is effect.

Include People with the Necessary Skills and Power in the Resolution of Problems

Although it is best for people to assert ownership of the problems that concern them, it is not always possible for everyone affected by a problem to be part of the problem-solving effort. What is more important is that the right people be involved—those who have the skills to resolve the problem and the power to make the resolution permanent. In most cases, finding and implementing a solution to a problem will require the engagement of a broad range of players and stakeholders.

Be Accountable for Ensuring Problems Are Solved

Although leaders are obligated to see that problems are solved, they are not obligated to solve problems they do not own. The important consideration in determining who should deal with a problem is who owns it and who is best placed to resolve it (i.e., usually one and the same person or group). The role of the leader, in most cases, is merely to provide the proper people with everything they need. As a result, the leader's focus is not so much on the problem as on the process.

If the owners of a problem turf it outside of their locus of control, the problem is unlikely to remain fixed for long. Therefore, leaders must make sure that problem-solving skills and processes are embedded in the organizational culture and that those who are attempting to deal with a problem have the wherewithal to take care of it.

Counterproductive beliefs and practices are significant barriers to the permanent resolution of problems. For example, despite what many leaders think, being committed to resolving problems is not nearly as important as being committed to using good problem-solving techniques and processes. These techniques and processes create the insights and skills necessary to deal with problems effectively and quickly enough to avoid long-term trauma.

ELIMINATING FIREFIGHTING ALTOGETHER

The best thing the leader of an organization can do is replace firefighting activities with much more productive behaviors. The research and work of Roger Bohm have been important in codifying what is wrong with most problem solving and in publicizing better methods (Bohm and Jaikumar 2000). To make problem solving truly effective, the leader needs to use tactical methods and strategic approaches and to alter the organization's culture.

> **Point To Ponder**
>
> *Firefighting is not a good problem-solving approach because it keeps the focus off the root issues and on the symptoms. In fact, the more firefighting a leader does, the more firefighting the leader has to do.*

Tactical Methods

The advantage of tactical methods of problem solving is that they can be put into place quickly and aid in dealing with problems in the short term while the infrastructure for the more lasting approaches is constructed.

Getting Help from Outside the Circle

It is often wise to have someone from outside the service or unit help with the response to problems inside. A person from outside will have a fresh view of the issues and will not be invested in the issues or the solutions under consideration. Leaders often refrain from using outside resources because they are uncomfortable with others knowing their problems or simply because they have not attempted this maneuver in the past. Yet, the more insight that can be obtained from those who do not own the issues, the more objective and effective the solutions are likely to be. In the new age, one of the expectations should be that leaders will call on each other as outside consultants in dealing with the deeper and more complex problems and issues that undoubtedly will arise.

Trying Something New

People have a tendency to do the same things while expecting different outcomes. They become attached to rituals and routines that are inherently problematic and refuse to face the challenge of learning new practices. Most problems in organizations occur because the members hold on to old practices that have become barriers to smooth functioning and effective performance. The leader of an organization, acting as a change agent, must begin at the fundamental level—by creating a good fit between form and function and establishing a culture that supports changes in behavior. Here again, it is by creating the right context for change and creativity to occur that leaders can most help reduce the impact of habit and make it possible for people to let go of past practices.

Triaging Problems

Problems are always occurring. The goal is to solve them as soon as possible so that they do not incubate greater problems. It therefore makes sense to sort through current problems quickly to determine which are normal or trivial and which are pivotal and likely to cause other problems. A conflict between two practitioners, for example, might create a bottleneck in the flow of work, especially if they sabotage each other's efforts. Resolving their conflict would therefore prevent a range of difficulties down the road, and so the conflict would appear high on the list of problems to be tackled immediately.

Strategic Approaches

Strategic approaches, because they are embedded in an organization's way of working and doing business, take longer to plan and implement than tactical methods.

Prioritizing Problems

Problems should be looked at as a normal part of organizational operations and their solution as a normal part of the leader's work. As much as possible, the leader should help the staff see problems as normal and develop categories for classifying problems according to their potential impact. Problems that affect staffing and the availability of clinical support resources, for example, would be treated as more urgent than office supply problems, and conflicts between departments would rank higher than conflicts between individuals on a given unit. Prioritizing problems is not intended to diminish the importance of any problem; it simply ranks them so that more critical issues are not left hanging.

Using Learning Scenarios

The leader of an organization is crippled if she or he is the only one to take on the responsibility of solving problems. The "mamma" syndrome, in which problems are seen as exclusively within the leader's jurisdiction, prevents the building of problem-solving processes into the system. Everyone needs to develop problem-assessment and problem-solving skills and the independence to take care of problems at the right time.

There is no way to avoid or eliminate all problems, and indeed problems are a sign of life in the universe. Once the staff understand this, the leader can use present or past problems as vehicles for teaching problem-solving skills. Through this kind of "scenario learning," the leader can help the staff alter their attitudes toward problems and can change the locus of control for solving them. The staff will be able to embrace problems as tools and develop the skills necessary to manage them to the organization's benefit.

Building a Problem-Solving Tool Chest

The solution of each problem should build the skill sets necessary to solve subsequent problems more quickly and easily. In a sense, each solution serves as a database for future problems. Codifying and recording approaches to specific kinds of problems increases the likelihood that recurrences will be solved in a similar fashion. Better still, it increases the likelihood that recurrences can be dealt with early enough to prevent their having a negative impact. In addition, banding together the strategies for dealing with particular types of problems creates a good framework for handling problems effectively.

Cultural Changes

An organization's attitude toward its own problems is as critical to their permanent resolution as any other single factor. If the organization refuses to see its own problems, nothing it does will ensure its ability to thrive in the long term.

Rejecting Patching as a Problem-Solving Approach

Focusing on situations instead of issues—or being sucked into situations and seeing the issues only from the inside—is sure to lead to failure. The best policy is to help the staff develop problem-solving skills so that they see clearly the problems that arise as part of their work and act as independent troubleshooters. Everyone who faces a problem wants the associated pain taken away. However, the pain is merely a symptom, and focusing solely on it will ensure that the underlying issues never hit the table. In other words, the patching approach to problems must be challenged and eliminated from the set of permissible approaches.

Making Problem-Solving Deadlines Irrelevant

Yes, it is true that problems cannot be allowed to go on forever. Rather than set deadlines for solving problems, however, the leader should embed a problem-solving methodology into the work itself. If the methodology is effective and problem solving is fostered by the organization's culture, deadlines will become moot. The problems that arise will not be avoided or treated as belonging to "the other guy" but instead will be looked at as opportunities for growth.

Do Not Reward Firefighting

In health care, a premium tends to be placed on those who can make critical decisions quickly and correctly. Health professionals with this ability are treated as heroes by every medical soap opera and documentary. Heroes make poor citizens, however, and require a great deal of ego feeding. In fact, they are not necessarily good models except in war and can cause more problems than they are credited with solving.

It is better to implement good problem-solving methods and mechanisms than to have staff use individualistic approaches. It is better to build an organization committed to problem solving than to reward good firefighters. Waiting for problems to manifest means being a day late and a dollar short—by the time the problems are addressed, most of the damage has been done. The preferred strategy is to anticipate problems and incorporate their resolution into the life and work of every member of the organization.

CONCLUSION

For a leader, transformation can be a way of life. It is a journey consisting of logical stages made up of specific actions and processes. At its best, the journey is rational, progressive, and purposeful (Table 8–1).

Leaders who accept the role of transformational coach must embrace and cope with the vagaries of these changing times. Through their role-modeling and commitment to self-direction and growth, they create a context for new expectations and new behaviors. Through liv-

Table 8–1 Personal and Group Stages on the Journey of Transformation

Stage	Personal	Group
Stage 1	Unlearning Letting go Reacting	Seeing change Acknowledging Resisting Mourning
Stage 2	Naming new skills Learning new skills Applying new skills	Discerning impact Finding meaning Experimenting Giving form
Stage 3	Reinforcing the new Evaluating behavior Teaching the new Extinguishing the old	Shifting expectations Relating in new ways Celebrating Taking ownership

ing the reality of change, they ensure that others are able to embrace their own changes and respond appropriately. In all their actions, they fulfill the aims of transformational coaching by remaining fully engaged with the staff and guiding them on the way to a productive future.

REFERENCES

Argyris, C. 1999. *On organizational learning*. New York: Blackwell.

Bohm, R., and R. Jaikumar. 2000. Stop fighting fires. *Harvard Business Review* 78, no. 4: 68–77.

Conners, R., T. Smith, and C. Hickman. 1994. *The Oz principle*. New York: Prentice Hall.

Porter-O'Grady, T. 1992. *Implementing shared governance*. Baltimore: Mosby.

Porter-O'Grady, T. 1994. Whole systems shared governance: Creating the seamless organization. *Nursing Economics* 12: 187–195.

Porter-O'Grady, T., and S. Finnigan. 1984. *Shared governance for nursing*. Gaithersburg, MD: Aspen Publishers.

Porter-O'Grady, T., and C. Krueger Wilson. 1995. *The leadership revolution in health care: Altering systems, changing behavior*. Gaithersburg, MD: Aspen Publishers.

SUGGESTED READINGS

Barthelemy, R. 1997. *The sky is not the limit*. Boca Raton, FL: St. Lucie Press.

Beer, M., and N. Nohria. 2000. *Breaking the code of change*. Boston: Harvard Business School Publishing.

Bell, C. 1996. *Managers as mentors: Building partnerships for learning*. San Francisco: Berrett-Koehler.

Califano, J. 1993. The nurse as a revolutionary. *Revolution: The Journal of Nurse Empowerment* 3, no. 3: 67–68, 108–110.

Clegg, B. 2000. *Creativity and innovation for managers*. Philadelphia: Butterworth-Heinemann.

Dotlich, D., and P. Cairo. 1999. *Action coaching*. San Francisco: Jossey-Bass.

Goffee, R., and G. Jones. 2000. Why should anyone be led by you? *Harvard Business Review* 78, no. 5: 63–70.

Holman, P., and T. Devane. 1998. *The change handbook*. San Francisco: Berrett-Koehler.

Kohles, M., W. Baker, and B. Donaho. 1995. *Transformational leadership: Renewing fundamental values and achieving new relationships in healthcare*. Chicago: American Hospital Publishing.

Kotter, J. 1995. Leading change: Why transformation efforts fail. *Harvard Business Review* 73, no. 2: 59–67.

Kurtzman, J. 1998. *Thought leaders*. San Francisco: Jossey-Bass.

Miles, R. 1997. *Leading corporate transformation*. San Francisco: Jossey-Bass.

Waldroop, J., and T. Butler. 2000. Managing away bad habits. *Harvard Business Review* 78, no. 5: 89–98.

Zohar, D. 1997. *Rewiring the corporate brain*. San Francisco: Berrett-Koehler.

Quiz Questions

Select the best answer for each of the following questions.

1. Accountability always:
   a. is externally generated
   b. is delegated from above
   c. is internally generated
   d. moves from the bottom upward

2. Accountability differs from responsibility in which of the following ways:
   a. They measure different kinds of processes.
   b. Responsibility is more results oriented.
   c. Accountability is measurable and responsibility is not.
   d. Accountability is defined in terms of outcomes.

3. In confronting change, most people find that their first response is to:
   a. personalize it
   b. feel excitement
   c. challenge the necessity for change
   d. refuse to change

4. In transformative learning, theory-in-use:
   a. consists of the conceptual foundations for an action
   b. is an automatic thought process related to an action
   c. is the theoretical validation of an action
   d. is a research-based response to a need

5. The first step in gathering staff together for the purpose of learning and adapting is to:

a. identify a good methodology to use
b. enumerate the rules of engagement
c. understand the stages of the change process
d. get to work on the problems immediately

6. The issue of resources plays a critical role in all problem solving. In dealing with this issue, leaders should keep in mind the following rule of thumb:

a. It is always possible to find more money if you look for it.
b. Providing additional resources is not the way to reach a sustainable solution.
c. Allocating more resources is necessary for solving problems.
d. Budgeting adequate resources is part of all planning.

7. In problem solving, leaders must remember that the one absolute unforgivable is to:

a. leave problems unresolved too long
b. create inadequate processes for resolving problems
c. lack a methodology for change
d. solve other people's problems for them

8. The coach is the chief:

a. facilitator
b. problem solver
c. learner
d. agent of change

9. When a coach is acting as a revolutionary, the most important task is to:

a. get action underway quickly
b. bring down existing structures as fast as possible
c. expand the circle of conspirators
d. construct an individual plan of action

10. In innovation coaching, risk is critical for success. What else is critical?

a. experimentation
b. planning
c. creating ideas
d. brainstorming

11. In undertaking tactical changes, the first thing the leader does is:

a. get out of the way
b. outline a process for change
c. direct the participants in their work
d. create a set of priorities

12. In managing strategic changes, the leader focuses on:

a. processes, elements, and tasks
b. priorities, learning scenarios, and problem-solving tools
c. context, functions, and solutions
d. vision, solutions, and outcomes

13. In facilitating cultural change, the leader avoids:

a. fighting, opposition, and conflict
b. directing, controlling, and disciplining
c. patching, setting deadlines, and fire-fighting
d. narrowing, limiting, and refining

CHAPTER 9

The Leader's Courage To Be Willing: Building a Context for Hope

Something unforeseen and magnificent is happening. Health care, having in our time entered its dark night of the soul, shows signs of emerging, transformed.

—Barbara Dossey and Larry Dossey

Chapter Objectives

At the completion of this chapter, the reader will be able to

- Review the sources of health care professional disenfranchisement.
- Describe the behavioral concept of willingness as it relates to the role of the leader.
- Describe a process for identifying and evaluating dogma in the health care system.
- Define the five essential qualities of will.
- Identify specific situations in which leaders can positively impact practice using the five essential qualities of will.

This chapter explores the concept of *willingness* and related concepts (e.g., *will, the will,* and *willpower*), the personal and organizational context in which willingness unfolds, and the factors that may erode its expression. It explains how the will of a person generally operates, how leaders can maximize their will, the evolutionary stages that a person's will goes through, and the purposes toward which a person's will can be directed. It also describes the five essential qualities of will (or willpower): courage, passion, energy, discipline, and trust. Finally, it presents eight strategies for facilitating willingness and associated assessment questions for leaders.

Why are health care workers, especially nurses, so discouraged? Where has all the hope gone? Job-related stress, emotional exhaustion, and feelings of depression, helplessness, hopelessness, and entrapment continue to fuel dissatisfaction and discouragement among all health professionals, even physicians and health care administrators. The combined assault of staffing shortages, excessive regulation, and reduced reimbursement has left a pall of apathy over the health care profession.

First, severe staffing shortages are challenging leaders to find quick solutions—a nearly impossible task. Second, state and federal regulations require health care leaders and workers to perform numerous procedural tasks to document compliance, with associated high costs in time and money. A recent article identified more than 30 regulatory bodies at the national level and a number of state licensing agencies (8 or more per state) that have jurisdiction over health care organizations. The complex laws and regulations generated by these agencies are often conflicting, and their benefit to the public is generally unknown.

The fact is that the regulation of health care would almost certainly be less extensive if health professionals were consistent in their practice and used value-based interventions exclusively. After all, it is not clear whether regulations passed to govern procedures are working as intended.

Yet, despite the problems in the nursing profession, the public has more regard for nurses than for any other type of health professional. Nurses have a powerful voice in their communities—perhaps even more powerful than they know. Consumers and politicians want to know what nurses think about prescription issues, ensuring access to care, and changing the health system to meet the needs of patients and their families.

Why are some leaders more successful than others in leading an organization through transformational change necessary to address staff shortages, reimbursement, consumer needs, and regulations? Why do some leaders fail to sustain their commitment to a change, letting it slowly subside or disappear altogether? Why are some people able to create an environment of hope and calm despite desperate or difficult circumstances? The answer can be found in the notions of *will* and *personal willingness*. Willing leaders are the co-creators of change. They recognize that no one person or no situation can take away their personal peace, joy, and sense of competence, and they transmit these feelings to others.

Owing to feelings of desperation, personal investment in the status quo, or a need for psychological preservation, some very knowledgeable leaders lose their willingness to take the initiative in making changes. Instead, they replace their willingness with an organizational mask, becoming what they think the organization or a powerful other wants them to be. Such leaders may be incapable of seeing the whole and acting on their vision of it. Willing leaders not only see the whole but also claim responsibility for creating their personal experience of transformational change.

A CONTEXT FOR HOPE

Leaders of quantum organizations can move only in one direction—toward building and sustaining the context for health care services and reinforcing expectations for a better future. These leaders behave in new and bold ways and see things from an optimistic and futurist perspective. Further, they are willing to do the work that needs to be done to meet patient needs, adhere to professional standards, and stay within the limits of available reimbursement. By their commitment to creating a hopeful context, they ensure that health care workers will be better able to do the work of healing and health promotion.

The degree of a leader's willingness to lead can be explained by the extent to which he or she possesses courage, passion, energy, discipline, and trust. By possessing these qualities in abundance, the leader is able to engender in others not only hopefulness but a greater willingness to provide service.

> **Point To Ponder**
>
> *Hope springs not from trying to remodel the past but rather from being willing to continually create the future with our colleagues to meet the changing needs of the community.*

WILL

Will (or willpower) has been defined as an inner power—a power over nature and over the self (i.e., self-control). Only the development of this inner power can offset the risk of our losing control of the tremendous forces at our disposal and becoming victims of our own achievements.

The terms *will* and *willpower* are usually used to refer to this inner power in the abstract, apart from the consideration of any individual person. The term *the will* is used when discussing willpower as evidenced by an individual person. In this usage, a person is said to have a will, and this will, typically viewed as the center of the

> **Key Point**
>
> *Will is the self-directing capacity of human beings—the internal body of personal power.*

person's self, is what exhibits willpower (or lack of willpower). Because the development of each person's will depends on the person's culture and the current circumstances, including political and economic factors, a person's will can be very powerful, very weak, or some degree in between these two extremes.

In coaching others, leaders should recognize that developed willpower has an enormous potential for creating and adapting to change. Once leaders gain an appreciation for how the qualities of willpower get expressed, they will be able to comprehend the dynamics of those whose will is less strong and understand their rational for pulling away. Reframing the work of leadership in terms of willpower can serve to create or rebuild hope and redirect others toward greater achievement and satisfaction.

Discovery of Will

This section explores the view that a quantum leader's will is critical to his or her leadership success. The leader needs to discover the essence of his or her will and to create the conditions for others in the organization to discover and honor their own will.

For each person, the discovery of his or her will encompasses the following five phases:

1. recognition that willpower exists
2. realization that one has a will
3. living one's personal will
4. recognition of one's soulfulness (an awakening of the self resulting from insight and self-exploration)
5. recognition that awakening the will can be risky and can even threaten paralysis

The simplest and most frequent way in which a person discovers his or her will is through determined action and struggle. When a person makes a physical or mental effort or actively wrestles with some obstacle or opposing force, the person feels a power, or inner energy, rise up inside.

Self-exploration, particularly investigation of one's will, does not appear to be widely embraced by those in leadership positions. Overworked and sometimes taken for granted, leaders must struggle with a number of issues before they are able to embark on an examination of their will. These issues include the following:

- Leaders often have a Victorian conception of will according to which it is associated with stern control over others.
- Most people are reluctant to change, particularly if it involves personal examination. Also, change requires time and patience—two commodities that are in short supply. It is easier to sit back and let others carry the ball.
- Leaders often do not want to pay the price for becoming more involved in change (or becoming less involved).
- Leaders are hesitant to discuss willpower and its characteristics with the executive team for fear of job loss.

Not surprisingly, the organization's culture strongly influences whether an exploration of willpower does in fact occur. The values, practices, and longevity of employees can facilitate or obstruct meaningful changes that foster a readiness to investigate the nature of willpower.

Initially, a person's will has a regulatory and directive function. Take the case of a rehabilitation patient. He knows what his legs are supposed to do and in which direction he is supposed to move, but, in addition to the normal power he uses to propel his legs, he needs the encouragement of the physical therapist, giving him the willpower to act. Without this encouragement, the patient's willpower would be weak or sporadic and might disappear altogether.

When individuals discover that willpower exists within themselves and realize that the will and the self are intimately connected, they become more oriented toward the self and concomitantly less oriented toward others and the world. Recognizing that the power to make changes is located primarily in the self and not in others, they are now free to use their willpower to choose, relate, and bring about changes in themselves and others. They feel a new sense of unlimited potential for action, whether this involves altering themselves or acting on the outside world.

Consider the prevalence of noise in patient care areas. It is well known that noise prevents patients from relaxing and resting, yet little is done to keep down the noise level.

Care providers know that they should be less noisy and also remind others of the importance of quiet, but only rarely will an individual with a high degree of courage speak up about the need for a restful environment. In other words, the will to act is usually missing or is not sufficient for action. Although solving the problem of noise would seem to be simple, the fact is that noise in patient care areas continues to be one of the most common causes of patient complaints!

Another example concerns the resistance of workers to changes in their work routines. They may believe that the current work routines are the best way to achieve the desired goals, but often they are merely fearful of what will happen to them after the changes are implemented. Thus, their fear rather than their will is driving their behavior. Overcoming resistance to change is a consistent theme in management literature, and efforts to guide leaders in developing the skills needed to foster change and innovation are well documented.

Given that any complex adaptive system exhibits self-organization, unpredictable interactions, and interdependencies, leaders need to learn to work with the natural energy of the system. They can learn this and overcome resistance to change more effectively by developing an understanding of will and willingness. It is helpful to note that will, despite the Victorian conception of it, is not about sternness but rather about the multidimensional directive and regulatory balances employed by an individual.

It is not difficult to let the easygoing side of one's nature take control and to allow internal or external influences dominate change when negative pressures exist. Such behaviors reinforce apathy and discouragement. Leaders need to take the trouble to oppose negative behaviors. They should not expect training of the will to be accomplished without the expenditure of energy and persistence required for the successful development of any other quality, physical or mental. Effort lies at the base of any worthwhile leadership activity and is a requisite for success.

> **Group Discussion**
>
> Identify at least two situations in which you thought about reacting to a problem situation but did not. Was your reluctance related to patient care, the behaviors of coworkers, organizational policy, or something else? Now that you have identified a situation that should be managed, how can each member of the group support you in summoning the courage to react in the future?

The Nature of Will

Because will is embedded in the self, self-exploration and the astute observation of colleagues is a starting point for gaining an appreciation of the significance of will for leadership. Self-exploration can help a leader

- control his or her own will
- identify areas needing development
- assess the application of willpower by others
- intervene in cases of inappropriate use

Awakening of the self requires insight, self-absorption, and struggle. In the journey through transformational change, leaders discover the power to make choices, relate to others, and bring about changes in themselves and others. As a result of the new insights they gain during this journey, leaders could withdraw their support for certain projects or change priorities. Both positive and negative actions can be conscious or unconscious, depending on the degree of self-examination. When self-examination is a conscious process, the effect on the individual can be profound, as the self shifts its orientation inward.

> ### Key Point
>
> *Are you willing to want what you get when it comes or to force yourself to get what you want? How strong is your will?*

Unfortunately, there are obstacles to and dangers in self-exploration of the will. All too often, leaders work to become who they think the organization wants them to be, preventing themselves from becoming who they really are. When this happens, they struggle and perceive themselves stuck in a persona that is not authentic, with the result that they feel impotent, apathetic, and insincere. The questions that leaders, not to mention other individuals, need to ask themselves are these: Are you willing to say yes—to act, think, and feel as you really are? Can you picture what this would be like? Would it not be joyful to do things because they reflect your will and are authentic rather than solely because the organization expects such behaviors?

By developing their will, leaders are better able to make decisions intuitively and rationally. By integrating their personal heart and objective mind, they become more authentic individuals and increase their willingness to act. Alternatively, if they act solely for reasons and values outside of themselves, they will continue to suffer and be disinclined to participate in the changing environment.

Further, denying one's personal will is a way of avoiding personal accountability. Assuming accountability, on the other hand, means never experiencing anything that is not a product of one's vision, mental model, or emotions. The self, not the external world, is the source of experiences. It follows that nothing can take away one's peace, joy, or sense of adequacy—each of these must be given up voluntarily.

Types of Will

Characterizing some of the types of will that people have can help clarify what will is. For example, it is relatively common to hear people described as having a strong will, a skillful will, or a good will. A brief account of each type follows.

To say that someone has a *strong will* is to say that that person has significant power or determination. A typical mistake is to think that strength of will is the essence of the whole will—that having a will means always attempting to get one's own way.

Someone who possesses a *skillful will* is able to achieve desired results with the least amount of energy. People who have this type of will must understand their own habits, goals, and desires and the relationships between these in order to use them skillfully.

A person with a *good will* is benevolent, has a high degree of integrity, and does not use his or her will to overpower or corrupt the will of others.

Essential Qualities

The notion that a person's will consists only of strength or weakness or goodness or badness is incorrect and can lead someone engaged in self-exploration in the wrong direction. Instead, for a person to exhibit will or willpower, he or she must possess a certain set of qualities, namely, courage, passion, energy, self-discipline, and trust (Figure 9–1). Leaders who are interested in increasing their expertise should use this set of qualities as a paradigm of will during periods of self-examination or when evaluating the behavior of others.

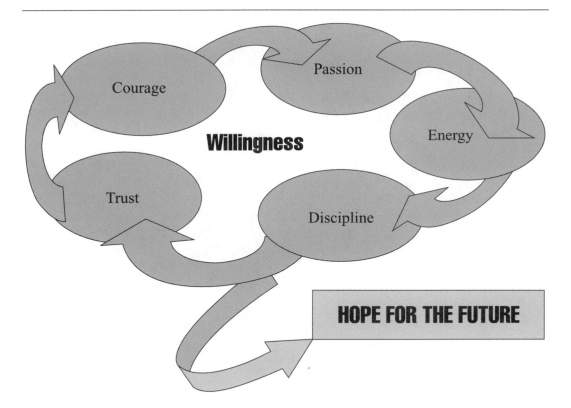

Figure 9–1 The Five Essential Qualities of Will Lead to Hope for the Future

Courage

Courage is that quality of mind or spirit that enables individuals to face difficulty, danger, and pain without fear and to act in accordance with their beliefs. Courage is required to stay the course during the shaking and shuddering of the chaotic stage of change and to

---

Group Discussion

After reading the following case study, identify the presence (or absence) of courage, energy, trust, passion, and discipline in the behavior of the nurse.

A staff nurse admitted a terminally ill patient and reported to her supervisor that she believed she had really made a difference in the care of the patient and in the final outcome. She also stated that she had required a total of two hours for the admission process—an hour in excess of the allocated time. The supervisor, in response, showed concern about the extra time used in the admission process and the additional expense for this type of care.

The staff nurse then explained the situation more fully. A female patient with terminal cancer, accompanied by her husband, was admitted for pain management and relief of abdominal ascites. She was scheduled for a fluoroscopy-guided paracentesis to relieve the fluid and to receive IV pain medication. The patient was exhausted and wanted relief from her discomfort. Also, in the course of the admission, the patient informed the nurse that she was ready to die, that she had fought hard and long enough and knew nothing could be done to extend her life. Her husband agreed.

The nurse asked the patient if she knew that draining the fluids from her abdomen would relieve the pressure temporarily but would leave more space for the fluids to collect again. The patient was told that she could be kept comfortable without the paracentesis and could be assisted to die as comfortably as possible. This approach was discussed with the physician, who gave it his approval. The patient and husband chose to have pain management only. The patient died peacefully two days later.

In discussing the case with her supervisor, the nurse argued that use of two hours for the admission process resulted not only in a desirable outcome but in an economic savings. True, the admission cost the organization an additional hour of RN time, but eliminating a fluoroscopy-guided paracentesis avoided the addition of approximately $2,500 in charges to a DRG bill. The organization was saved this entire amount as the reimbursement for the patient was fixed. Thus, the nurse maximized the quality of the care while minimizing the organization's costs.

manage resistance to change in order to reach new levels of knowledge and performance. It is also required to tolerate paradox—to function while holding two competing forces inside. Courageous individuals also tend to be creative, daring, and trusting of their intuition, whereas individuals who lack courage are cautious, to put it politely (Exhibit 9–1).

Courage often does not emerge until the pain of not doing something exceeds the fear of doing it. The fear that we feel when we encounter an unfamiliar pathway and must enlarge our thinking is a signal that we are on the brink of learning. It is like traveling in a foreign country and being seized by a vague fear and the instinctive desire to go back home. Similarly, during periods of change, we experience an instinctive desire for the protection of old habits. At that moment, we are tense but also porous to learning.

> **Point To Ponder**
>
> *To know what is right and not to do it is the worst cowardice.*
> —Confucius

Numerous explanations for the lack of courage exist. Most point to fear of the unknown or discomfort with what is happening. Fear is paralyzing and brings out the worst in people—their most basic instincts, those for self-protection and survival. Yet healthy fear—the kind of fear that enhances the acquisition of new knowledge—needs to be valued, reinforced, and fostered.

To create a more hopeful culture, leaders need to assist others in finding the courage to deal with the type of fear that causes imperviousness to learning and shuts down the capacity for connectedness. Believing in others and remaining patient while they endure and experience the process further supports their personal growth and accountability.

The Nike slogan "Just do it" calls individuals to jump out of the comfort zone and into the fringe of the unknown. Leaders need the same "just do it" attitude. This does not mean acting impulsively and without a plan but instead doing the best that one can given what one knows and expects at that particular time.

As an example, although the perceived conflict between financial viability and professional standards will probably continue

> **Point To Ponder**
>
> *There is nothing more difficult to take in hand, more perilous to conduct, or more uncertain in the success, than to take the lead in the introduction of a new order of things.*
> —Machiavelli

Exhibit 9–1 Qualities Associated with Willingness and Reluctance

Willingness	Reluctance
• Courage	• Fear
• Passion	• Apathy
• Energy	• Lethargy
• Self-discipline	• Self-indulgence
• Trust	• Skepticism

forever, decisions still need to be made. Leaders must often "just do it"—make a decision that balances standards and reimbursement. Developing the courage to make such decisions is about letting go of what others think you should be and boldly showing the world who you are. Courageous leaders

- face their fears
- explore their vulnerability
- lean toward risk
- celebrate failures
- never give up!

Group Discussion

Reflect on a situation in which you were at your wits' end and finally reacted. At what moment and for what reason were you inspired or forced to respond? In the future, will you react more quickly? Why or why not?

Passion

Creating a sense of passion and willingness in employees requires leaders to institute employee incentives that are based on patient satisfaction and to empower employees to do what is right for the patients. The goal is to create an organizational culture that turns employees and patients into thunderous evangelists for the organization. This type of culture is very different from the traditional organizational culture, in which:

- The employees are expected to manipulate patients into using a select group of providers in a particular geographic region.
- Employee productivity is closely monitored.
- Policies are strictly enforced.

Energy

Energetic individuals are vigorous and active, with a capacity for serious effort. Such individuals also have an intensity of will capable of overcoming opposing forces, like an athlete in competition. This intensity of will is a form of power and needs to be recognized and used positively. The energy required for optimal willingness is never limitless; rather, energetic individuals learn to temper and manage their energy expenditure, balancing high-energy times with quiet times.

In contrast, low-energy individuals are apathetic, uninterested, or burned out. Some are fearful of getting involved or becoming too hopeful because of past disappointments. For these individuals, the lack of a clear, defined sense of self is often at the root of their inaction. If they see themselves as disempowered, which many of them do, their stagnation is reinforced. What low-energy individuals need is assistance in reentering the unfolding processes of life. In particular, they need to assess their goals, focus on the future and on what is positive and working, and accept that human beings are inherently imperfect.

Self-Discipline

Self-discipline is personal willingness to adhere to standards and meet responsibilities. It is the ability to check impulsive actions while persisting in selected activities. Self-discipline is regulation of one's own behavior, not that of others. Without self-discipline, a leader with a strong will acts impulsively and unpredictably, negating the positive spirit of leadership willingness.

When leaders develop self-discipline, they are better able to focus their attention and minimize impulsive and scattered activities. Their inner concentration grows, allowing them the steady control and clarity of action and thought they need to gain the support of colleagues.

Trust

Developing trust between colleagues requires congruence of values, nonpossessive warmth, effective communication, and empathy (i.e., the ability to understand the perceptions and feelings of others). It also requires knowledge that the shared values are ethically sound and that the work of the care providers is truly intended to further the public's interest. The trust that has been built up between colleagues is reinforced when everyone consistently behaves in accordance with accepted patient care standards and uses resources wisely, shares information appropriately, and discusses new ideas openly.

A leader with a fully developed will, characterized by courage, passion, energy, self-discipline, and trust, almost cannot help but create a positive and encouraging context in which employees are expected to practice within professional standards and values. This type of leader also instills a sense of hopefulness in all members of the organization, increasing the chance that together they will bring about a better and more meaningful health care future (Exhibit 9–2).

Exhibit 9–2 Attributes of a Willing Leader

- *Openness to change.* Willingness to approach changes in staffing, organizational structure, and roles with a positive attitude while maintaining a focus on patient care. Willingness to be a co-creator of change rather than a defender of the past.
- *Tolerance for diverse perspectives.* Willingness to look at multiple reasonable alternatives while giving up the role of patient advocate. Willingness to acknowledge that some situations may not be acceptable but are a major part of one's work life and must be handled patiently.
- *Focus on value.* Willingness to educate others to understand evidence-based approaches as the new context for providing health care services.
- *Awareness of the larger system.* Willingness to move between micro and macro views of issues—from the patient to the team to the department to the organization to the community to the state to the world and back.

Hope

Hope is the feeling that what is wanted can be had or that events will turn out well. People find it difficult to be hopeful if they do not think things are going satisfactorily. They become less inclined to get involved and less willing to do the right thing, because it does not seem to matter. When the qualities of will—courage, passion, energy, self-discipline, and trust—are present, a beacon of hope emerges to begin a positive cycle of behaviors. Discouraged and disenfranchised workers start to see new opportunities and develop a new willingness to focus on the present and future, leaving the past behind.

Group Discussion

The following questions are posed for reflection. Examine behaviors related to all five categories: courage, passion, energy, self-discipline, and trust. Are some behaviors more prevalent than others? How can you improve behaviors in each category? Finally, develop a plan to incorporate the desired behaviors into the interview process for new employees and in the annual performance review competency set.

Courage

- Is there evidence that members of the organization are able to share their values and ideas in a nonthreatening manner?
- Is there evidence that members are able to stand their ground in defending their values and ideas?
- Are the members brave enough to ask the right questions?

Passion

- Is there evidence in the organization of a strong and vocalized commitment to ideas? To projects?
- Is there evidence that all employees take great pride in their work?
- Are there groups or projects in which enthusiasm is lacking? If so, which are they?

Energy

- Does the organization's leader exhibit vigor and vitality when managing projects?
- Does the leader's opinion dominate the ideas or actions of others?
- Are employees willing to participate in organizational group activities, social events, and/or committees?

> **Group Discussion (continued)**
>
> **Self-Discipline**
>
> - Does the organization's leader regulate his or her activities appropriately?
> - In managing projects, does the leader act impulsively?
> - Are meetings or programs well thought out and implemented with little chaos?
>
> **Trust**
>
> - Is the organization's leader honest, forthright, and candid with others, or does the leader tell half-truths, damaging the trusting bond between leader and colleague?
> - Are team members open and honest with each other?
> - Do team members rely on each other?

STRATEGIES TO FACILITATE WILLINGNESS

Once leaders understand the nature of will, they are in a position to facilitate willingness as a means of achieving their goals. Below is a discussion of strategies that incorporate the qualities of courage, passion, energy, discipline, and trust. Note that these do not exhaust the strategies for increasing the willingness of employees but constitute a beginning upon which to build.

Removing the Dogma Brick Wall

So much health care is done routinely and automatically, with little thought to its rationale. As science advances, new technologies and practices emerge and become popular. These and the older technologies and practices should be examined to ensure that the highest quality care is being provided at the lowest cost. Examining tech-

> **Point To Ponder**
>
> *Any competent manager can direct men and women who are already motivated to achieve. A great leader can do the same for those who are tired, discouraged, and fearful.*
>
> *—Alan Axelrod, Elizabeth I CEO*

nologies and practices demands significant courage, for it can involve challenging the system and its players. It also requires openness to new ideas and the recognition that change *is* (i.e., change is inevitable and should not be avoided).

In surveying health care for the purpose of making improvements, leaders should not look first to see what additional products, services, and providers will be needed in the future but rather review the current situation to identify non-value-adding services for elimination. This approach, besides helping to create excess capacity for future needs, revalidates what is important in health care. All too often, practices become integrated into the system and continue to be used long after their rationale is lost or forgotten. "We have always done it this way" is not a good reason to keep on using a nonbeneficial practice.

For one thing, we have not always done it this way. At one time only physicians were allowed to take blood pressures, insert nasogastric tubes, administer IV bolus medications, and write prescriptions. Now aides, technicians, and nurses perform these same tasks. The fact is that health professionals, especially physicians, often hesitate to relinquish technical tasks that the state practice act does not really require them to perform.

This is cause to wonder, for example, how and when the task of taking and recording blood pressure came within the purview of nursing assistants—or, better still, the responsibility of the patient! An individual somewhere, someplace was willing to question whether it was really appropriate for physicians to own this chore. Courage is needed to examine current practices, give up what is not appropriate, and retain what is. Further, this type of examination needs to be done with passion for the essence of the profession, not for personal recognition or benefit.

Group Discussion

Dogmas, or unquestioned beliefs, exist in every organization and in every culture. Following are three examples that might exist in a health care organization: (1) Nursing is women's work. (2) Nurses wear white. (3) Patient registration takes place at the front entrance of the facility.

Identify at least three practices based on dogma in your current organization. Begin with the policy and procedure manual in your department. Can you suggest any changes that would improve organizational efficiency?

Unquestioning adherence to authority and tradition is a well-known barrier to the development of knowledge. Although authority and tradition provide a seemingly stable foundation, in fact blind faith is problematic and can be detrimental to survival. Continuing progress in nursing and other areas of health care thus warrants an examination of all dogmas and a release from those that are without foundation.

There are dogmas that pertain to professional roles as well as procedures and practices. Efforts to delineate the boundaries of each profession need to be ongoing. Those responsible for delineating the domains of the various health professions must look at the received wisdom (conventional beliefs) within each profession, the profession's knowledge base (science), and the profession's application of that knowledge (art). The practices of any professional health care worker go beyond science as traditionally conceived to include, for instance, the use of intuition and the therapeutic use of the self. Likewise, the emerging principles that pertain to building relationships and partnerships beg for inclusion into the health care disciplines.

The real work of quantum leaders is to deconstruct the dogmas of traditional Newtonian science and transform current organizational underpinnings to reflect the essence of complexity science. The realities of current organizations—the great number of connections and relationships between the many elements and the inherent capacity for change or adaptation—demand a better explanation than can be delivered by the linear thinking characteristic of Newtonian science.

Unlike the mechanistic Newtonian paradigm, complexity science affirms that no leader is an island. In other words, the achievement of desired outcomes in a system is beyond the talents of any one individual. Instead, outcomes result from the relationships between individuals. Although the abilities of a single individual are important, they are not completely useful until the individual establishes relationships and works together with other individuals. Thus, the attention of leaders shifts from individual performance to appropriate patterns of interrelationship.

Strategies for minimizing dogma include these:

- Examine and assess the value of at least three current practices each month. Retain or eliminate each practice depending on its value.
- Believe in the value of process so strongly that at least three employees gain the same appreciation each month.
- Approach difficult situations in which there is personal impact with the same enthusiasm as situations that do not affect you personally.
- No matter how long current practices have been used, be willing to examine others.
- Review prevalent dogmas in a patterned way. Commit to making no change impulsively. Instead, first talk with colleagues to ensure that every proposed change makes good sense.
- Know that colleagues share concerns about long-held practices and believe there are better ways as well but may not be quite ready to address the issues. Patience is needed!

Continuous Learning

High-quality health care services can be delivered only by educated, compassionate, and skilled care providers. Further, such providers need to maintain or increase their competence levels through continuing education. Following through on a commitment to professional growth, however, can be incredibly difficult in an organization steeped in reorganization. Everyone's energy is channeled into the redesign and maintenance of the new context, making continuing education hard to pursue. The quantum leader must therefore support the acquisition of new knowledge and skills by employees while at the same time sustaining the reorganization efforts. Following are some ways for a leader to ensure that continuous learning becomes part of the organization:

- Create and maintain a culture that fosters continuous learning.
- Recognize that new knowledge is essential for all to survive.

- Participate enthusiastically in continuing education and share the knowledge you gain with colleagues.
- Support continuous learning consistently, namely, through every budget cycle and challenge throughout the year.
- Identify and trend performance measures that support the value of continuing education.

Minimizing Professional Antagonism

In hierarchical, departmental organizations, the work groups tend to become competitive and adversarial. In health care organizations, for example, nursing and nonnursing departments continually battle for resources and position.

In addition, nurses have been reported to "eat their young." A recent panel of student nurses working in a particular health care organization identified the nurses who coached and mentored them in a positive way and those who reinforced their novice status in the presence of others. One student freely shared why she would not select that organization for employment: She had been assigned a preceptor who was a nationally recognized nurse expert but who was avoided by students because of her intimidating behaviors and perceived intolerance.

Antagonism between new employees is often because of the possession of poor interpersonal skills by supervisors, preceptors, and colleagues. In nursing, it is the nurses (the staff and the nurse manager) who have the greatest impact on nurse stress, not nonnurse coworkers. Thus, in this regard, nurses truly are their own worst enemies—and consequently the solution may lie within nursing rather than outside the health care system. Nurses need to care for each other—just as they do for their patients. They need to be their brothers' and sisters' keepers. The leader's role in reducing professional antagonism is to do the following:

- Bring issues into the open for discussion and minimize behind-the-scenes dialogue.
- Realize that relationships can truly be therapeutic. Expecting collaboration is the only way to develop the culture and context for high-quality, low-cost patient care services.
- Address issues as they arise.
- Stay focused and remain objective.

Meeting the Needs of Employees

There are two categories of employees: those who have jobs and those who have careers. Those with jobs report to work, perform their duties as well as possible, and go home at the end of their tour of duty to get on with their lives. In contrast, those with careers not only do the necessary work but plan where they are going in their chosen profession and participate in professional activities outside of the workplace.

Not every person is seeking a career. Some individuals are satisfied with a job that is meaningful and fairly compensated. Expecting to motivate all employees to commit to a career is unrealistic. It is especially ill-advised to dangle cash before professionals as a way of inducing desired behaviors and changes. This strategy is based on the assumption that people are motivated only by material gain and is likely to lead to a health care work force that is indeed petty and greedy. It is also based on the assumption that individuals act independently of their social institutions and that social systems are nothing more than the sum of individual actions. This is a shallow notion of human decision making and ignores the way our values and actions are conditioned and constrained by social relations.

> **Group Discussion**
>
> The assumption that people working in health care are shallow, single-minded, materialistic, and socially unfettered is consistent with Newtonian science. These beliefs support the practice of attracting new employees by giving them sign-on bonuses. Do you agree or disagree with this rationale? What are the effects, positive and negative, of this approach to recruitment on quality, productivity, and cost? What types of reward and recognition practices would be consistent with complexity theory? What are the effects of these reward and recognition practices on quality, productivity, and cost?

The world of work today is very different from what it was in the past. Workers used to stay with one company or organization for a lifetime, whereas now workers may have several career pathways, and mobility rather than promotion is the symbol of advancement. The notion of loyalty needs to be redefined to reflect the marketplace of the 21st century. Loyalty to an organization may have been appropriate at one time, but now loyalty to one's core values is more suited to the way work is organized.

Leaders need the courage to recognize this phenomenon and ensure that both types of employees—job holders and career seekers—are valued and treated fairly. The organization must meet not only the needs of the customers but also those of the individuals it employs. The presence of employees from different generations and with different values requires leaders to use multiple strategies, such as these:

- Create a compensation system that recognizes the multiplicity of employee values and needs. In addition, the system should support retention and guide employees to new opportunities when the organization's needs change, the required job skills change, or the employees' desires change. Become a partner with employees in managing their work and planning for the next position.
- Be vigilant and persistent when implementing and maintaining an appropriate compensation system and recognition and reward program.
- Stay focused and committed despite resistance from those who would like the current compensation system and recognition and reward program to remain unchanged.

Providing Value-Based Services

What one does and what difference it makes are the key issues for all providers. If an organization provides 1,000 services and only 25 make a difference, then the other 975 services must be considered for elimination—even if the 975 services have billing codes that render them reimbursable.

Provider accountability for contributions to patient care outcomes is a missing piece of health care. All professional care providers must focus their actions on achieving desired outcomes and only implement interventions that have a basis in science or a realistic chance of benefiting patients.

The measurement of health care outcomes is gradually becoming more meaningful and reflective of patient needs. Unfortunately, indicators are often looked at in an order that fails to take into account the basic goal of health care—health improvement. For example, productivity measures are typically examined prior to clinical outcomes. If productivity targets are exceeded, increases in productivity are mandated without consideration of their potential impact on care provision.

Nonetheless, consumers of health care services expect that the services received are based on logic and scientific knowledge and that the intended outcomes are likely to occur. Further, they view the primary goal of health care organizations as providing effective clinical services, not making a profit. The problem for these organizations is how to provide value-based, high-quality care that is affordable and at the same time make money (this is different from making as much money as possible).

Given the constraints caused by balanced budget initiatives, leaders are often caught in a cost-quality balancing act and are not always sure how to achieve value-based care. No clear solutions are on the horizon for the ailing health care system, certainly no financial relief of any significance. This raises the question whether we can afford to spend money on quality initiatives. Ethically, the answer is a resounding YES! And that is the public's expectation as well.

Perhaps it would be helpful to reframe the quality question as a value question. Value is determined by the three elements of cost, quality, and service (Malloch and Porter-O'Grady 1999). Cost is driven by the available resources, which are currently very limited. Quality is partly determined by the outcomes of care. Service is a matter of the time and type of care provided. Thus the question becomes, Are health care leaders obligated to provide value-based services to patients and family members? The issue of spending money on quality is now linked to both cost and service.

Achieving value-based health care faces an additional challenge: drawing conclusions about quality initiatives and return on investment when there are multiple factors involved. A further complication is the extensive use of a type of cost-benefit analysis that is not sensitive to health care objectives. If the benefits of a program can be priced in dollars, then a cost-benefit analysis will be able to identify the alternative with the largest benefit-to-cost ratio. However, many decisions involve benefits that are not easily quantifiable in monetary terms or otherwise, such as psychological benefits and environmental benefits (clean air and water).

Health care leaders and providers are now required to examine services using the value equation and make decisions accordingly. If resources are limited, leaders must ask whether every patient sign and symptom requires intervention, particularly if minimal or no improvement in the patient's clinical condition is the likely outcome. Paying close attention to the health improvement value of health care services is an incredibly difficult challenge for providers and leaders schooled in the doctrine that increasing access to health care and growth in the health care system were absolute goods. Unfortunately, accountability and control were absent from the cost-based payment system, and the results are well known—exhaustion of resources. Health professionals are currently challenged to move from "rich" care to "wise" care.

Another value-related issue of interest is productivity. Because business still operates under questionable assumptions regarding productivity—that the more hours employees work, the more productive they are; that the faster employees work, the more they accomplish; and that the more employees are paid, the more motivated they are to be productive—leaders are challenged to better understand the reality of employee productivity (Exhibit 9–3). Health professionals in this country are working more hours than ever before and getting less done. In fact, Americans have the dubious distinction of being first in the number of hours worked each year. The U.S. Department of Labor, Bureau of Labor Statistics, noted only a slight increase in productivity from 1960 to 1990, and the productivity increase in the last 10 years is attributed to technological advances, particularly the development of the Internet.

Health care employees are burning out faster than the replacements are coming in, yet they are still being pushed to become more productive. They are working 12-hour days, are commuting up to 2 hours a day, and are held by an electronic leash to the office. Their opportunity to relax is almost nonexistent.

Contrary to popular beliefs, we need to learn how to slow down our thinking at times, not speed it up. Time for reflection and contemplation of ideas and issues is sorely missing in health care. The never-ending checklist is always present and demanding attention.

Exhibit 9–3 Myths and Truths about Employee Productivity

Accepted Notions

- If employees work more hours, they will be more productive.
- If employees work faster, they will be more productive.
- If employees are paid more, they will be motivated to work harder and produce more.

The Reality

- Employees perform optimally for 6 to 7 hours and may be able to work longer in a burst of energy or inspiration, but then they must rest.
- Employees need balance; they need a life outside of work.
- Slower, intuitive thinking is often more effective in solving problems than mental agility.
- Studies show that, in Germany, where individual performance is not rewarded with pay increases, productivity is often higher than the United States.
- Employees are most productive when their employers pay them *equitably* and then do everything possible to help the employees put money out of their minds.

Source: Data from C.B. Johnson, When Working Harder Is Not Smarter, *Inner Edge*, Vol. 3, No. 2, pp. 18–21, © 2000.

Further, experts report that pay is *not* the chief motivator for productivity. In general, employees desire to do meaningful work most of all, next they desire opportunities for collaboration through group decision making, and then they want equitable pay.

What drives people to work at their best? How can health care leaders revitalize the lost passion of employees? What are the retention strategies that will support the rebuilding of a hopeful culture? Interestingly, the answer is simple. When employees believe their work is meaningful—productive in the sense of producing beneficial results—then they will be motivated to work harder and will experience a renewal of passion and hopefulness. Productivity is not only about quantity; it is also about quality.

Optimizing employee performance takes on a whole new meaning in this context. All human beings have a need to express their uniqueness and their talents in the work they do and be recognized for their contributions (Exhibit 9–4). Therefore, employees are typically motivated by jobs that develop their skills and expand their minds, demand individual initiative, involve working on teams, benefit others, and spark a desire to make a difference in the world. Jobs that have these characteristics possess what Cedric Johnson (2000) called *fruitfulness*—work flows from one person to another in a way that is both respectful and valued. To ensure that health care work possesses fruitfulness, leaders need to do the following:

- Continually examine services, measures, and systems to assess their impact on patient outcomes. Retain those that improve patient outcomes, and eliminate those that have no effect or a negative effect.
- Believe that hope can be restored to care providers through restoring value to the work they do.
- Believe intensely that individuals will give their best when treated like adults.
- Be alive and be committed to doing what is best for patients.
- Consistently expect only value-adding services to be delivered to patients. Publicly recognize individuals who are able to focus on value, and guide those who require assistance in eliminating unnecessary and non–valued-adding work.
- Believe that all health care providers intuitively know that restoring value to work is the right path but have not been able to translate their perceptions into practice. Believe that most, but not all, will eventually make the transition. Believe that the health care system will not only support but will require increases in the value of health care services. Know that colleagues support caring, healing work that makes a difference.

Becoming Mentally Fit

Some care providers appear tougher than others. In fact, their "toughness" might be a kind of mental fitness resulting from their sense of commitment, perception of control, and ability to view change as a challenge. Mental fitness involves taking responsibility for one's reactions to adversity. Through this kind of fitness, individuals can prevent emotional exhaustion and turn stressful events into meaningful challenges.

Mental fitness is helpful for handling role modifications and reductions in the work force. Employees who lack mental fitness often develop an attitude of learned helplessness. For example, if they are laid off, they react with anger, believe getting laid off is beyond their control, blame themselves, and generally feel helpless. Their helplessness triggers a downward spiral of self-defeat in which they see themselves as increasingly unable to get ahead.

Exhibit 9–4 Optimizing Performance: Productivity or Fruitfulness?

Productivity

- Productivity is mechanistic.
- In a productivity-driven organization, employees are treated like machines and judged on the quantity of their output.
- The predominant concern is getting more "bang for the buck."
- Efforts to increase employee motivation are dependent on external sources, pay, benefits, etc.

Fruitfulness

- Fruitfulness is humanistic.
- Fruitfulness involves a respectful, holistic view of each person that recognizes values, beliefs, and expectations.
- Fruitfulness honors the inner need of each person to express his or her uniqueness and talents and to develop and expand.
- Fruitfulness engages the inner selves of employees and causes them to grow and be sustained naturally and enduringly.

Source: Data from C.B. Johnson, When Working Harder Is Not Smarter, *Inner Edge*, Vol. 3, No. 2, pp. 18–21, © 2000.

Goal setting, mental imagery, emotional mastery, and positive thinking are all part of the mental conditioning that is necessary to overcome this helplessness and survive substantial changes. The mentally fit alter the perception of stress and mobilize effective coping techniques, lessening the trauma of stressful events. In fact, they transform these events into opportunities for increased meaning in life. Leaders who are mentally fit learn to manage the context of the work as well as the specific content of their discipline.

Mental fitness among leaders is associated with leadership resilience and leadership agility. As leaders become more mentally fit, they also become more resilient, decreasing the probability that they will experience burnout. Many leaders, particularly those at the vice-presidential level, work persistently to support and guide the chief executive in clinical matters in addition to meeting their own responsibilities. The relationship between the head of the nursing department, for example, and the chief executive is not only intense but typically requires more from the nurse, who is likely to be continually providing feedback about the impact of decisions on patient outcomes and care provider satisfaction. Not surprising, the nurse leader, if lacking in mental fitness, will be prone to burnout.

Leaders who are downsized experience a much greater emotional and psychological impact than typically has been acknowledged, and their ability to deal with such trauma is minimal at best. For one thing, the skills needed to handle disappointment are seldom taught in educational programs. Therefore, downsized leaders spend considerable time second-guessing past decisions and become reluctant to make decisions for fear of further emotional insult. If they get follow-up counseling, it is directed toward helping them cope with their behaviors rather than preparing them for future disappointments. Becoming mentally fit, on the other hand, is a matter of learning to expect, anticipate, and plan for job-related disappointments and defeats and taking a proactive approach to managing one's personal destiny (Exhibit 9–5).

Exhibit 9–5 Planning for Position Elimination

- Recognize that no position is forever, nor should it be if the work of the organization is changing to meet the needs of the marketplace.
- Consider other roles that might be of interest in the future and begin to develop skills in the relevant areas.
- Discuss your interests with your immediate supervisor, request assistance in continuing to meet current expectations, but also be prepared for changes. (*Note:* Although it may be difficult to discuss role changes, open and honest communication is always the best approach.)
- Retain control of your career—avoid letting other factors control you.

Leadership agility is the ability to respond quickly and appropriately to input from employees and colleagues, the actions of competitors, and developing crises. Leaders with this ability are better able to manage the stress of situations and to calculate the odds of success or failure. Once they acquire agility, along with resilience and mental fitness, leaders will be in a good position to handle their responsibilities without becoming exhausted and incapable of experiencing the pleasures of their work. They also will be in a good position to appreciate the virtues of mental fitness and understand its importance for the organization as a whole. To ensure that the organization's entire work force is mentally fit, leaders should do the following:

- Create a culture that recognizes that good and not-so-good events occur, understand that employees need support when things do not go well, and provide the necessary support to those who require it.
- Develop a personal commitment to help others acquire mental fitness, resilience, and agility.
- Continually strive to increase their own mental fitness and create the culture that requires others to do the same.
- Extract hope and energy from the mission of health care.
- Establish a program of self-examination and self-renewal.
- Recognize that no individual is an island and that each person needs relationships, support, and feedback.

Balancing the Use of Time

The transition into the Information Age has left many people with far too many activities on the to-do list and too little time to accomplish them. Leaders must therefore guide employees toward looking at time use in a different way. No individual will ever have enough time for all of the things that he or she would like to do. Time management strategies may assist employees in eliminating nonproductive or nonessential tasks, but the employees will still need to find a good balance between the things that are truly important to them. More specifically, they will need to achieve an equilibrium between the activities of work and personal activities so that they can find joy and pleasure in both.

Some progress has been made in creating more balance between work and personal life, but more needs to be done to minimize the burnout and keep employees from feeling discouraged and disenfranchised. When organizations identify balancing work and personal life as a goal, they tend to focus on the time at work. An organization might develop initiatives to help employees have flexibility in work hours, for example, but at the same time it might leave vacancies unfilled and ask employees to do more with less. It does not matter that the employees have flexible hours if they also have to work 5 or 10 more hours each week. Because they are not much better off as a result of the initiative, the employees will view the message as ambiguous. In addition, management might then perceive the employees as ungrateful, causing the employees to feel that the executives just do not get it.

Achieving a balance between work and personal life is a never-ending process for both leaders and employees. Employees need tools to do their jobs well and to help them feel successful, and they need recognition and reward systems that measure and acknowledge their accomplishments. Leaders need to build a culture of respect for employees and their accomplishments. When people feel successful, leaving the workplace at the end of the day is easier both physically and mentally, as the shadow of work does not hang over their heads.

Leaders also should help employees feel successful in other aspects of their lives. Sometimes the support needed might seem like it falls outside the leader's jurisdiction. However, quantum leaders recognize that no individual ever enters the door of the organization and leaves all personal issues behind. They understand that personal issues will impact any employee's ability to work effectively and that assisting the employee might be critical to the team's success. Employees have a wide variety of needs that change as their lives change. Few have the personal skills to achieve and maintain balance. A strong mentoring program not only produces better employees but also can teach the skills needed to balance work and personal life.

Once employees feel supported and successful in the workplace, they are better able to reduce or eliminate time-wasting activities and behaviors, such as gossiping. Certain attitudes and emotional states can act as hidden consumers of time. These include defensiveness, selflessness, and boredom. Defensiveness is a common problem. Reacting to criticism by uttering sharp remarks or lashing out in defense of one's actions creates an atmosphere of irritability and anger and can affect everyone in the environment for some time to come. Time spent in angry rumination is wasteful at best.

Selflessness, not selfishness, can be a time waster as well. Saying yes to every request is not realistic. Learning to say no on occasion will let the individual take back some of the time he or she has been losing. The hardest part, of course, is getting beyond the guilt.

Boredom is another time waster that is not often recognized. Boring tasks often cause individuals to waste time procrastinating. If a task is extremely boring to an individual, it most likely could or should have been delegated.

The strategies below should be used by leaders to help themselves and employees balance their work and their personal life and avoid activities, behaviors, and emotions that consume time to no good purpose:

- Recognize that everyone has the capacity to balance his or her use of time better.
- Focus on balancing time use as an opportunity for increasing meaningfulness and not as an opportunity for increasing control and regimentation.

- Share the reality that time is short, desires are many, and every person engages in a never-ending struggle to close the gap.
- Be persistent in examining personal activities for balance and avoid the tendency to shift back to being task focused.
- Be persistent in coaching others in how to balance work and personal life.
- Believe that colleagues know that a good balance between work and personal life results in higher productivity and greater job satisfaction.

Increasing the Focus on Patients

It is no secret that the locus of control for health care services should be the patient, not the provider. Yet in spite of all of the efforts to create patient-focused care delivery systems, few patients would agree that they are in fact the focus of services or in control of anything. In explanation, they could cite facts such as these:

- Providers continue to prescribe treatments without discussion with the patients.
- Visiting hours are still in effect.
- Appointment times for services are based on Monday through Friday schedules.
- Patient procedures and their scheduled times are determined by providers without input from patients or families.

Leaders have plenty left to do to transform the health care system into one that is truly based on the will of the patient. A good place to begin is the Internet, which should be pushed as a proactive means of assisting consumers in interpreting health care information. Other strategies leaders should use to increase the patient focus of health care include these:

- Find the courage to continue the journey to creating a better system. Avoid the tendency to believe that the system is as consumer focused as it can be.
- Recognize that personal experiences as a patient can be invaluable for learning the truth about health care service delivery.
- Remain committed and focused when complaints override positive feedback. Resist the temptation to retire from health care.
- Never stop asking patients to share their experience of the health care system. Learn from them and share the information gained with other health professionals to improve the system.
- Believe that every health professional possesses courage, passion, energy, and self-discipline but may need reassurance and encouragement to exhibit them fully.

Becoming Politically Competent

Political competence encompasses the ability to accurately assess the impact of public policies on one's domain of responsibility and the ability to influence public policy making at both the state and federal level (Longest 1998). Politically competent leaders are aware of relevant regulations, laws, proposed acts, and certification procedures and are able to remove or mitigate outside barriers to the delivery of services. They also work within the organization to define issues affecting the delivery of patient care services and identify internal policies or procedures that should be altered.

However, these are but the first steps. The leaders need to ensure that all members of the organization have a degree of political competence, are able to address concerns in a timely manner, and are able to suggest possible solutions. The point-of-service staff experience the real concerns and successes that occur at the delivery of services, know when things do not go well, and can offer recommendations for change. Their input is needed not only in the executive suite but, in many cases, in the legislative arena as well. Strategies for increasing the political competence of the organization as a whole include the following:

- Develop the ability of all employees to share information about system effectiveness. Be aware that the empowerment of employees, if not guided, can result in chaos.
- Recognize that empowerment can light a fire throughout the organization. When a person's personal contributions are valued, the fire in that person's heart is fueled.
- Patiently guide employees to communicate and share information. Never give up trying to ensure that the information necessary for identifying and implementing improvements is available to the members of the organization.
- Pay close attention to the desired outcomes of care as well as to the processes used to achieve them. On the other hand, never circumvent necessary processes for the sake of efficiency.

RELIGHTING THE LAMP

Nursing and health care have always been hard work. But in today's health care environment, it is harder than ever. There are cutbacks in funding, difficult government regulations, and the worst nursing shortage in history. All these add up to challenges to work more effectively than ever and to achieve job satisfaction in an atmosphere of tremendous pressure and shrinking support. Cost-saving measures may be crucial to an organization's survival, but to caregivers, they mean stress, frustration, and attrition.

With job stress high and morale at an all-time low, interdepartmental tensions have grown to epidemic proportions. With fewer nurses on staff and with the budgetary scalpel cutting deep, nurses are expected to do more with less—work more shifts, attend more and sicker patients, and perform a broader range of duties. And they are expected to do all this with greater sensitivity, patience, and empathy. It is ironic that the emphasis on patient satisfaction in health care comes at a time when the pressures are making high-quality care next to impossible—when safe care has become the motto of many nurses (Buckley and Walker 1989).

Although the above quotation was written more than 10 years ago, it is still applicable today, partly because of the cyclical nature of health care and the recurring need to create health care services that are congruent with the demands and resources of the marketplace. We have much to learn about the health care system's cycle, but the basic needs are always the same—to meet current challenges, to learn from the past, and to continue to create new and better methods to integrate technology, information, and the wisdom of providers and leaders.

The words of Florence Nightingale offer hope and gentle reminders for all health care workers. Her perceptions are consistent with the public and political consciousness of today, namely, that public health and human caring are supremely important. Further, as in her time, many are now calling for reform of basic social and health care practices. In our era, for example, there are many critics of our society's response to the needs of the homeless, the medically indigent, those who are HIV positive, those who are living with AIDS or another incurable or chronic illness, and those who are relatively powerless or neglected, including pregnant women, children, and the elderly.

> **Point To Ponder**
>
> *If there is light in the soul,*
> *There will be beauty in the*
> *person,*
> *If there is beauty in the person,*
> *There will be harmony in the*
> *house,*
> *If there is harmony in the house,*
> *There will be order in the nation,*
> *If there is order in the nation,*
> *There will be peace in the world.*
> *   —Chinese proverb*

Consider these themes from Nightingale's writings:

- Basic caring and healing practices must be restored.
- The moral, the spiritual, and the metaphysical must be reintegrated.
- The knowledge and values of women—the sacred feminine healing spirit—must be allowed to play an essential role in health care.
- Healing professionals must recapture their sense of "calling."
- The public's requirement of personal and professional caring competencies and commitments must be honored.
- The wisdom of connected oneness and wholeness—the interrelationship between person, nature, environment, and health—must also be honored.

Aren't these same themes relevant today? Is there any doubt that the transformative journey we are on dates back at least to the 19th century? As Watson (1999) noted, our work should be about relighting the lamp and helping our colleagues to reintegrate and reconnect in order to restore the professional wholeness that was wounded during the recent modern era.

CONCLUSION

The Age of Complexity encompasses exponential increases in information, technology, and interaction between diverse people and cultures, confirming that our world is truly global. In addition, despite the fear that many people feel today, the complexity of this new age can be a source of hope. The speed of change, the blurring of work and home life, and the new global relationships will enrich each one of us directly or indirectly.

In this next era, leadership thinking will be more humanistic and more sensitive to the complex interrelationships in the world. Hope in the future and willingness to transform bureaucracies into self-renewing organizations is but another aspect of the journey of lead-

Group Discussion

"In our rush to reform education, we have forgotten a simple truth: Reform will never be achieved by renewing appropriations, restructuring schools, rewriting curricula, and revising texts if we continue to demean and dishearten the human resource called the teacher on whom so much depends. Teachers must be better compensated, freed from bureaucratic harassment, given a role in academic governance, and provided with the best possible methods and materials. But none of that will transform education if we fail to cherish—and challenge—the human heart that is the source of good teaching" (Palmer 1998).

The above comments by Parker Palmer, noted educator, are about the current state of the education system. With these words in mind, answer the following questions: In what way is the state of health care similar to the state of education? Is it possible that health care already has enough financial resources and that the solution to the problems in the health care system is to rearrange funding, reduce bureaucracy, and increase involvement? Are there other important strategies that need to be part of the solution? How do the concepts of will and willingness apply to the current situation in health care?

ers into and beyond the millennium. To accomplish their goals, the leaders will require courage to do the right thing, passion for the work of healing, energy to stay the course, self-discipline to remain focused, and trust that others are partners in the process. Finally, they must be steeped in the belief that the future will be indeed better because it is they who have designed it.

REFERENCES

Buckley, C.D., and D. Walker. 1989. *Harmony: Professional renewal for nurses.* Chicago: American Hospital Publishing.

Johnson, C.B. 2000. When working harder is not smarter. *The Inner Edge* 3, no. 2: 18–21.

Longest, B. 1998. Managerial competence at senior levels of integrated delivery systems. *Journal of Healthcare Management* 43: 115–135.

Malloch, K., and T. Porter-O'Grady. 1999. Partnership economics: Nursing's challenge in the quantum age. *Nursing Economics* 17: 299–307.

Palmer, P.J. 1998. *The courage to teach: Exploring the inner landscape of a teacher's life.* San Francisco: Jossey-Bass.

Watson, J. 1999. *Postmodern nursing and beyond.* New York: Churchill Livingstone.

SUGGESTED READINGS

Buerhaus, P. 1998. Milton Weinstein's insights on the development, use, and methodologic problems in cost-effectiveness analysis. *Image: Journal of Nursing Scholarship* 30: 223–227.

Huber, C. 1998. *The key: And the name of the key is willingness.* Murphys, CA: Keep It Simple Books.

O'Malley, M.N. 2000. *Creating commitment: How to attract and retain talented employees by building relationships that last.* New York: Wiley.

Zimmerman, B., C. Lindberg, and P. Plsek. 1998. *Edgeware: Insights from complexity science for health care leaders.* Irving, TX: VHA.

Quiz Questions

Select the best answer for each of the following questions:

1. Which of the following is not among the reasons that health care workers report disenfranchisement:
   a. staff shortages
   b. excessive regulations
   c. loss of patient respect
   d. job stress

2. The fully developed will:
   a. creates an enormous potential for change
   b. requires significant coaching and mentoring
   c. is inherent in all leaders
   d. avoids expressing authentic feelings

3. From the perspective of a leader, the will emerges through several phases of discovery. In the most important of these phases, the leader:
   a. evaluates colleagues' perceptions of the leader's degree of willingness
   b. informs his or her supervisor of his or her intention to explore the concept of will
   c. makes an attempt to identify areas in which personal growth is needed
   d. recognizes the will as a unique and describable phenomenon

4. Among the obstacles to a leader's exploration of his or her will, the most common is:
   a. peer pressure to avoid additional work
   b. organizational pressure to conform to established practices and norms
   c. lack of time
   d. lack of knowledge about exploration of the will on the part of the leader's supervisor

5. Passion as an essential quality of will is expressed in the following way:

a. Employees share their values and ideas in a nonthreatening manner.
b. People in the organization take pride in their work.
c. In decision making, the leader's opinion dominates the opinions of others.
d. Power is distributed equally among all leaders.

6. Dogmas obstruct the transformation of the health care system for which of the following reasons:

a. Policies require too much time to review.
b. Employees are allowed to retain jobs that no longer are needed.
c. The boundaries between professions continue to remain unclear.
d. The use of resources is not always related to patient outcomes.

7. Regaining balance between work and personal life requires courage to do the following:

a. Create new compensation systems to recognize the differing values of employees.
b. Pursue change with zeal until satisfactory human resource policies are created.
c. Accept that employees are interested in the recommendations of the leader.
d. Remain focused on creating change.

8. Value-based services differ in several ways from the kind of services most commonly delivered. Which of the following would not be affected by the transformation to value-based services?

a. quality of the services
b. research base of the services
c. license of the provider
d. available reimbursement for the services provided

9. Leaders who are mentally fit are better able to manage the complexity of the health care system. Which of the following is *not* a benefit that mental fitness bestows on leaders?

a. ability to handle the disappointment of not being selected for a position
b. ability to take responsibility for one's actions and one's reactions to adversity
c. increased sensitivity to the situation of employees who have been laid off
d. ability to avoid confrontations and the discussion of pertinent issues

CHAPTER 10

The New Spirit of Leadership: Becoming a Living Leader

I am being driven forward
Into an unknown land.
The pass grows steeper,
The air colder and sharper.
A wind from my unknown goal
Stirs the strings of expectation.

Still the question:
Shall I ever get there?
There where life resounds,
A clear pure note
In the silence.

—Dag Hammarskjöld

Chapter Objectives

At the completion of this chapter, the reader will be able to

- Describe the personal needs that relate to self-care and development as a leader and as a person.
- Construct a personal plan for self-direction and self-development that addresses professional, personal, and spiritual needs.
- Distinguish between the various competing aspects of life as a leader and understand the creative skills necessary to manage the leadership role and make a difference.
- Understand how to set time aside in a format that permits deepening of the spiritual journey.
- Enumerate 10 spiritual rules for personal growth that incorporate the principles of chaos and complexity.

Much of the life of a leader is invested in taking care of others and the system that encompasses them. The demands on the energy and resources of the leader are tremendous. Without a sense of spiritual centering and integrity, the leader will not have adequate support, for much of the needed support must come from within. The leader must have self-discipline, resolve, insight, and a sense of direction to prepare for the tough experience of empowering others to manage their own lives. The leader must also focus on her or his resources and enter into a process of self-reflection, centering, and nourishing his or her spirit. This chapter describes the elements and processes associated with leadership self-care and support, including spiritual and personal routines.

Leadership is more than a set of learned skills. Effective leaders possess a deep comfort with themselves and an engagement with life that is generative and harmonizing. They exhibit an excitement and a way of embracing life that are encouraging and hopeful to those they lead. They have a depth of commitment and a reservoir of spirit and energy that are inspiring, along with a sense of being fully in touch with who they are and what moves them. At the same time, effective leaders appear never fully content, as though on a journey or in search of something still just out of their reach that is driving them on.

Leaders who are more than just effective—who qualify as great leaders—have an understanding or acceptance that some deep force runs through all existence and gives it form and life and direction as yet mysterious. This force comes in many forms and goes by an unlimited number of names, but it operates regardless of what it is called. Great leaders sense, indeed feel, this force and at some point are driven by an awareness of its movement within. In the lives of most great leaders, a question arises about what they would do in response to the call deep within, and they respond by moving in concert with this force and by making out of it whatever they can. In short, they commit to the great "yes" of their lives and as a result are driven to do great and meaningful things.

This "call" is not just reserved for the great of the world; it is actually part of the greatness that is in each of us. Regardless of the place we occupy in society, moments of opportunity, risk, and commitment surround us. We all experience the sense that a call is being made to our own greatness. We all possess gifts and strengths that determine our uniqueness and that, when fully expressed, can have a valuable impact on our own lives and, at least by reflection, on the lives of others. We each simply need to be aware of the stirrings of the force within and to act in concert with it. Our awareness of the force does not simply happen, however; it comes out of the insight born of a spiritual discipline (Figure 10–1). Spiritually grounded leaders undergo a cycle of interactions that evidence their ongoing commitment to personal growth and development.

CHAOS AND THE CALL TO LEADERSHIP

In these times, it is difficult to find enough moments of peace to think reflectively about anything. The times seem filled with activity, change, and movement, responses to ever-increasing demands for the new and different. As we leave the Industrial Age and move into the Age of Technology, we can sense the significance of the changes in understanding, work, relationships, and life itself. All the science fiction we have read appears to be coming to life before our very eyes.

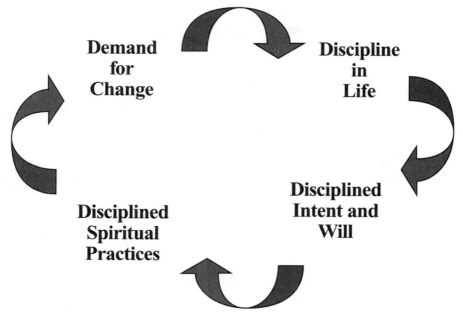

Figure 10–1 The Cycle of Spiritual Discipline

The pace of change has in fact picked up during the past 20 years as we have gotten closer to leaving the old age behind forever. Our movement into the new age tempts us with the loss of all the beliefs and practices that characterized the Industrial Age, especially the linearity and vertical orientation of our thinking, which had a defining influence on all our social institutions and practices, from science to government and religion.

The unidirectional and linear notions associated with the Newtonian view of the universe have now been refuted. The quantum theorists, for example, have proved that life cannot be understood in terms of unilateral and vertical action. The chaos of the universe has a rhythm and flow that move multidirectionally, and through the cloud of chaos can be seen a discrete and elegant simplicity that defies the chaos that created it.

These realities confound and confuse us. They disrupt our sensibilities and our rituals and routines. They create incongruities in our beliefs and understanding. The uncertainty they cause makes us disquieted and anxious. The confidence we garnered from settling on a set of practices and beliefs that brought order to our lives has been undermined. Yet we are not sure what to replace those practices and beliefs with. We hunger for

> **Point To Ponder**
>
> *The spiritually centered leader focuses each eye separately: one eye focuses on the close-up realities and vagaries that must be addressed now, the other focuses on the farthest horizon of the future.*

some certitude and some sense of the absolute that can guide our thinking and acting, but finding these tools of life is turning out to be extremely difficult.

> ### Key Point
>
> *Chaos and the loss of certainty provide an opportunity to let go of those things that are inherently changing and passing. Chaos is a fundamental element of the spiritual discipline, severing us from our false certainty about what can never be certain, refocusing us on the journey, and allowing us to hear the journey's call to adapt and grow.*

There is a tremendous backlash associated with the loss of certainty. Groups on the political far right express a high level of anger and anxiety and call for a return to fundamental beliefs and historic practices as a solution to the loss of certainty. The problem with this approach is it does not engage with the facts that have been recently revealed by science and research—facts that will not disappear because they are disconcerting and incongruous with what we think should be true.

Change is always a challenge to human beings. It presents us with the task of confronting ourselves and everything that defines our lives. It reminds us that life is forever in movement and is more journey than event. Truth is also more journey than event. We want truth to be immutable so as to avoid the discomfort, uncertainty, and unclarity associated with change and to keep from having to question the premises of our actions. Absolutism removes control over our lives from our hands and puts it someplace outside of us. It frees us from the obligation to own what we know and how we must change, and it limits the experience of "noise" that accompanies all aspects of life. The surrender of control to an external absolute eliminates the pain, challenge, risk, and suffering that arise out of the struggle to cope with the vagaries of existence.

> ### Group Discussion
>
> The group participants each recall a serious tragedy or overwhelmingly painful experience that they thought they would never recover from. They then discuss with the other participants what it was that moved them on, got them past the pain, and enabled them to reengage with life and make a difference once again.

It is into this fray that the leader enters, attempting to engage with the vagaries of life and incorporate the uncertainties of the experience into the work of adaptation and growth. The leader finds comfort, not in the safe haven of an unchanging external reality, but in staying the course and deepening his or her own personal journey. The spiritually aware leader recognizes that being available to the challenges and opportunities embedded in the eternal process of change is critical to personal growth. By connecting to the experience of change and demonstrating growth within his or her life, the leader encourages others to continue on their own journey of development.

Chaos is pervasive throughout the universe. Yet, to understand the chaos, it is important to visualize the simplicity that lies at its center. Touching that center brings confidence and order to an individual's life and encourages experimentation and engagement. It is hard work, however, to move through the clouds and shrouds of the chaotic experience to land at the center—the place where the elements of chaos converge and create the mosaic that represents inherent order. Endeavors to get to that place make up much of the work of leadership.

Following are some principles that can illuminate the conditions of participation in change. These help in explaining the proper role of leadership in a world defined by chaos and complexity:

- The universe is a work in progress, still unfolding, yet in creation moving everything in it forward in a web of energy and understanding.
- Chaos and complexity are the essential characteristics of the universe. The universe cannot be understood independent of its own complex reality.
- Everything in the universe is self-organizing. The patterns, webs, and intersections of life create a mosaic of intense goodness of fit that reveals the ultimate connection between all the elements of the universe.
- People, too, are part of the universal network of relationships and are co-creators in the ever-constant unfolding and self-organizing activity.
- Organizations (systems), as smaller reflections of the universe, are self-organizing, complex, and adaptive entities in which people purposefully express their creativity, energy, and meaning together.

Quantum science has revealed many of these principles in its attempt to understand the physics of the universe. From the moment of the "big bang" to the present, all aspects of the universe, including those that involve life, operate within the context of the principles of chaos and complexity.

The leader's role is to apply these principles in the organization. This includes showing a willingness to act in concert with quantum design—that is, engage with chaos and harness its implications. The traditional institutional and vertical views of work and relationship are inadequate for understanding how to lead and implement changes. Instead, a "whole systems" view must underpin the work of the leader and inform the actions and priorities of the organization's members.

Leaders of organizational units, such as services, departments, and divisions, must recognize that rather than merely leading their units, they lead the whole organization from the perspective of their units. Most leaders see their primary responsibility as making their units operate as effectively as possible. Although this is a laudable goal, no unit can thrive if the other units do not. Thriving requires an intersection of actions, each advancing the others and together ensuring the health of the whole. All the leaders of units are working to harmonize the efforts of everyone in the organization in an array of connections that together advance the organization's mission. Chaos and complexity are simply the normal context for all work and relationships, and therefore the leaders must use their understanding of chaos and complexity in every element of their work.

SELF-MANAGEMENT AND CREATIVITY

Newtonian physics and Darwinism, as Margaret Wheatley (1992) points out, suggest that the universe is a cold mechanical process, and that life is harsh, hierarchical, accidental, and beyond the ability of human beings to affect. This view of the universe as mechanistic and indifferent or even hostile is inaccurate. Subsequent work by quantum scientists has revealed that the universe is an exploring, experimenting, adapting process that is continuously and endlessly in the act of creation. Potential, change, adjustment, and becoming represent the character of existence, indicating that life is more challenging and dangerous than previously imagined. Because all things are essentially related, no action is without a wide-ranging influence. In particular, each person's behavior has an effect on the processes of life everywhere. The well-known fact that small events can have large effects far away—encapsulated in the notion that the gentle flapping of a butterfly's wings in China can influence the unfolding of a hurricane in the Atlantic—is a reminder of the interconnectedness of everything.

For leaders, the implications of these newer notions are profound. Leaders, by the smallest of their actions, can have a significant impact on others at every level in the organization. By their behavior, which is under constant scrutiny, they create the organization's culture and build the framework for responding to the challenges and uncertainties of a world forever in flux. They exemplify the normalcy of change by embracing and engaging with it and responding with acceptance and adaptation.

It is important for leaders to fully live up to the expectations of their role. If a leader is not personally disposed to live in the potential, he or she cannot ask others to live there either. Leaders must demonstrate in their leadership practices a personal pattern of response to life's calls. For example, the universe delights in exploration and transformation, and leaders must exhibit in their behavior the enthusiasm of experimentation, challenge, and engagement (Figure 10–2). Indeed, they must be the living representatives of this dynamic. Following is a discussion of some issues that leaders need to consider to live and lead in accordance with the realities of life.

Life is joyful. If the leader of an organization is not excited, neither will the other members be. The leader creates the context for work and relationships. If the mental model of the leader implies that life is hard and treacherous, it will be hard and treacherous in that organization. The leader must believe that life is exciting and full of adventure so that everyone feels that they are being invited on a journey of discovery and transformation. Otherwise, the environment will be rife with the fallout of what the leader does believe about work and relationships.

Time must be allowed for reflection. Leaders need to spend time thinking about their role and the context of their role. No leader can be in touch with what is influencing his or her work if there is no room in the

> ### Point To Ponder
>
> *Rather than being harsh and unforgiving, life is full of opportunity. All it asks is that you desire it enough, work at it the right way, patiently build your personal resources, then grab it when it calls. Whether good things happen to you depends more on you than on the good things.*

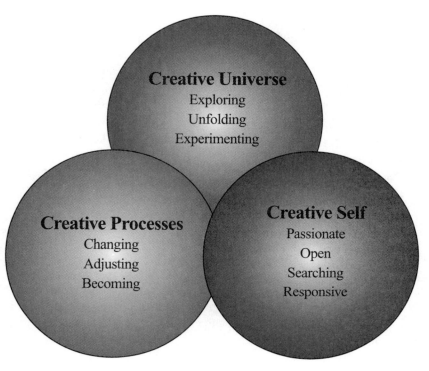

Creative Universe
Exploring
Unfolding
Experimenting

Creative Processes
Changing
Adjusting
Becoming

Creative Self
Passionate
Open
Searching
Responsive

Figure 10–2 The Creative Spirit

day for personal reflection. Call this activity what you will—meditation, deliberation, or some other term—it leads to renewal, insight, engagement, and reenergizing response. Both the external and internal elements of life's changes are considered in a way that has meaning for the leader. The focus is on the person of the leader and that individual's own life issues, priorities, challenges, and growth.

Group Discussion

The group participants each reflect on three words that describe their fundamental beliefs about life. Each participant then presents his or her words to the group, spending no more than two minutes to explain what they mean. All the words are written randomly on a flipchart. At the end of the session, each participant looks at the composite of words and on a second flipchart writes the one word that best describes what he or she sees or feels about all the words on the first flipchart. When all the participants have finished, that page represents the prevailing spiritual culture of the group.

Leaders are co-creators. Leaders know that things do not simply happen by accident or without meaning. They are always seeking to discern the relationship between specific actions and their significance. Sorting through the vagaries of change to find its prime movers and intersections is a part of the work of transformation. People do not make change. Change is. People give change the form it will take and link it to all the elements that will either constrain it or facilitate it. By "seeing" the inner life of change and identifying what it is trying to reveal, leaders attach to it the factors that give it form and meaning for those it will impact. Knowing this, leaders act as co-creators, operating in concert with the change, digging for its meaning and impact, and working with others to determine the most appropriate response.

> **Point To Ponder**
>
> *If leaders have no idea what drives them, how can they expect anyone else to know? Self-knowledge is the beginning point of self-direction.*

Chaos is always the route to order. Leaders know that chaos is a constant. They also know that order is generated from chaos. Looking at the simplicity that lies at the center of complexity, leaders search for the connections that the chaos is breaking up or reformatting on a way to the very next stage of the change journey. They tie the forces at work to the mission, purposes, and direction of the organization in order to "fit" the pieces together to converge around the change. Leaders recognize that chaos is a requisite of order and are thus better able to accept chaos as an element in their own lives. They also recognize that chaos is normal and to be welcomed as a part of life. Further, they embrace chaos before expecting others to engage with their own experience of chaos.

Leadership is a contract with possibility and opportunity. Leaders understand that experience is simply the application of potential to present circumstances and that their role is to give substance to the changes occurring by making them real for those they lead. In other words, they translate the potential reality into language that has meaning for the staff in their present situation. In addition, they put the staff's current experience into a much broader context by treating it as a stage, a milepost, on a longer journey. By operating with this frame of reference, they are able to help the staff understand the context of their work and actions. Here again, leaders must live in the embrace of the potential, always seeing it ahead and translating its implications into language the staff can understand. As has been repeatedly noted, leading is a way of life, not just a skill set.

Life gets messy before order shows up. Living with mess is hard for many people. We desire logical, rational, and visual order and are usually able to manage our lives so as to obtain such order. The problem is that while we are busy establishing and maintaining order, life is getting ready to put sand in its gears. Another way of saying this is that in our desire for order we sometimes treat the journey of life as a stationary condition that can somehow be fenced off by an unchanging set of self-created parameters. The journey, however, soon reasserts itself, sometimes dramatically, as when it brings down our neatly constructed world of supposed impervious order. This type of disruption reminds us of the impermanence of order and the essential character of the journey that is life, which is to move from where we currently are through a process of change, challenge, and, hopefully, growth. The movement does not occur in a straight line, however, and messiness is one of the reminders that we need to continuously adapt.

Leaders must preserve their identity. All living things seek to preserve their identity and sustain themselves. Leaders are no different. Yet leading is demanding work and can lead to "burnout" and to damage of one's personal integrity. Living in the world means finding a place in the world. For leaders, it means recognizing that they occupy a space that is influencing all the surrounding spaces. How well they live in their own space, respond to the demand for movement, address personal issues, and confront the challenges to growth determines their ability to impact others through their personal leadership. Leaders cannot help others adapt to what they cannot adapt to. The paradox of identity is that persons must change in order to maintain their identity. Leaders must adapt in order to assist others in becoming reconciled to their own changes.

We all participate in the evolution of each other. We all have an impact on others—there are no foreigners on life's journey. Everything everywhere ultimately connects to facilitate change at every level. The rules, processes, and conditions of growth are ever changing and cannot be counted on to act in the same way at different times and places in the change cycle. The leader knows this, understanding that synthesis rather than analysis, fluidity rather than solidity, principle rather than law, and focus rather than function are the real operating conditions of life. Discernment is a more valuable gift than definition. Direction is more important than location. These truths merely indicate how different the workings of change are from our linear expectations. We confront the patterns and movements of change in our responses to life, but change continues regardless of our responses. Our success in the journey of life depends mostly on the congruence of our responses and our recognition that we are fundamentally interdependent.

Leadership work is important and influential and thus requires care and concerted effort. The personal engagement of leaders in their own journey, for example, is a means of demonstrating to others that they have an obligation to confront the challenges presented by change and also a means of guiding them in their attempts to adapt to change. On the other hand, leaders who have not attended to the personal issues of adaptation and have failed to sustain their insights, courage, and creativity probably will be unable to help others gain the self-understanding and discernment they need to meet their own challenges successfully.

CREATIVITY AND INNOVATION

We are born creative. No matter what else or who else God is, the spirit of God is the force of creativity. Artists, musicians, writers—creators of every type—all make reference to some deep source of power from which flows the energy of creativity. Yet, although creativity is inextricably linked to the life force in each of us, many of us talk of creativity as something we can own or control and manipulate. We treat it as external to ourselves and profess to think we could do so much more if we only could get hold of it. We fail to realize that we all have it—it is a part of who we are. We do need, however, self-awareness and discipline to access it and to give it form and direction.

There is a direct relationship between creativity and discipline. Creativity needs its own time. We need to allow it the space to take form and to have expression. Rarely is it acci-

Key Point

We are all creative. We are, however, naturally creative in different ways. Although creativity is deeply hardwired within each of us, it is malleable enough to be expressed in almost any way we choose. The only requirement is that we do decide to do something with it, as it can wither and die if left unattended.

dentally revealed and exposed. If it is visible, it is because it was made visible, disciplined by the action that brought it forward and molded it into a format that could be experienced and then shared with the world, for all to marvel at and enjoy (Figure 10–3). For its expression, creativity demands a format and also a context. By setting a specified time and place for its expression, we provide the discipline necessary for the elements of creativity to converge and produce something of value. The products of creativity could not exist without the work of creativity, and we should appreciate the latter as much as the former.

At the same time, creativity demands release from the slavishness of routine and the straightjacket of habit, rote, and ritual. Only within the chaos of experience can the elements of creativity converge. Further, the format for its expression must be allowed time and space to emerge. Forcing creativity into prescribed structures of expression will limit its ability to take shape. This does not mean that no format is required. There is no pottery without the potter's wheel, no painting without a canvas.

It is difficult to live creatively. There is always some reason not to. We have all made comments about creative people who seem eccentric, even weird. Because they appear to live fully in their own world or to walk their own way, they make us feel funny or uncomfortable. In general, we experience uncertainty and unease if people fall outside our definition of what is appropriate, and because creative people tend to operate outside the parameters of normal behavior, we wonder whether getting in touch with the creative in

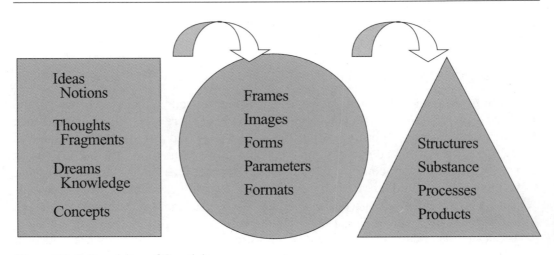

Figure 10–3 Requisites of Creativity

ourselves will make us become like them. The answer, of course, is that creativity does not have a look and a walk, and that we can connect with our creativity without changing in every way possible.

It is important to recognize that leaders cannot get the best out of those they lead if they cannot touch the best in themselves. This means they need to develop an awareness of who they are and how their essential self gets expressed in the normal course of living each day. Leaders must understand that their spiritual part is frequently expressed in their most creative moments. Getting in touch with one's own creative center means discerning the spiritual values that lie within as well. For creativity to find expression, of course, requires discipline and habit and the meeting of certain conditions.

Finding the Source of Creativity

A person's creativity does not simply appear on demand. The person has to search for it and then develop ways to give it expression. The best way of getting in touch with it is to set aside a regular time during the day to focus on nothing but the inner self. Journaling is a helpful tool in this endeavor, for regularly writing down one's thoughts establishes the habit of focusing on the creative and bringing it out into the open. The process need not be complicated or demanding. The goal is to write from one to three pages about whatever comes to mind at the moment. No one need see what was written, as the purpose is merely to make sure that something has been done. In time, the act of writing begins to touch a deep part of the self, and expressing what lies within becomes easier. How long it takes to achieve fluency depends on how many blocks are standing in the way.

Everyone possesses an internal auditor that makes judgments about what is written or spoken or thought and decides whether it is appropriate or not. Often the auditor appears just as the person is about to get in touch with his or her creativity and prevents the expression of ideas on the grounds that they are, for example, not right, appropriate, good, or normal. This review and approval function is the person's own creation. A good way to bypass it is to commit to the process of daily writing and go wherever it leads. In time, the auditor will disappear and be replaced by a sense of freedom and openness, which is the groundwork for creative expression.

Journaling is a way of meditating that is often easier than the more defined forms of meditation. What often happens is that the wisdom that lies deep within emerges through the process and finds expression in a language that can inform, inspire, and guide. It is a chance for the "inner voice" to assume an outward form, deepening the meaning of our lives and perhaps moving us in a new direction.

Spending Time with the Child Within

As Jung and many contemporary psychotherapists have revealed, we each have a child embedded deep within us that will reside there throughout our lives. This child is the enthusiastic, joyful, excited part of ourselves that embraces life fully and without reservation. It is only when we are wounded by the behavior of others or by negative experiences that our inner child loses touch with the primordial joy that typifies the experience of the spirit. And even when the child loses touch with the joy of life, it continues to seek it until it finds it again, renewing itself in the process.

The creative process often, if not always, meets up with this inner child. There are many who say that it is impossible to get in touch with one's creativity without confronting this inner child and giving it a voice. Indeed, it is this voice that is the expression of creativity. Further, because the inner child, by its very nature, is not bound by the rules and parameters of adulthood, these are rendered powerless to limit the expression of creativity. However, whatever the child is feeling, whether pain or joy or some other emotion, will emerge as a part of the journey to the place of creativity, and until they are expressed and dealt with in a meaningful way, the creative expression will remain blocked at the very place where it resides. That is why we must take up our unfinished business with this child (the pains and hurts of our life experiences and journey to adulthood) to free the creativity within.

Group Discussion

Getting in touch with the unrestrained child within is critical to touching our own creativity. The participants should each take a moment to reflect on a childhood episode in which they did something that was different or even unique (at the time)—in a word, creative. Those who wish to should tell their story to the rest of the participants. During each story, the listeners write down what each perceives as the key elements of the story. The group then discusses these elements and considers whether they are present in creativity regardless of age or time. Finally, the participants identify ways in which they will incorporate these elements into their own efforts at touching their individual creativity.

Through the process of journaling, a person will typically arrive at the door of creativity but be prevented from entering by the remnants of past pain. In verbalizing these on the daily pages of the journal, the person can get them out of the way and open the route to creative expression. In some circumstances, working on the issues with a professional or other trusted person may be a necessary step in the journey to freeing the inner child and releasing the creativity residing there.

Opening the Gates of Creativity

When we complete the journey to the center of our being, we find a deep well of creativity—a place filled with things that can be used as vehicles for creative expression. We are all artists of one kind or another. Some of us are creative with our hands, some with our heads, some with our hearts—all of us with something. By using our regular set-aside time to explore different avenues, we can find that form of creative expression that most resonates with our inner self. Some people, of course, may discover more than one form. In any case, in order to give shape to our creativity, we will need to release the energy that lies within the urge to create. Creativity always seeks a way out into the world, and once touched and released, it cannot be contained and must find expression, enriching the life of everyone it touches and connecting all of us in ways we cannot even imagine.

Creativity is expressed in symbols and images. Even the wordsmith has a vision before forming the vision into words. Leaders also express their creativity through the construction of a vision. They then present this vision to others as evidence of their commitment to make some difference, to cause something to happen that will enhance the life experience of everyone.

In this dynamic, leaders recognize that the critical ability is the ability to be available to the creative force without attempting to master it. Creativity is a mystery and requires awareness instead of readiness. The creative force must first be seen before it can be expressed. Further, to give it form, the creative mind must be attentive to what it might be saying. Form comes as a product of good discernment and the discipline of translating the creative force into words or substance.

> **Point To Ponder**
>
> *The creative leader recognizes that what is critical is being available to the creative force, not mastering it.*

Creativity leads each of us inward and then onward. We must spend time in the "inward place." As Georgia O'Keeffe and Brenda Ueland caution us, we must spend time watching the flowers, puttering around in the imagining, idling, seeing, forming stuff that lives within. Leaders will have to identify the activities that guide them to the creative place within. Each of us can recall where we got our best ideas. For some, it is the shower stall; others, the car; still others, the bathroom. Wherever the ideas come, the creative force is always seeking expression; we need only be aware of where and how it operates.

Overcoming the Fear of Being Wrong

Many artists and psychologists have noted that the opposite of love is not hate but fear. It is fear that closes the door to the creative—indeed, to most of life. Fear is a mental door that keeps the spirit imprisoned and unaware. How much faith is an expression of fear and as a result narrow, ritualistic, and rigid? How many people neurotically seek the spiritless road, comfortable in their own rightness but devoid of life and joy?

Fear, like a trap from which there is no escape, imprisons the heart and keeps it from experiencing the fullness of life. It closes the mind and shuts the door on life. It is the ultimate indicator of nonengagement. It keeps people from reaching out toward those very things that will advance their experience and reduce the chance that fear will rule them. It is all too common to see people failing to confront fears that are impacting their expression of life—or to see someone struggling to avoid something infinitely less painful than the life of fear the person is living.

There is virtually nothing about fear that is redeeming. Yet much of the relationship that so many people have with life is tinged by their accommodation to their own fears. In addition, the structures of 20th-century organizations are largely grounded in the concept of fear. In hierarchical organizations pervaded by the culture of "bossism," the negative power of the boss is what keeps people in line, and the power that managers wield is often articulated in the language of control and punishment. It is no wonder that changing the way the leadership role is perceived and expressed is so difficult. To make the necessary changes and remove fear from organizational life, leaders must therefore confront the history of the role and people's perception and experience of it.

Being wrong is an essential constituent of creativity. In fact, creative people spend more time being wrong than being right. The road to rightness is paved with experimentation, innovation, mistakes, and redos. In fact, in systems language, success of any kind is simply the culmination of sufficient error. When the right amount of error has occurred and a sufficient amount of learning in relationship to the error has been obtained, then success emerges. Mistakes are the signposts of the journey toward achievement. The only error that is untenable is the error repeated. An error repeated indicates that no learning occurred and the error's lesson was missed.

> **Key Point**
>
> *Being wrong is not a defect. We learn as much from our errors as we do from our successes. The critical issue is to learn from any error what it is trying to teach us so that we do not repeat it or stay imprisoned in a never-ending cycle of repetition and decline.*

Mistakes are to be embraced by the organization as the tools of growth. The more fully that error is incorporated into the expectations of work, the fewer errors are present and the more certain the leader is that the right errors will emerge. By celebrating error, the leader takes the fear out of it and puts it into the right category—the category of devices for determining where people are on the journey toward their goals.

Confronting personal fear and fear in the workplace is a challenging process (Exhibit 10–1). So much of human experience is defined by fear that it becomes nearly impossible to push it out of people's lives and experience. From regulation to accreditation, there are plenty of opportunities to be afraid of something or someone in a way that limits creativity and engagement with life. So many folks worry about whether they will "get in trouble" because of projects or activities with which they might be associated. For example, instead of thinking about how their behavior enables the organization to deliver high-quality services, health care workers waste their time worrying about whether they will offend someone or do the wrong thing or, God forbid, cause a patient's death.

Of course, the probability of any one person doing sustainable damage is very low. People in an organization are generally incapable of permanently jeopardizing its integrity and functioning unless they have that goal as their evil intent. Of late, much work has been written on fear in the workplace and how unnecessary it is, not to mention detrimental to performance and even dangerous. One of the main goals of leadership should be to drive fear-based behavior out of the workplace and replace it with the commitment to relationship and creativity.

How much of the fear present in the workplace is there because of the fear of management? If the leaders have not resolved their own fear issues, are these issues affecting their relationships with others and impacting the organization as a whole? If their language is

Exhibit 10–1 Overcoming Fear

Sources of Fear	**Ways of Overcoming Fear**
• Parents	• Meditation
• Teachers	• Risk-taking
• Peers	• Therapy
• Self	• Focused action
• Authorities	• Confrontation
• Religion	• Surrender-embrace
• Events	• Medication
Means of Identifying Fear	
• Self-awareness	
• Therapy	
• Reflection	
• Input from others	
• Trauma	

laced with fear-based terminology, are they helping to create an atmosphere of anxiety and suspicion?

Fear-based behaviors—judging, blaming, pointing fingers, complaining, and so on—kill innovation. There is simply no place for it to emerge. The job of the leader is to eliminate fear-based behaviors by giving *them* no room to emerge. The leader begins this process by making sure that his or her own fear issues have not tainted the environment. By focusing on fear issues and grappling with their presence in each individual's life journey, the leader has a good chance to create a workplace of trust and joy and creativity.

> **Point To Ponder**
>
> *Fear kills all creativity.*

Confronting the Core Negativity Within

As we move through life, we collect flawed mental models, negative stereotypes, and unsupported generalizations. These become deeply embedded in our consciousness and are reflected in our attitudes and behaviors. They often surface in our self-talk and our conversation with those closest to us. Although the generalities we employ are usually inaccurate, even groundless, we still fall back on them in the midst of stress or during periods of difficulty. Following are a list of examples (to which each of us could add):

- I *always* do this.
- No one likes me.
- I'm going to die of . . .
- I'll always be poor.

- I can't study.
- I've never been able to . . .
- I'm just not good at . . .
- It's too late for me to do . . .

How many of these phrases have we caught ourselves saying at some time or other? Most people are surprised that this type of language is so pervasive. Think about how limiting and just plain incorrect these statements are. The challenge for every leader is to look carefully at his or her own language and assess the extent to which it is laced with negativity. The fact is that most leaders use (and hear) more negative language in a day than any other type.

Group Discussion

The participants discuss the content of their self-talk—the things they say to themselves when they are alone. What are the words used? What are the themes? Are the comments primarily positive or negative? The participants then share their self-talk words with each other. Taken as a whole, is the group's self-talk supportive and encouraging or negative and punishing?

Most of our negative ideas and images are untrue, including those that pertain to our own abilities. If we really could not do most of what we imagine cannot be done, we could not do what we have, most of us, already done. The majority of our core negatives come from outside ourselves—from parents, friends, religion, society. On top of these we add other negatives based on our experience. Eventually we have so many that they cannot help but impair our relationships and degrade other aspects of our lives.

What is important to remember is that negative beliefs are just that—beliefs. They are also obstacles blocking the enriched experience and the creative endeavors everyone is capable of. They shut the door on awareness and limit the places where talent or opportunity can make a positive change in our lives. Further, they give us all an excuse not to address challenges: No matter what we do, we will not succeed anyway.

Sitting on the sidelines of life, we can join others in spreading negativity. When we see others struggling to be creative, we can assure them that they will not succeed and thus need not strain themselves. The most threatening person to a negativist is the person who has agreed to engage with his or her negatives and take on a creative task and follow wherever it will lead. This person creates a risk that the negativist will see someone achieve all that the negativist has failed to do and thereby make the role of negativist very uncomfortable.

Leaders struggling to fight their own negatives should remember that affirmation is the enemy of negativity—that affirmative beliefs are just as viable and powerful as negative beliefs, only they have more mileage. They also need to replace the negative terminology they have used in the past with affirmative language, demonstrating their commitment to a different set of images and mental models, raising the level of the dialogue in the organization, and creating a healthier organizational culture. Here are some examples of affirming language:

- I am very good at . . .
- I've always been able to . . .
- You're an excellent . . .
- I am a brilliant . . .
- I am challenged by . . .
- It's great fun to . . .

If leaders fight the urge to blurt out a negative comment and substitute an affirming statement, they will be able to notice the different results. Language and behavior are themselves strong change agents. De Bono's (1996) research shows that positive statements, even when untrue, can become true through changing behavior over time.

The transition to a more positive culture does not happen overnight. The bombardment of negative images and generalizations that most of us have undergone eventually turns negativity into our second nature. Leaders therefore have to make the overcoming of negativity a focused part of their leadership work. In order not to get sucked into the drama of constant negativity, they must have a way of exploring the sources of their own negativity and lack of creativity, past and present.

For leaders, getting in touch with their own journey means being willing to look squarely at themselves and at how their nature affects their relationship with and leadership of others. How much do they understand about negativity and what causes it? What overwhelms their creativity? What affects their ability to embrace innovation? What personality characteristics keep them from relating to the elements of life that challenge or frighten them? How can they help others reflect on their attitudes and behaviors if, as leaders, they have no mechanism for doing that in their own lives?

Leaders cannot ask others to go to places they themselves are not willing or able to go. They thus need to routinely engage in reflection to gain essential insights about themselves, including whatever internal obstacles are blocking their own creativity, engagement, and courage and decreasing their ability to guide others and help them overcome the many challenges they will face on their individual journeys.

EXERCISING THE SPIRIT

We all know how important it is to exercise the body. Almost all medical literature about longevity tells us that exercise is an essential part of our lives. Regular exercise leads to good health and lifelong productivity, and failure to exercise is one of the major causes of untimely death (Exhibit 10–2).

Stretching the Spirit Within

Each person's spirit—the source of creativity, energy, and engagement and seat of the self—has precisely the same need for exercise. When the spirit is not exercised, it becomes weak and flabby and fails to grow. A weak spirit cannot provide the meaning that people

Exhibit 10–2 Exercising the Spirit Within

Requisites	Obstacles
• Setting aside time daily	• Fear
• Exercising regularly	• Tiredness
• Being self-disciplined	• Distractions
• Using a specific format or method	• Laziness
	• Excuses
	• Other commitments
	• Family responsibilities

need and look for in their lives. In the case of leaders, a weak spirit limits their effectiveness and makes them lose direction. When that happens, their enthusiasm is diminished and they cannot motivate others to embrace the challenges of change. They then become depressed and subject to all and any of the diseases of the spirit. Without exercise, both the muscle (spiritual strength and creativity) and the immune system (moral courage and focus) of the spirit cease to operate effectively. They become susceptible to spiritual infections, such as evil intent, lack of direction, poor decision making, depression, and lack of focus.

Most leaders who want to pursue self-development read motivational or spiritual books. Reading these books can pique their interest in spiritual matters, even to the point of moving them to discuss spiritual topics with others. It does not, however, ensure that they grow spiritually. In fact, reading often prevents people from growing spiritually by keeping them at a certain level of interest. Reading never calls people to do the deeper task of stretching their spirits in a way that actually changes their lives. Touching the spiritual energy within requires regular discipline—and focus!

Developing an Exercise Routine

Every leader needs regular spiritual workouts every day. The stress caused by confronting so much change requires a regular recess for recentering and refocusing on the meaning that drives the work of leading. This daily period of reflection and connection to one's spiritual energy should last at least 15 minutes. Of course, each leader must adjust the routine and time based on his or her individual needs and circumstances. The length of the period can be extended as the leader develops more skill and as the spirit increases its tone and strength. It is recommended that the leader gradually work up to spending 30 minutes on spiritual exercises each day.

A large body of research indicates that a spiritual workout should encompass five specific steps: deep breathing, a spiritual warm-up, spiritual stretching, spiritual strengthening, and a spiritual cool-down. Here is one approach to establishing a regular routine of reflection and spiritual centering (Exhibit 10–3).

Deep Breathing

At the beginning of every exercise routine, you will need to transition from one level of energy to another lower level. You will also need to move from a primarily external

Exhibit 10–3 A Spiritual Exercise Routine

Deep breathing. Transitioning from a high energy level to a lower one.

Spiritual warm-up. Reading a selection from a source that has special relevance.

Stretching the spirit. Reflecting on an incident or theme.

Strengthening the spirit. Applying knowledge and experience to gain wisdom.

Spiritual cool-down. Breathing, letting go, and choosing a thought to keep for the day.

---

focus to looking inward. Deep breathing is a technique that helps you make the necessary journey.

Deep breathing facilitates the transition from a high level of energy to a lower level. In a relaxed position, you will slowly but continuously breathe deeply through your nose. After each inhaling, hold your breath for a second, then let it go fully out through your mouth all at once. You will need to do 10 to 20 of these before you begin to feel the relaxation unfold. The routine should be slow and continuous, completely unrushed, allowing you to peacefully and quietly relax yourself and refocus your attention on yourself and the reflective work you are about to undertake. Every time you sit down to do your reflective work, you should begin with deep breathing, as it sets you up for the steps to follow.

Spiritual Warm-Up

The next step is to read a brief selection from a source that has relevance to your own life or experience. The reading is meant to move your spirit and mind into a reflective mode. By making the transition to a quieter, more peaceful perspective, you become ready to begin the journey to an intensive spiritual experience. This exercise should last anywhere from three to five minutes.

Stretching Your Spiritual Energy

You can use a real-life event or situation to center your attention on a particular theme or aspect of life. For example, you might choose an event that exemplifies the theme of the selection read during the warm-up. Using an actual incident or circumstance as a focal point is designed to narrow the reflective work so that it fits within the workout period but will still be illuminating. This exercise, like the warm-up, should last three to five minutes.

Strengthening and Focusing the Spirit Within

During reflection, a question or series of questions will arise. These might concern an aspect of your life or experience or a component of your role, relationships, or work. At this point, you apply your knowledge and experience to learn about yourself—about your issues, relationships, problems, and concerns—and gain wisdom.

This is where the heavy exercise occurs. Your response to your insights has an important impact on your choices, approach, method, and focus for the day. The insights you obtain during this strengthening exercise may accumulate over a number of days and eventually come together to clarify what course you should take in dealing with a challenge, problem, or issue. You should spend 5 to 10 minutes (and no more than 10 minutes) on this part of the workout.

Cooling Down

The spiritual workout is concluded with a brief period of breathing and letting go. This exercise brings the workout to a close and transitions you back into your daily activities. You should choose an important thought or moment in the reflection to remember and keep with you for the rest of the day. You might even write it on a small card. Writing down important thoughts or memorable moments allows you to recollect them at any time during the day and to apply them whenever and in whatever way appears right. This finishing exercise should take between 2 and 3 minutes.

Quiet Please

A quiet place is necessary for proper exercise of the spirit. Unlike the body, which can be toned by exercising to vigorous music and enthusiastic encouragement, the spirit needs quiet to be stretched and strengthened. The quieter it is during spiritual exercises, the better the results.

Finding and maintaining quiet can be difficult. Some people even feel initial anxiety in a quiet place. Today, distraction is the name of the game, and we have become conditioned to continuous assaults on our consciousness. For leaders, the very work of leading forces them into a host of relationships, conversations, processes, and problems that leave no time for consideration and reflection.

> **Key Point**
>
> *Spending time with ourselves is the most valuable and most difficult thing we can do in life.*

Focusing on our spiritual resources is inner exercising. The better we get at it, the deeper we go and the more we desire the joy and peace that come from going deeper. Regular spiritual reflection leads to a surprising yet extremely satisfying calm, accompanied by a deep sense of peace and contentment. The secret to discovering this place is the quiet and calm that surrounds us when we undertake our exercise routines. Each workout should be done in a quiet place and at an available time (i.e., a time free of other commitments), and preferably the same time and place should be used for all the workouts.

A wide variety of spiritual resources have emerged over the history of humankind. The warm-up exercises, for example, can be drawn from a broad selection of spiritual works. The goal of spiritual exercising is to stretch the spirit through a variety of growth experiences and challenges that fall inside and outside of the person's usual spiritual context. These experiences and challenges instigate growth by pushing the person to employ a diverse set of spiritual resources as a tool kit.

The notes written during the spiritual cool-down act as "memory joggers" to help connect the person's experiences to the wisdom gained through the exercises. In the midst of daily activities, the spirit will periodically generate windows or moments of perception that will affirm the insights that arose from that day's reflection. The notes from a particular exercise session can also serve as a doorway back to the work done during that session, allowing the wisdom gained to continue to play a role in meeting life's challenges.

The Importance of Exercising Every Day

Regularity is the key to good spiritual work. It is recommended that these exercises be done first thing in the morning or as early as possible in the day. Although morning is best, exercising the spirit is valuable any time it is done. As mentioned, exercising for 15 to 30 minutes a day is enough for the benefits to accrue.

If a leader does the exercise routine suggested here every day, he or she will begin to see a difference in the areas of feeling, acting, and thinking. The leader will have more energy, experience more enthusiasm, exhibit more creativity, and feel more centered. As a result, the leader's work relationships will improve, among other positive consequences. As the spirit uses better strategies to handle stress, anger and tension will ease and then dissipate, sleep will come more easily, and worry will begin to lessen. After faithfully completing a full 100 days of regular workouts, the leader will almost certainly be able to see dramatic changes in his or her life.

> **Key Point**
>
> *In developing self-awareness, the discipline of regular reflection can make an important difference. Progress is always variable, but no progress will be achieved if the process is not a regular habit.*

The First 100 Days

The leader should make a commitment to do a set of daily exercises for 100 days. This commitment is meant to help the individual continue the workouts long enough to experience some of the benefits of reflection and begin to seek out other sources and methods of spiritual strengthening. The spiritual energy of every person matures in its own fashion, and by the time the workout routine is well established, the leader's spirit will thirst for further spiritual experiences. Indeed, the leader will come to find that he or she cannot live without them.

SPIRITUAL INTELLIGENCE: TEN RULES OF THE ROAD

Leadership is not simply a set of skills but a whole discipline. As such, it requires a commitment to constant growth and self-development. Leaders, in living the role, not only direct the process of change and adaptation but exemplify adaptability, modeling it for others. This means that personal change, maturation, and development make up a fundamental part of the life of any leader. Consequently, leaders are always involved in reaching for the potential within the self.

Following is a discussion of some basic themes that thread through the life of a leader. These themes underscore the fact that leaders, in virtue of their role, are on a journey of exploration and growth (Exhibits 10–4 and 10–5 and Figure 10–4).

1. The leadership role demands courage. For leaders, risk is a pervasive fact of life. Leaders live in the potential, by definition a place of great risk. They have a responsibility to translate the potential into real experiences in a way that helps others see how the journey of transformation impacts their own roles. Leaders are always alerting the staff to the meaning and requisites of their work and the direction it must ultimately take to have value. Thus, they are sometimes required to live on the cutting edge, pushing against the walls of reality, forcing the staff to confront their own perceptions and behaviors, and challenging them to create their own futures. Leaders frequently appear to be running counter to the prevailing sensibilities and must confront the noise that their actions create, holding strongly to what is right and necessary in a way that advocates for these things in the face of the noise—certainly a challenging reality but a requisite of the role.

> **Key Point**
>
> *A leader is never "off" while in the leadership role. The leader is always under the scrutiny of others while at the same time trying to turn every moment, every interchange, every experience into an opportunity to make a difference in the lives of those he or she leads.*

2. Caring for the self is the first priority. Leaders are not self-sacrificing, long-suffering, passive personalities who mindlessly implement the organization's directives. Instead, they have a strong sense of self and are fully in touch with their own motives and intentions. They are clear where they are in relationship to what motivates action and response, and they always act on the basis of their understanding of this. They also recognize that they cannot address the needs of others if their own neediness is greater. Therefore, they realize that they require time for

---

Exhibit 10–4 Ten Spiritual Rules of the Road

1. The leadership role demands courage.
2. Caring for the self is the first priority.
3. Setting a few focused goals and achieving them is preferable to setting and failing to achieve a broad range of goals.
4. Prayer is a tool of leadership.
5. Challenge and change are normal features of the universe.
6. The universe is full of creative and transforming energy as well as mystery.
7. Leaders need to seek out others who are committed to change and growth.
8. The goal of leadership is to connect to the journey of transformation.
9. Judgment is an enemy to the spirit within.
10. You can't love your creation if you don't love the creator.

Exhibit 10–5 Requisites of the Spiritual Journey

- A desire for truth
- Self-love
- Creativity
- The support of others
- A disciplined process
- Ability to see life itself as a journey

reflection, opportunities for self-development, and the skills necessary for dealing with critical growth issues. It is only through self-understanding that leaders can help meet the needs of others.

3. Setting a few focused goals and achieving them is preferable to setting and failing to achieve a broad range of goals. There is nothing more debilitating than setting a host of goals and not meeting them. Thus, it is wise to set a small number of goals and commit to achieving these. Being less ambitious will ensure that the focus does not get lost and that significant progress can be made. Personal development is a work in progress and will require a lifetime commitment.

Focusing only on key issues of self-development makes it possible to resolve them and move on. Not every behavior or habit can be altered at the same time. Leaders need to be

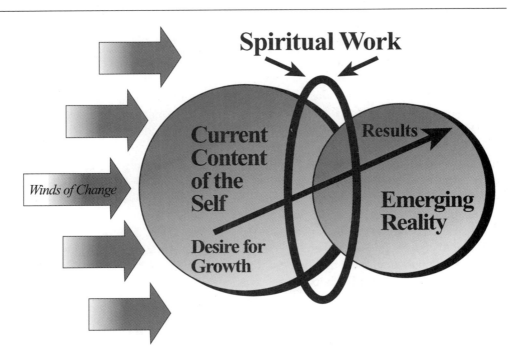

Figure 10–4 The Journey of the Spirit

kind to themselves and not expect progress on every front. Small successes can serve as the foundation for significant change and as the means for attaining ultimate goals.

Leaders need to be similarly kind to those they are helping to change. They should assist them in setting priorities so that they can better succeed in revising their behaviors and practices. By being realistic and not expecting too much, leaders can turn success into a way of being. Success does much to alter attitudes and re-energize performance, changing both the milieu and the spirit of the work.

4. Prayer is a tool of leadership. Although there are as many religious traditions as there are leaders, prayer is central to all of them. Whatever their convictions, leaders should know that prayer has been determined to have a great impact on the quality of decisions and the comfort with which challenges are faced. Prayer is simply a reflection of a reality beyond one's own. It harnesses the spiritual forces within and without to help create the stamina required to carry on. It centers the mind and calls it to focus in a way that leads to new insights and deep, strong relationships.

Prayer ensures the constancy necessary to any meaningful effort and links the effort to the forces needed for something to happen. It encourages and strengthens the individual, realigning the individual's energy to fit the requirements of the task. It helps keep things in perspective and pulls the mind and heart back to the journey, putting the work into a life framework rather than an event model. In prayer, the issue or situation takes on broader and deeper implications and gets connected to a whole range of intersections that give it meaning and call people back to the larger picture. Prayer renews, strengthens, encourages, and connects people in a way that ensures their faithfulness to the effort and to each other.

5. Challenge and change are normal features of the universe. Stability is equivalent to death. Change is the normal state of existence. The role of leaders is to walk the tightrope between stability and chaos, tending to favor the latter. Chaos is a sign of life in the universe and pervades human experience. Realizing this, leaders do not expect stability to last for long. Any stability they find is simply a resting point on the journey to the next place.

Opposition, including the clash between differing interests, is part of change. Thus, leaders are always prepared for opposition and contrary arguments, practices, and behaviors. Indeed, the techniques of managing relationships encompass ways of challenging people's mental models. Leaders begin by clarifying their own perceptions, roles, and commitments and then challenge others to make their own commitment to fostering change and meeting the challenges that arise on the journey.

6. The universe is full of creative and transforming energy as well as mystery. Regardless of their personal belief traditions and perceptions, leaders need to understand what this means at the individual level, for they must be able to harness the internal energy of the staff and the external energy embedded in all transformation. This combined energy reflects a resonance with change that itself can keep people focused and directed. Leaders need to appreciate that influence and the wisdom that is often evident in the demand for change.

Because everything is always in motion, everything that the leader does and creates somehow reflects change and adaptation. A particular change does not happen for its own sake. It is a reflection of a grand concert of changes that, when connected together, co-create the next stage of the universe. Leaders, along with everyone else, are participants in this universal dance or exchange of energy, and by understanding this fact, they can deepen the meaning of their work and change efforts. Becoming aware of the wisdom guiding the universe is the first step in discerning meaning and value in the individual efforts of all who are contributing to the transformation.

7. Leaders need to seek out others who are committed to change and growth. Companionship on the journey of leadership is a great gift—but only if the companions are of the right kind. There are those who for some reason are committed to making the journey of life difficult and rocky. They want others to be in their condition. They obstruct the processes of transformation and suck the life out of the experience of leadership.

These people should be avoided. Leaders need as much support as they can get in doing the work of leadership. They should expect colleagues and friends to be as committed to personal and organizational transformation as they are. The work of leadership takes a lot of energy and demands the support of good people who can clarify the work and stimulate the person doing it. Leaders must seek out those who are themselves well motivated and can act to advance rather than limit the leadership role. Like-

> ### Key Point
>
> *Sometimes all that is possible is to embrace the mystery, the unknown, of a situation and allow it to be beyond reach or understanding for a while. Going with the flow of an experience helps position the leader to discern something different or new and advances the leader's insight and experience in a way that simply cannot be controlled or managed.*

wise, they must break their relationships with people who are somehow driven to try to discourage them or deflate their energy. The work is tough enough as it is.

8. The goal of leadership is to connect to the journey of transformation. When surrounded by the challenges of leadership, leaders can lose sight of the fact that change is normal and that people cannot keep from changing. The issue, thus, is not whether they will transform but how they will change and what condition they will be in at the end of the change cycle.

People can change by design or by default, and it is part of the leadership role to help them change by design—to guide them on the journey of transformation rather than let them be carried down the rapids. Working with people through their own tough times, however, can skew a leader's perceptions and obscure the fact that change is unavoidable. Therefore, leaders need to get away from their work occasionally or talk to colleagues in order to reaffirm their commitment to leading change and reestablish their connection with the journey and their vision of the future. Indeed, this is an essential part of leadership— staying grounded in transformation.

9. Judgment is an enemy to the spirit within. How many people have been sacrificed on the altar of judgment? Other than in courts of law, judgment is usually destructive. The appraisals that people make of their own activities are usually negative and have the effect of suppressing their creativity. The appraisals of others can be just as negative and just as counterproductive.

People's judgments reflect their feelings about what they are judging, and their judgments obviously are formed by their values and prejudices, fears and uncertainties. People rarely see things as they really are but instead make what they observe into shadows of their own biases. In addition, judgments about actions are often more concerned with the agents than with the actions themselves. An action or performance, for example, might be condemned just because the person who did it was assumed to be unskilled or inept or to lack the right to do it. Everything has value when seen in a valuable way. Even negative behavior can have meaning if it is understood.

> ## Point To Ponder
>
> *Judgment is always finally destructive. It puts up a barrier in consciousness that prevents leaders from seeing the potential at their disposal. It keeps them stuck in the present and the superficial, unable to dig to a deeper place where meaning resides and truth can be found.*

Leaders should avoid making their own judgments, about themselves or others, and should not seek out or pay attention to the judgments of others. They should instead try to see things within their actual context and from a perspective generated from within that context. Judgments are generally loaded with fear content, and fear disables and limits human responses and kills the creative urge. Leaders must do everything in their power to eliminate judgment to allow others to respond inventively to the demand for change.

> ### Group Discussion
>
> As a group, the participants brainstorm the ways in which judgment obstructs progress. They then brainstorm impeding judgments and place these on a flipchart. Their next task is to discuss possible approaches to use to prevent the various mechanisms of judgment from taking control of a leader's consciousness. Finally, the participants enumerate the characteristics of the judgment process, identify clues that someone is habitually making judgments and acting on them, and discuss ways in which the tendency to make judgments might be managed or avoided.

10. You can't love your creation if you don't love the creator. No person can love another in a healthy way if the person feels unloved or even without the right to be loved. This is as true for leaders as for anyone else. How many people have aspired to hold formal leadership positions because they are still seeking from others the love they could not get from their parents? How many actual leaders have a greater neediness than those they lead? How many are looking for satisfaction in the adulation and dependencies that can be accompaniments of the leadership role? How many leaders keep a tight rein out of the fear that they will lose control and no one will love them because they failed to do their job or cannot own the glory?

There are many who seek the leadership role not solely out of a desire to make a difference. Instead, they are there because of their own need to shine, to be noticed, and to get from their position what they could not get elsewhere: recognition, reward, and love. They do not realize that if they cannot find satisfaction within themselves, they will not find it in the leadership role either. Nor do they understand that they must first love themselves before they can expect to get from the role what it truly has to offer. Unfortunately, others often have to pay the price for their ignorance.

> **Point To Ponder**
>
> *You simply cannot love another for long if you cannot love yourself first.*

These 10 themes are the givens around which the leadership role is built. Consequently, they can serve as a personal template for leaders as they struggle to make sense of their role and find the center within that informs each of them about their own issues. In addition, leaders who embark on a spiritual exercise regimen of the sort described above can incorporate a personal assessment of the individual implications of these themes into their initial workouts (or periods of reflection).

BECOMING SELF

All creation is good. There is simply no other way to evaluate it. Life appears because it wants to. Life wants life. Life seeks fullness, expression, identity, emergence, and flowering. In every aspect of creation, it appears as though life wants to live. The evidence is to be found in all of its acts of self-creation, change, adaptation, and growth.

Life's drive toward self-organization is a fundamental feature of the universe, and it has operated from the beginning of existence as we know it. We simply needed the right science, the right moment, and the right perceptions to be able to grasp these facts.

Francisco Varela, a famous biologist, coined a term for life's creation of more life out of itself. He named this process *autopoiesis,* which means "self-formation." He affirmed that life is unique in having the ability to create itself—to continue to generate more life.

> **Key Point**
>
> *Life wants life. Life seeks fullness, expression, identity, emergence, and flowering. In every aspect of creation, it appears as though life wants to live. The evidence is to be found in all of its acts of self-creation, change, adaptation, and growth.*

The process of autopoiesis is continuous and cyclical. And it is generative in that life enlarges itself, growing the options and the potential and the fullness that make it what it has become at any moment in time. Life cannot stay the same. It complicates and diversifies itself, constantly becoming something more than it was.

The journey of life is an experience without boundaries. It moves in all directions and offers choice without limit. Once a selection has been made, however, boundaries emerge, forcing the selection to take form, to be lived fully in the form that it takes, expressing the reality that the selection now represents. Yet, paradoxically again, the boundaries themselves, while disciplining the selection into form and action, allow choice to move in a new direction and seek options that could not have arisen without the discipline imposed by the boundaries.

Each person must find the way into this mosaic of simplicity and complexity that best exemplifies the person's own journey. This self-referencing process, in which the discipline of choice requires living consistently with any selection made, operates at every level of the universe. For instance, the patterns or "habits" of role can appear anywhere, from the operation of scientific laws to the simplest routines of human behavior. This self-referencing also influences how we see the world, because it affects what our eyes see and what form our seeing will take in our lives. Our self-perception informs our world, not usually the other way around. We begin to create what makes sense to us, and the limits and permissibles embedded in our personal worldview create boundaries around whatever it is that supports our worldview.

Self-referencing tells us a lot about how we change, grow, and adapt at every level, from the personal to the societal to the systematic to the universal. As Teilhard de Chardin, the famous Jesuit paleontologist eloquently pointed out, we are co-creators of the universe, working in concert with the energies and forces of creation to engage with the requirement to keep creating. Each component of life is working within its parameters, intersecting with others, and interacting with the components it most directly touches. Together, all the components operate in a way that ultimately changes everything in an endless cycle of creativity and growth.

It is this paradox of boundary and intersection that is critical to the role of the leader. Nothing in life operates outside of this paradox. Each boundary intersects and interacts in a dynamic way with every other boundary in a dance that ultimately causes each of them to change. The energy of life comes out of this complex interaction of cross-secting boundaries moving in a constant flux of relationship that transforms each of them singly and collectively. Such are the physical laws of the universe and conditions under which leaders must act out their role.

Life evolves in a context of co-creation. No one acts independently of anyone else. Indeed, there is no real independence but only interdependence, and this fact gives both form and direction to the role of the leader. Leaders are always working to understand the interdependence of situations, circumstances, and people. They know that, in the workplace, everything has an impact on everything else. Yet, every person is acting out of his or her own space, doing the work that is expected. It is the aggregation of all of the elements of the work and the efforts of the workers that, when brought together, makes something sustainable happen.

Leaders live life in the white spaces—the boundary land—between people, places, and processes. They do their work in the context of the potential future to which the confluence of their efforts will ultimately lead. They read the signposts of the journey by identifying the elements of the journey and the forces that, when aggregated, tell the story of direction and process. At the same time, they are working to evolve, to respond to the demand for personal change. In short, they are managing both the journey and their personal experience of it.

Each member of the organization must be able to do the same thing. The main leadership task is to make it possible for all members to have an awareness of this work, know its implications for their personal journey and the collective journey, and respond to the demand for change by applying their creativity.

The leaders of an organization must also see the undercurrent of linkage that exists every place in the organization. To achieve this goal, they need to be highly receptive and be able to hear the sounds of the universe in the language of persons, movement, and self.

LISTENING FOR THE SOUNDS OF CHANGE

Perhaps the most important and, at the same time, most difficult skills for a leader to obtain are listening skills, including those needed to hear the sounds of direction and change. We are always getting ready to speak or respond even as we listen to someone else talk. In short, much of the time we are not really listening.

To exercise good leadership, leaders must listen from the very core of their being. They must listen to the sounds of change and to the more spiritual sounds of life, hearing themes as well as words, seeing intent as well as message, determining direction as well as impression. Listening deeply is essential for adapting to the vagaries of the journey and meeting its challenges. By being able to hear themes and undercurrents, leaders are able to anticipate events and take the right action at the right time.

No one can listen deeply without preparation and development of their listening skills. Leaders must assess their level of attention to the words and actions of others as well as their focus on the ebbs and flows of the work. They must ask themselves about their readiness to respond to the issues affecting health care and their ability to detect the trends, including economic trends, that will impact its future.

Deep listening comprises contextual listening and content listening (Exhibit 10–6). Both are critical. The purpose of contextual listening is to become aware of the surrounding circumstances—the external events that affect what work people do and what resources are available to them. The purpose of content listening is to hear what people are saying, understand what it means, and grasp its implications. The deep listener listens to content while maintaining an awareness of the context, at the same time recognizing that what people say is always influenced by their beliefs, experience, perspectives, and prejudices.

Exhibit 10–6 Contextual and Content Listening

Contextual Listening	Content Listening
• Circumstances	• The message
• Conditions	• Components
• Framework	• Players
• Environment	• Truth
• External factors	• Perception
	• Issues

Listening with a broad frame of reference provides the listener with an accuracy gauge—a way of placing what is seen and heard within a context that validates, challenges, or alters its meaning.

Leaders develop an inner ear through reflection and self-awareness. They must understand their own perspectives and perceptions—those things that might skew their ability to hear with openness and acuity—to hear the voices of others accurately. If leaders cannot hear their own notions, values, fears, and prejudices and give them a language and a place in the journey, they will be unable to incorporate incoming information into their knowledge base, undermining their ability to lead effectively.

> **Key Point**
>
> *It is important not only to listen to the words of the message but to listen for the intent, value, passion, focus of the message, and the speaker's relationship to what he or she is communicating. By listening deeply, the listener gets the message and the meaning as well.*

Leaders who have not yet done deep spiritual and personal work will still have filters in place that adjust messages from the outside to their comfort level or even block messages that are not congruent with their beliefs and values. By modifying what is heard, these filters reduce the leaders' ability—and the ability of the entire organization—to respond appropriately and effectively to the messages.

By using their inner ear to access their beliefs and attitudes, leaders can become alert to the same dynamic going on in others. They can then perceive more completely the struggles, uncertainty, barriers, and challenges embedded in the utterances they hear and also understand better how information is received and used by the staff as they attempt to deal with the realities affecting their own work and relationships.

Spending time in quiet self-reflection is a proven way of enhancing one's ability to listen deeply. If leaders can get past their self-constructed barriers to self-knowledge, they will be able to see behind the words, read into the language, and look beyond the present, all gifts that, among other things, will help then create a more accurate profile of the issues they face.

FINDING SPIRIT IN THE CHAOS

Art and nature have always had an impact on the human spirit. The culminating beauty of a mountain vista or a symphony orchestra has the power to move the spirit and bring great contentment. Yet each of those is the fractal image of smaller units of what would otherwise be seen as chaos. Imagine looking at the mangle of the infrastructure of a forest or listening to each individual instrument playing its own music. Clearly, only when the elements of the forest or the symphony aggregate can the beauty of the collective intersections be revealed and fully enjoyed.

It is the ability to see the whole and recognize its beauty that inspires the spirit and deepens the character. Further, although the art of Mandelbrot sets (mosaics created when aggregated chaos reveals the order within) can be enjoyed to a degree, the addition of human consciousness, as occurs in the art of the human spirit, intensifies the experience and raises the level of appreciation.

The human story and the art and spirit of life are filled with metaphors, contradictions, challenges, myths, and created scenarios. Using patterns of self-similarity and self-discord, artists and mystics are creating in ways that stimulate, challenge, and resonate with our humanity. By experiencing these convergent and divergent realities, we can fathom our connection to each other and to the universe and can grow in ways that intensify and enrich our lives.

The art of chaos can also have an impact on the way in which leaders address uncertainty, diversity, and variability. Leaders must come to prize divergent and convergent realities at the same time. Suspending the expectation to see order right away is the first step toward appreciating what complexity has to offer. By looking broadly at problems and opportunities, leaders can understand what they are and what they entail, whereas examining them too closely would obscure their meaning. Standing on the balcony of experience gives leaders the chance to observe both actions and their context and to perceive a reality that might otherwise make no sense.

The ability to see things broadly, one of the foundations of wisdom, takes time to acquire. It is only after observing enough from the balcony that leaders can develop the depth of insight and understanding needed to put everything into its proper context. Leaders, like other people, frequently get stuck in their own experience and are co-opted by their attachment to it, making it impossible for them to place it in a broader frame. By keeping unattached to any particular position, leaders can see every event, situation, or issue from outside and can also link it to other elements of the system invisible from inside. There is no indictment intended here of the perspective of those inside an issue, for example. The point is to celebrate the distance and wisdom of the leader coming from the outside and thus able to place the issue into a context that gives it meaning.

The ability of leaders to operate in this way is enhanced by personal work directed toward putting life in perspective—that is, seeing it as part of a chaotic and complex world (Figure 10–5). Spending time reflecting on the mystery of life and integrating this fact into their lives gives leaders a firm center and leaves them confident and composed.

We have, all of us, seen leaders of this type and observed with interest and not a little awe how balanced they appear, even in the midst of a notable crisis. Their ability to see around, through, or beyond the crisis inspires us, especially when their insight stands the test of time. Having gained a deeper perspective (really, a broader one), these leaders show how everything, even a crisis, fits into the multiplicity that is life and experience.

THE COMPENSATIONS OF IGNORANCE

Paradoxes and koans are forever there to challenge each of us in our certainty. There is clearly more that we do not understand than there is that we know. Much of what is written in this book, while true at our current level of understanding, will soon enough be no longer true. The authors can recall the commitment they brought to previous books and the energy with which they articulated the truth of the time, only to note how much has changed and how little of what was written 20 years ago is as true today.

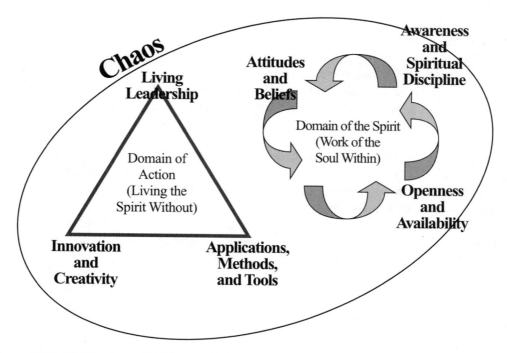

Figure 10–5 The Realms of Spirit within the Chaos

Still, every generation, through its work, builds the foundation for the next. No work is an end in itself; no process or experience simply comes to a dead halt. Each piece is part of the mosaic of revelation that got us to today and will get us to tomorrow. This longer term perspective must inform the leadership role. Even in the midst of a vital crisis or critical life event, leaders must use the fabric of complexity to put the circumstances in a larger frame of reference, for this frame of reference better reflects the reality of the time than do the experiences and stresses of the event itself. It is so easy for leaders to get sucked into an event and allow it to become the center of their reality, losing all sense of its place in the course of events.

Koans keep us from putting temporal and spatial boundaries around our lives and experience. They invalidate our parameters. The minute something makes sense to us or becomes clear, the intersections of our clarity take us back into the chaos to the next level of intellectual or perceptual challenge. Rather than a negative, this feature of reality keeps us always on the edge of creativity and discovery. It also reminds us that there is no place to rest (at least for very long) and nothing that is an end in itself.

The challenge for leaders and others lies in the engagement with the flow of life. If religious or intellectual beliefs become strongly entrenched, they can serve as the barriers to subsequent discoveries, insights, or revelations. As has been said, truth is a journey, not an event. It is a lived dynamic, not simply a fact of life.

None of us can know everything. Even those of us who are well educated come to understand how little we know of all that is knowable. Further, our quest for knowledge is a delusion if we think of knowledge as a thing. Knowledge is not a thing but rather a dynamic—a revelation bound up in the time and circumstances that make it available. Although it is valuable, knowledge is not an end in itself. Nor is it ever complete. In mathematics, when equations are carried out to the third decimal, they reveal a particular product. When carried out to the sixth decimal, they reveal a different product. This process can continue ad infinitum.

> **Point To Ponder**
>
> *Truth is a journey, not an event. Honor those who are seeking truth, avoid those who have found it.*

In decision making, the issue is not the total quantity of information possessed but whether there is enough information to make a decision. In no case will more information eliminate all of the risk associated with choosing. Indeed, the collection of information can be pursued for so long that any action that would have been effective becomes untimely.

Leaders must recognize that the leadership role is rife with risk, just like every other aspect of life. The demands of the time are part of a broader canvas that resists comprehension, and every decision sends into motion effects that will never fully be known.

In considering a particular decision, leaders need to be concerned about two things: Is it the right decision for the time, and does it set a direction that fits the circumstances of the journey? In short, do the signposts appear to validate the decision? If they do, that is the best indicator that the decision is the correct one. After all, the overarching goal is to make decisions that, over time,

> **Key Point**
>
> *For leaders, the issue is not how much information they have but how much they need in order to act. No amount of information will eliminate all risk, and beyond a certain point gathering more information will reduce not the risk, but the timeliness of any action taken.*

take the organization and everyone in it to a better place where knowledge and the quality of life are advanced. Thomas Edison made 90 attempts before the light bulb went on. After which failed attempt should he have stopped? All 90 were necessary to the journey of light, and we can be thankful for every one of them.

MYSTERY

For leaders today, perhaps their most notable need is to be re-enchanted by a sense of mystery. In every area of life, the more questions get answered, the more questions get raised. Indeed, the explicit lesson of chaos and complexity is the profound inscrutability of it all.

Despite the advances of science and the discoveries of medicine, we still are largely in the dark about the nature of the universe and the things that it contains. The billion-dollar effort to decipher the human genetic code was a seminal event in the course of human history. Of course, besides finally revealing the code, what it did was to open the door to a whole new project: identifying the billion or so proteones that do the work of the genes and discovering how the genes perform their myriad tasks through these proteones. Collating and codifying the proteones will be a tremendous undertaking, yet it is the work demanded by the revelations of the genome project. One level of complexity leads to an even deeper and broader level of complexity.

Wherever there is progress, there is a temptation to become arrogant and controlling. We are easily lured into thinking that what we are doing is magnificent and grand—that we are creating the future of humanity. Because we know so much, we become deluded by our knowledge, giving it more credence and more importance than it merits. If history has taught us anything, it is that we are essentially ignorant. That is to say, what is unknown is infinitely greater than the combined knowledge we humans have garnered on our short journey through time.

In the United States, our enthusiasm and egotism often insulate us from the depths of our ignorance. Being so busy making discoveries and applying them in different and exciting ways, we have little time to set aside for contemplating the fathomless mysteries that remain and feeling awe at the very small part we play in the unfolding of the universe. It is this awe for the unknown, this respect for the mystery of life, that is so important to leaders in the midst of the chaos of transformation. Leaders need to be able to put their efforts into perspective as the Industrial Age gives way to a new age—one filled with promise but, as of yet, lacking much substance.

> ### Point To Ponder
>
> *The wonderful thing about mystery is that it relieves us of the obligation to know everything. It allows us to appreciate the uncertain, the unformed, indeed, the journey of life. Mystery opens us up to discernment and discovery and moves us away from definition and control. It deepens our appreciation for the experience of life rather than the management of life.*

Leaders today, besides regaining a sense of mystery themselves, face the additional challenge of deepening the appreciation of staff for the chaos and complexity that pervade the universe. They can do this by engaging with change directly and exemplifying in their behavior an awareness of the mystery in all movement. By not knowing, by not having all the answers, by being uncertain and exploring alternatives, leaders demonstrate their vulnerability to the effects of complexity. They also create a safe space for staff to express their own uncertainty, discomfort, anxiety, and excitement. A further consequence is that leaders and staff together, through their appreciation for the mystery of their journey, will come to realize that they are about important things—that they are all participating in a larger project as co-creators and that what they do makes a difference, sometimes apparent, at other times unknown, but an inexorable difference nonetheless. And this is the centerpiece of the mystery.

SYNTHESIS AND SYNERGY

Finally, leaders need to be reminded that the work of leadership itself is filled with mystery. We have all done apparently unimportant things that, we later discovered, had a profound impact on someone else. In some secret way, quietly and steadily, our words or actions thoroughly changed that person's life. Caught up in the moment, a leader might see an act as inconsequential—and as a single act it might be. When connected to some other reality, it can take on a new form and new dimensions and significantly impact another's life.

Spiritual forces are embedded in all reality, and mystery is present in all aspects of life. Everywhere, unknown influences, relationships, and intersections exist just beneath the surface of the actual and operate synergistically to continue the movement of change. Because some of these have no form or are not yet perceived, their effects can sometimes be traumatic. As part of their role, leaders are always looking for the unseen, the intersections, the goodness of fit between the elements of chaos and change. By looking for the linkages and connections, reading the signposts of the journey, looking within or behind motives, they are able to give language to the experience and the journey. Being disciplined to see the whole and to distinguish the contribution that the whole makes to the parts and vice versa, they are in a position to appreciate the greater mystery to which everything relates, to be awed by its implications and moved by its inscrutability.

> **Point To Ponder**
>
> *The imagery of complexity pervades the world, from artwork to zebras. The order embedded in complexity—an order made visible as a mosaic of intersections and interactions—reflects the synthesis and seamlessness of creation and the connections within and between everything.*

There are always missing pieces. We may be tempted to think that by discovering those pieces we will unravel the ultimate secrets of the universe and will know everything we need to know. Of course, this is just plain foolishness. Every secret unlocked reveals a host of new secrets not yet addressed—meaning that the process of discovery is endless. Understanding this, leaders see and experience their role as the journey it really is. All of the parts of the journey intersect in visible and invisible ways, and the array of interactions and intersections necessary to the experience of life is also the work of life and the raw material for the work of leadership.

Operating within the context of their own journey, facilitating the experiences of others, and finding and defining the relationships between the elements and forces of movement and change, leaders are faced with the challenge of seeking and seeing the synergies that will allow them to pursue their work and support the collective work of the organization. In harnessing these synergies, they represent for everyone in the organization the action of creation, complete engagement with life, and the full embrace of the mystery of complexity.

> **Key Point**
>
> *Any knowledge that we gain forms the foundation for the next mystery. Inscrutability will outrun understanding as long as there is life.*

REFERENCES

de Bono, E. 1996. *Masterthinker*. New York: New Star Media.

Wheatley, M. 1992. *Leadership and the new science*. San Francisco: Berrett-Koehler.

SUGGESTED READINGS

Anderson, T. 1997. *Transforming leadership*. Boca Raton, FL: St. Lucie Press.

Arnold, W., and J. Plas. 1993. *The human touch*. New York: Wiley.

Barnum, B. 1995. Spirituality in nursing. *Nursing Leadership Forum* 1, no. 1: 24–30.

Clegg, B. 2000. *Creativity and innovation for managers*. Philadelphia: Butterworth-Heinemann.

Etzioni, A. 1993. *The spirit of community*. New York: Crown.

Fulmer, W. 2000. *Shaping the adaptive organization: Landscapes, learning and leading in volatile times*. Chicago: AMACOM.

Halil, W., ed. 1999. *The infinite resource*. San Francisco: Jossey-Bass.

Hawley, J. 1993. *Reawakening the spirit in work*. San Francisco: Berrett-Koehler.

Jacobsen, M.E. 1999. *Liberating everyday genius*. New York: Ballentine.

Jaworski, J. 1996. *Synchronicity: The inner path of leadership*. San Francisco: Berrett-Koehler.

Lappé, F.M., and P.M. Du Bois. 1994. *The quickening of America: Rebuilding our nation, remaking our lives*. San Francisco: Jossey-Bass.

Leider, R. 1997. *The power of purpose*. San Francisco: Berrett-Koehler.

Leonard, D. 1998. *Wellspring of knowledge*. Boston: Harvard Business School Publishing.

Lindin, W., and K. Lindin. 1993. *The healing manager*. San Francisco: Berrett-Koehler.

Quinn, R. 1996. *Deep change: Discovering the leader within*. San Francisco: Jossey-Bass.

Sen, A. 1999. *Development as freedom*. New York: Knopf.

Tiller, W. 1997. *Science and human transformation: Subtle energies, intentionality and consciousness*. San Francisco: Jossey-Bass.

Quiz Questions

Select the best answer for each of the following questions.

1. Most great leaders can recall a time when:

    a. situations made them what they became
    b. all greatness was simply chance and mystery
    c. they felt a deep call within to leadership
    d. they thought that leadership was simply learned

2. The spiritually focused leader emphasizes the importance of:

    a. the here and now
    b. the longer and more distant road
    c. keeping focused on the emerging issues
    d. only focusing on the future

3. Chaos is always the route to:

    a. order
    b. complexity
    c. uncertainty
    d. mystery

4. We all participate in each other's evolution because:

    a. all things are ultimately interconnected
    b. the universe acts independently on all other creation
    c. we have been made masters of creation
    d. genomics shows that we are essentially the same

5. Creativity is expressed in:

    a. art and music only
    b. the scientific process
    c. politics and society
    d. symbols and images

6. There is virtually nothing about fear that is:

    a. unnecessary
    b. redeeming
    c. invalid
    d. just

7. Exercising the spirit requires:

    a. prayer
    b. a fixed approach
    c. a regular routine
    d. a guru

8. According to the 10 spiritual rules of leadership, leaders must have the ability to:

    a. point in the proper direction
    b. see all issues with clarity
    c. embrace the needs of others
    d. take risks

9. A major enemy of the spirit within is:

    a. anger with others
    b. the tendency to make judgments
    c. lack of regular reflection
    d. lack of strong relationships

10. A fundamental tenet of the universe is that:
a. all life is self-organizing
b. all things can ultimately be understood
c. all action is rational
d. all change is impermanent

11. There is no more important ability for leaders to develop than the ability to:
a. direct
b. act
c. listen
d. take risks

12. Leaders, for those they lead, represent:
a. the respect for the mystery that is present in all aspects of life
b. the hardships that attend every action
c. the challenges that arise out of all action
d. the internal logic that guides all creation

Quiz Answers

**CHAPTER 1—A NEW VESSEL FOR LEADERSHIP:
NEW RULES FOR A NEW AGE**

1(d), 2(b), 3(a), 4(b), 5(a), 6(d), 7(c), 8(c), 9(a), 10(b)

**CHAPTER 2—THRIVING IN COMPLEXITY:
TEN PRINCIPLES FOR LEADERS IN THE COMING AGE**

1(d), 2(b), 3(a), 4(a), 5(c), 6(d), 7(b), 8(c), 9(c), 10(a), 11(b), 12(d)

**CHAPTER 3—THE LEADER AS PEACEMAKER:
MANAGING THE CONFLICTS OF A MULTIFOCAL WORKPLACE**

1(c), 2(b), 3(a), 4(d), 5(c), 6(b), 7(a), 8(a), 9(b), 10(d)

**CHAPTER 4—LIVING LEADERSHIP:
VULNERABILITY, RISK TAKING, AND STRETCHING**

1(d), 2(a), 3(d), 4(b), 5(b), 6(c), 7(c), 8(a), 9(b), 10(c)

CHAPTER 5—HEALING BROKENNESS: ERROR AS OPPORTUNITY

1(c), 2(c), 3(d), 4(c), 5(a), 6(d), 7(b), 8(b), 9(a), 10(a)

CHAPTER 6—EMOTIONAL COMPETENCE: A VITAL LEADERSHIP SKILL

1(b), 2(a), 3(d), 4(b), 5(c), 6(a), 7(d), 8(a), 9(d), 10(a), 11(c)

**CHAPTER 7—TOXIC ORGANIZATIONS AND PEOPLE:
THE LEADER AS TRANSFORMER**

1(a), 2(a), 3(b), 4(d), 5(b), 6(c), 7(a), 8(d), 9(d), 10(a), 11(a), 12(b)

**CHAPTER 8—TRANSFORMATIONAL COACHING:
LEADING THE MEMBERSHIP COMMUNITY**

1(c), 2(d), 3(a), 4(b), 5(b), 6(b), 7(d), 8(c), 9(c), 10(a), 11(a), 12(b), 13(c)

**CHAPTER 9—THE LEADER'S COURAGE TO BE WILLING:
BUILDING A CONTEXT FOR HOPE**

1(c), 2(a), 3(d), 4(b), 5(b), 6(d), 7(a), 8(c), 9(d)

**CHAPTER 10—THE NEW SPIRIT OF LEADERSHIP:
BECOMING A LIVING LEADER**

1(c), 2(b), 3(a), 4(a), 5(d), 6(b), 7(c), 8(d), 9(b), 10(a), 11(c), 12(a)

Index

A

Accident, 162
Accountability, 105, 171, 180, 251–252,
    260–264, 292
Action, 104–106
    learning tools, 271
Actual reality, 43–44
Adaptability, 268, 270
Adaptation, 352–353
    continuous, 285, 286
Adverse event, 162
Advocacy, 241–242
Agenda for action, 104
Aggregation, 55, 69–75
Agility, 320
Agreement, formalizing, 110
American College of Physicians, 160
Antagonism, 96–99, 314
Antisocial behavior, 236–237
Argyris, Chris, 267
ARIA
    action, 104–106
    antagonism, 96–99
    invention, 101–104
    resonance, 99–101
Attitude, 212
Authority structure, 229–231
Autocatalysis, 14
Autopoiesis, 14
Awareness, 309
Axelrod, Alan, 174, 311

B

Balance, 199, 212–213, 225–228, 239–240,
    321–322
Barker, Richard A., 207
Behavior, 111–113
    assessment, 193
    management, 244
    value-adding, 252–253
Berwick, Donald, 160
Biotherapeutics, 17
Blame, 95–96, 97–98, 152–153
Bohm, Roger, 293
Boredom, 321
Breakdown, 162
Breathing, deep, 346–347
Burn out, 317

C

Career
    entrapment, 234, 235–236
    entrenchment, 234, 250
Care provider disenfranchisement, 161
Caring, 323–324
Caring for self, 350–351
Caucusing, 110
Challenge, 352
Champions, 280
Change, 6–7, 36–37, 42, 288, 352–353
    complexity, 67–70
    dynamics of, 289

Change—*continued*
  leading, 9–13
  openness to, 309
  opportunities for, 133–134
  service patterns, 169–170
  sounds of, 357–358
Chaos, 26–28, 64. *See also* Complexity
  diversity and, 56–58
  language, 14
  leadership call and, 330–333
  route to order, 336–337
  spirit in, 358–359
  understanding, 43–46
Character, 201
Charter development, 278–279
Chemotherapeutics, 17
Child within, 339–340
Chunking, 54
Clarity, 282–283
Cleveland, Harlan, 125
Clockware, 24
Clumping, 55
Coaching, 130–131, 276–277
  innovation, 281–285
  upward, 209
Co-creation, 336, 356
Cognition, 192
Collective mindfulness, 137,
      141–142
Communication, 109
  open, 83, 142–145
  technique, 112
  technology, 2
Community
  consciousness, 243
  culture, 50
Companionship, 353
Compassion, 195–196
Compensation, 104
Competence, 192
  emotional, 187–217
Complexity
  adding value, 52–54
  change, 67–70
  communication, 137–141
  creation and, 58–60
  disequilibrium, 64–67

diversity, 56–58
equilibrium, 64–67
image of, 363
language, 14
leader's focus, 274
local health care, 49–52
revolution, 69–75
simple systems and, 54–56
system functions, 60–63
thriving in, 41–43
understanding, 43–46
whole of parts, 46–49
Component-centered behavior, 62
Component systems, 55–56
Computer chip, 5
Concerns, defining, 109
Conflict, 57–58
  sources of, 81
  unresolved, 91
Conflict management, 79–80
  avoiding unnecessary, 82–89
  growth and, 80–82
  identity-based conflict, 89–96
  transformation and, 80–82
Confucius, 307
Conspiracy, 279
Control, 118
Control design, 5
Coordinated behavior, 127
Courage, 306–308, 350
Creative fruits, 285
Creativity, 334–337
  child within, 339–340
  core negativity, 343–345
  environment for, 130
  error and, 58–69
  expression of, 341
  fear and, 341–343
  innovation and, 337–345
  opening, 340–341
  requisites of, 338
  source of, 339
Creator, 354–355
Cultural alterations
  changes, 295
  strategic approaches, 294
  tactical methods of, 293–294

Culture, 12–13
  corporate, 243
  importance of, 51–52

D

Deadlines, 295
de Chardin, Teilhard, 356
Decision making, 69, 207
Decision tree, 5
Dehumanization, 175–177
Demands, impossible, 180–181
Demeanor, 112
Department of Labor, Bureau of Labor
     Statistics, 317
Developmental freeze, 176–177
Devil's advocate, 212
Devolution, 121
Diagnostics, 18
Dialogue, 273, 275
Differences, human, 94–96
Differentiation, 103
Discernment, 55
Discipline, 163–164
Disequilibrium, 64–67
Dishonesty, 238–239
Dissipative leadership, 190
Dissipative structures, 14
Diversity, 56–58, 95, 132–133, 233, 309
Dogma, 311–313
Double-loop learning, 270
Downsizing, 319–320
Dreyfus and Dreyfus skill acquisition model, 209
Drucker, Peter, 28
Dyer, Wayne, 200
Dysfunction, 226–227, 251

E

Ego, absence of, 120
Elizabeth I, 138
Emergent leadership, 189
Emotion, 192
Emotional competence, 187–188
  benefits of, 203–209
  character, 201
  development of, 209–213

holism, 188–189
incompetent behaviors, 212–213
integrity, 202
intelligence, 201
leadership, 189–191
leadership risks, 202–203
measurement of, 216–218
motivation, 189
nature of, 191–202
nonverbal, 197–198
team, 213–216
Empathy, 201
Employee
  dysfunction screening, 251
  needs, 314–315
  unmotivated, 233–236
Employment
  insecurity, 203
  skill sets, 2–3
Empowerment, 248
Enlightenment Age, 7
Equilibrium, 64–67
Error
  care provider disenfranchisement, 161
  creation and, 58–60
  disclosure, 160–161
  excellence and, 157–158
  foolishness and, 153–154
  health care providers and, 156
  inevitability of, 152–153
  learning from, 342
  mandatory reporting of, 159–160
  opportunities, 151–152, 161–164
    dehumanization, 175–177
    failure to own products, 170–173
    failure to shift services, 165–170
    impossible demands, 180–181
    providers as capital, 177–180
  perfection expectation, 156–157
  public reaction to, 158–159
  recognizing, recovering from, 154–156
  remediation vs. discipline, 163–164
  tolerating, 212
Evolution, 266–267, 337
Excellence, 157–158
Exercising spirit
  cooling down, 348

Exercising spirit—*continued*
  focusing, 347–348
  quiet, 348–349
  routine, 346–348
  stretching, 345–346, 347
Expectations, 282
Experimentation, 284–285
Experts, use of, 113

F

Facilitator, 26
Failure to thrive, 269
Fear, 101, 341–343
Feedback, 202–203
Fiber optics, 8
Fit, 55, 56
Follett, Mary Parker, 134
Foolishness, 153–154
Ford, Henry, 169
Fractals, 13–14, 25–26
Fragmented leadership, 173
Future, journey into, 45

G

Game playing, 88
Global consciousness, 243
Goal setting, 83, 105, 351–352
Growth, 80–82

H

Health care, 156
  local nature of, 49–52
  team-based, 170
  technological change and, 15–16
  value-based, 168–169
Health services deconstruction, 34
Heterarchy, 5
Heterogeneity, 57
Hidden agendas, 88–89, 110
Hierarchy, 5, 284
Hilfilker, David, 156
Hiring
  bonuses, 177
  focused, 204–205

Hock, Dee, 145
Holism, 188–189
Holographic leadership, 63, 173–175
Hope, context for, 300–301
Horizontal organization, 48, 265
Huang, Chungliang Al, 240

I

Identity-based conflict, 89–91
  ARIA, 96–106
  finding differences, 94–96
  parties in, 91–92
  relationship establishment, 96
  time, patience, 92–93
  trust building, 93–94
Identity characteristics, 92
Impulse control, 200
Inconsistence, 238–239
Individual errors, 161–162
Industrial Age, 2–4, 5, 7, 9, 20–22, 28, 63, 118, 131
Information
  availability, 42
  conflict, 85
  essential, 87–88
  exchange, 112–113
Information Age. *See* Technology Age
Innovation, 55, 337–345
  coaching, 281–285
  way of life, 282
Inspirational behavior, 125–126
Institute of Medicine, 156, 159
Institutions, 47
Integration
  elements of, 288
  leadership, 190–191
  making work, 285–290
Integrity, 202
Intelligence, 192, 201, 262
Interaction conflict, 85
Interactions, 60–63, 73–74
Interdependency, 22, 32–33, 275
Interest-based conflict, 86, 92, 93, 106–111
  resolution process, 107
  resolution stages, 108
Interests, 102
Internet, 7, 16–17, 134

Intersections, 60–63
Interventions, 106–107
Interviewing, 206, 251
Invention, 101–104

J

Journaling, 340
Joy, 334
Judgment, 123–124, 353–354

K

Kellner-Rogers, 126
Kelly, Kevin, 24, 46, 55, 57
Knowledge, 42, 120–122, 129–131
Koans, 359–361
Kouzes, 132

L

Lateral thinking, 61
Leadership
  call to, 330–333
  effectiveness, 191
  fragmented, 173
  holographic, 173–175
  models, 2–4, 20–21
  types of, 189–191
Leader, tasks of, 19
Learning, 277
  continuous, 313–314
  organization, 267–271
  scenarios, 294
Life journey, 355–356
Linear thinking, 13, 60–61
Listening, 246, 357–358
  critical, 138
Longest, Beaufort, 172
Lundin, Kathleen, 228, 241, 243
Lundin, William, 228, 241, 243
Lynch, Jerry, 240

M

Machiavelli, 307
Mainstream activity, 289–281

Maps, 268
Marketplace practice, 166–167
Mediation, 109–111
Medical therapies, 11
Meeting
  open, 143, 144
  setting, schedule, 112
  time, location of, 144
Mental boundaries, 135
Mental fitness, 318–320
Mentoring, 130–131
  toxic, 237–238
Middle Ages, 7
Mindfulness, 197
Miniaturization, 8
Mintzberg, Henry, 23
Mistakes, 59, 162. *See also* Error
  inevitability of, 152–153
Momentum, maintenance of, 104
Money, 284
Motivation, 37, 189, 201, 207
Mutual appreciation, 89
Mystery, 361–362

N

Needs, 102–103
Needs management, 181–182
Negativity, 94, 343–345
Negroponte, Nicholas, 46
Network, informal, 28–29
New age, 1–2. *See also* Technology age
  organizational levels in, 72
  seven imperatives, 16
Newtonian principles, 2, 4–5, 6, 18–19, 57,
  313
Nightingale, Florence, 324
Nonverbal communication, 197–198
Nut Island, 216

O

O'Keeffe, Georgia, 341
Openness, 194, 309
Opportunity, 336
Optimism, passionate, 198
Options, 17

Organization
   chart, 47
   consciousness, 243
   levels, 72
   models, 5
Orientation, outside information, 207
Outcome, 15, 21
Outpatient treatments, 18
Outside assistance, 293
Overtime, mandatory, 232–233

P

Pace, 2
Paradigmatic moment, 69
Paradox, 27–28, 359–361
Partnerships, 17
Passion, 308
   balance and, 199
   optimism, 198
Patching, 295
Patience, 279
Patient focus, 322
Patient-provider relationship, 17
Pearson, Carol, 155
Perfection expectation, 156–157
Performance, 53
Performance Measurement Matrix, 128–129
Personal boundaries, 135
Personal life, 239–240
Pharmacotherapeutics, 17
Planning, 22–24
   for error, 60
   succession, 205–206
Playing field expansion, 103–104
Point of service, 29, 31, 48, 50–52, 67–68, 69
POLICE acronym, 3
Political competency, 322–323
Political skills, 172–173
Porter-O'Grady, Tim, 245
Positioning, 98
Possibility, 336
Posturing, 98
Potential reality, 44
Power, 120–122
   abuse of, 232–233
   issues, 89

Prayer, 352
Presence, 196–197
Prioritizing, 109, 294
Privacy, 134–136
Problem definition, 105
Problem solving, 275, 290–292
   tool chest, 294
Process design, 5
Product ownership, 170–173
Productivity, 206–209, 317–318, 319
Profitability, 169
Projection, 99
Purpose, 53

Q

Quality initiatives, 316
Quantum rules
   balance, 24–26
   change, 36–37
   chaos, paradox, 27–28
   competition and, 32–33
   health care, 15–16
   health care timing, 17–18
   informal network, 28–29
   interdependence, 22
   leadership changes, 18–20
   leadership models, 20–21
   planning, 22–24
   relational thinking, 13
   structure, 13–15
   swarmware, clockware, 24
   system linkage, 29–31
   time compression, 33–35
   work value, 15
Quantum theory, 5–7
Quantum thinking, 19–20
Questioning, 138–140, 154
Quiet spiritual exercise, 348–349

R

Randomness, error and, 59–60
Reality, 6–7
   actual vs. potential, 44
   new, 127–128
Recognition, 231–232

Reflection, 334–335
Reflexive reframing, 99–100
Regulation, external, 171–173
Reinforcement, 270–271
Relational design, 5
Relational thinking, 13
Relationship
    building, 289
    consciousness, 243
    management, 263
    new, 131–137
    skills, 136–137
    Technology Age, 132
Relaxation
    balance, 212–213
    imbalance, 239–240
Reluctance qualities, 307
Remediation, 163–164
Reputation assessment, 217
Resiliency, 126, 198–199
Resolution process, 95–96, 107–109
Resonance, 99–101
Resources, 276
Resources management, 181–182
Respect, 249
    lack of, 233
Responsibility, 260–264
Revaluation, 177–180
Revolution, 69–75, 266–267
    argument for, 278
Revolutionary, leader as, 277–281
Rewards, 177, 231–232
Rilke, Rainer Maria, 136
Risk, 28, 60
    emotional competence, 202–203
    taking, 118, 124–126
Rothman, 89–90, 96

S

Safety, 162
Schroedinger's Box, 7, 43
Secretan, Lance, 130
Selectivity, 291–292
Self-awareness, 193–194, 201, 243–245, 260
Self-control, 200, 201, 309, 334–337
Self-disclosure, 136

Self-esteem consciousness, 243
Selflessness, 321
Service decisions, 69
Simplicity, 67
Social skill, 201
Socrates, 217
Solutions, 110
Spiritual boundaries, 135
Spiritual discipline, 331–332
Spiritual intelligence, 349–350
Spiritual journey, 351
Spiritual rules, 350–355
Spiritual warm-up, 347
Stability, 64
Staff
    messages, 283
    ratios, 176
Staffing
    accountability, 180
    evidence-based, 178–179
    patient needs, 179–180
    patient outcomes and, 178
    revaluation of, 177–180
Statement of objectives, 102
Strange attractor, 14
Strategy, 279
Stress, 226–227
Stretching, 118, 126–127
Structural conflict, 83–86
Structural integrity, 32–33
Structural supports, 289–290
Structure, 13–15, 25, 50, 69
Success, 280
Survival, 243
Sustainable change, 269
Sustainable solutions, 275
Sustainable value, 54
Sutcliffe, Kathleen, 198
Swarmware, 24
Syndication, 145–147
    business in, 146
Synergy, 362–363
Synthesis, 55, 362–363
System, 47, 48
    components of, 61–62
    context of, 74–75
    decisions, 69

System—*continued*
errors, 161–162
functions, 60–63
linkage, 29–31
simplicity, 54–56

T

Taguchi rule, 68–69
Talent, experimenting, 284–285
Taylor, Frederick, 2
Team
conflict, 87–89
decisions, 69
dysfunction, 215–216
emotional competence, 213–216
health care and, 170
leader, 211, 277
managing needs and resources, 181–182
Technology, 43
Technology Age, 1–2, 7, 9, 131
lateral thinking in, 61
Tension, 64–67
Thinking, critical, 140–141
Time
balancing, 320–322
compression, 33–35
importance of, 288–289
lack of, 273–277
Tinkering, 124
Toxic behavior, 228–229
authority structure, 229–231
minimizing principles, 242–253
reward, recognition, 231–232
Toxic organizations, 223–225
sources of, 230
Toxic stereotypes, 238
Transformation, 10, 72–73, 80–82, 243, 249–250, 353
causes of, 266
coaching, 259–260
cycle, 8
dynamics, 9
learning and, 290
mission of, 283
organizing for, 272–273
personal elements of, 287
worker, 264–266

Transition, 7–9
Treatment, unfair, inequitable, 87
Triage, 293–294
Trust, building, 93–94, 109, 309
Truth, 247

U

Ueland, Brenda, 341
Uncertainty, 94
Uniqueness, 88
Unit decisions, 69
Unmotivated leader, 37

V

Vagueness, 87
Value, 207
action and, 245–246
adding, 52–54, 252–253
conflict, 84
focus on, 309
knowledge, 194–195
sustainable, 54
what is, 167–168
Value-based health care, 168–169, 316–318
Varela, Francisco, 355
Vertical structure, 60, 229–231, 265
Visual tools, conflict management, 86
Volition, 192
Vulnerability, 117–118, 119–120, 260
choice of, 147
cycle of, 122–131
knowledge, 129–131
new reality and, 127–128
results evaluation, 128–129
risk taking, 124–126
strategies for cultivating, 142–147
stretching, 126–127
value of, 122–124

W

Weick, Karl, 198
Western medicine, 11
Whole systems thinking, 13
Will, 299
courage and, 306–308

discovery of, 301–303
energy and, 308–309
essential qualities, 305
hope, 310
nature of, 303–304
passion and, 308
self-discipline, 309
trust, 309
types of, 304–305
Willingness, 299
qualities, 307
Willingness strategies
balancing time, 320–322
continuous learning, 313–314
dogma and, 311–313
employee needs, 314–315

mentally fit, 318–320
patient focus, 322
politically competent, 322–323
value-based services, 316–318
Willpower, 299
Work
balance, 212–213
force reductions, 175–176
imbalance, 239–240
life, reality shift in, 4
value of, 15

Z

Zulu, 89